Principles of
Pharmacoeconomics

Third
Edition

J. Lyle Bootman, Ph.D.
Raymond J. Townsend, Pharm.D.
William F. McGhan, Pharm.D., Ph.D.

W HARVEY WHITNEY BOOKS COMPANY

Principles of Pharmacoeconomics/[edited by] J. Lyle Bootman, Raymond
    J. Townsend, William F. McGhan.
        p. cm.
    Includes bibliographical references and index.
    ISBN 0-929375-270 (alk. paper)
    1. Chemotherapy — Economic aspects. 2. Pharmaceutical industry.
3. Pharmaceutical policy. I. Bootman, J. Lyle. II. Townsend, Raymond J.
III. McGhan, William F.

Library of Congress Control
Number: 2004104338

HARVEY WHITNEY BOOKS COMPANY
8044 Montgomery Rd., PO Box 42696, Cincinnati, OH 45242 USA
www.hwbooks.com

Table of Contents

Preface

During the next decade, the development of new therapies will be stimulated by an increased understanding of disease processes at the genetic level and the application of biotechnology discoveries. The use of these new clinical agents in practice will be increasingly determined not only by their effectiveness, but also by the cost of the technology and the impact on patients' quality of life. In essence, the rising costs of health care will force decisions to be made regarding both the effectiveness of the technology and the overall cost implications. Therefore, the purpose of this book is to present various techniques, tools, and strategies to evaluate the economic contribution of specific drug therapies at a policy level and for individual patient needs and preferences. This information is relevant for researchers, practitioners, administrators, and students in health care. However, the major audience for this book is the introductory student. It should not be considered a text for the advanced level student of pharmacoeconomics.

Additionally, we hope that this book will further stimulate pharmacists, physicians, and others to generate more pharmacoeconomic research and reports to more adequately apply these principles to the prevention and treatment of disease. We believe that pharmacoeconomics as a discipline will not become a part of the mainstream of pharmacy education and practice until application of the research data takes place at the patient care level. The "genomics era" has great potential to enable practitioners to customize therapy, furthering the need for pharmacoeconomic analysis. The application of pharmacoeconomics to clinical practice and pharmaceutical care will be crucial to pharmacy's success in our future healthcare delivery system.

This book could not have been completed without the administrative assistance of the University of Arizona College of Pharmacy staff, especially Dr. Amy Grizzle, to whom we owe a great deal of gratitude for her organizational and editorial assistance. We also thank our families, colleagues, and friends for their support, love, and above all, their understanding as we completed this task.

J Lyle Bootman • Raymond J Townsend • William F McGhan

Contributing Authors

Jacob Abarca PharmD MS
Assistant Research Scientist
College of Pharmacy
Center for Health Outcomes and
  Pharmacoeconomic Research
University of Arizona
Tucson, Arizona
Chapter 16

Deborah E Atherly MPH
Graduate Student
Pharmaceutical Outcomes Research and
  Policy
School of Pharmacy
University of Washington
Seattle, Washington
Chapter 14

Judith T Barr ScD
Director
National Education and Research
  Center for Outcomes Assessment
Associate Professor
School of Pharmacy
Bouvé College of Health Sciences
Northeastern University
Boston, Massachusetts
Chapter 8

J Lyle Bootman PhD
Dean and Professor
College of Pharmacy
University of Arizona
Tucson, Arizona
Chapters 1, 2, 18

J Gregory Boyer PhD
Assistant Executive Director
Accreditation Evaluation and Research
Accreditation Council for Pharmacy
  Education
Chicago, Illinois
Chapter 7

Kathleen M Bungay PharmD
Research Scientist/Assistant Professor
The Health Institute
Tufts–New England Medical Center
Boston, Massachusetts
Chapter 7

Jesse L Cooke Jr BA
PhD Candidate
Pharmaceutical Health Services
  Research
University of Maryland
Baltimore, Maryland
Chapter 10

Stephen Joel Coons PhD
Professor
Pharmacy Practice and Science
College of Pharmacy
University of Arizona
Tucson, Arizona
Chapter 6

Michael Dickson PhD
Professor
College of Pharmacy
University of South Carolina
Columbia, South Carolina
Chapter 2

Jean Paul Gagnon PhD
Director, Public Policy
Aventis Pharmaceuticals
Bridgewater, New Jersey
Chapter 13

Jacqueline S Gardner PhD
Professor of Pharmacy
Faculty, Pharmaceutical Outcomes
  Research and Policy Program
School of Pharmacy
University of Washington
Seattle, Washington
Chapter 9

Jan D Hirsch PhD
Assistant Professor of Clinical Pharmacy
  and Family and Preventive Medicine
School of Pharmacy and Pharmaceutical
  Sciences
University of California
San Diego, California
Chapter 12

Nelda E Johnson PharmD
President
Outcomes Research & Design, Inc.
Houston, Texas
Adjunct Associate Professor
College of Pharmacy
University of Illinois
Chicago, Illinois
Chapter 12

Robert M Kaplan PhD
Professor and Chair
School of Pharmacy and Pharmaceutical
  Sciences
University of California
San Diego, California
Chapter 6

Deborah S Kitz PhD
Principal
Broshar Consulting, LLC
Horsham, Pennsylvania
Chapter 4

Lon N Larson PhD
Windsor Professor of Science
Professor of Pharmacy Administration
College of Pharmacy and Health Sciences
Drake University
Des Moines, Iowa
Chapter 3

Dell B Mather PharmD
Vice President of Pharmacy
Ancillary Care Management
Eden Prairie, Minnesota
Chapter 14

William F McGhan PharmD PhD
Professor of Pharmacy and Health Policy
Director
Graduate Program in Pharmacy
  Administration
Philadelphia College of Pharmacy
University of the Sciences
Philadelphia, Pennsylvania
Chapters 1, 4, 18

W Mark Moore PharmD
Director of Admissions
Assistant Professor
School of Pharmacy
Campbell University
Buies Creek, North Carolina
Chapter 13

C Daniel Mullins PhD
Professor and Chair
Pharmaceutical Health Services Research
School of Pharmacy
University of Maryland
Baltimore, Maryland
Chapter 10

David B Nash MD MBA
The Dr. Raymond C and Doris N
  Grandon Professor of Health Policy
Chairman
Department of Health Policy
Thomas Jefferson University
Philadelphia, Pennsylvania
Chapter 12

Jane T Osterhaus PhD
Wasatch Health Outcomes
Park City, Utah
Chapter 11

Gene Reeder PhD
Professor of Pharmacoeconomics
College of Pharmacy
University of South Carolina
Columbia, South Carolina
Chapter 13

Lisa A Sanchez PharmD
President
PE Applications
Highland Ranch, Colorado
Chapter 17

John J Schrogie MD
Vice President
Peri-Approval Research Services
Omnicare Clinical Research
King of Prussia, Pennsylvania
Chapter 12

Kevin A Schulman MD
Professor of Medicine and Business
  Administration
Director
Center for Clinical and Genetic Economics
Duke Clinical Research Institute
Vice Chair for Business Affairs
Duke University Medical Center
Durham, North Carolina
Chapter 15

Gerald E Schumacher PharmD MSc PhD
Professor of Pharmacy
Bouvé College of Health Sciences
Northeastern University
Boston, Massachusetts
Chapter 8

Grant H Skrepnek PhD
Assistant Professor
College of Pharmacy
University of Arizona
Tucson, Arizona
Chapter 5

Paul E Stang PhD
Executive Vice President
Galt Associates, Incorporated
Blue Bell, Pennsylvania
Adjunct Associate Professor
University of North Carolina
Chapel Hill, North Carolina
Chapter 9

Andy S Stergachis PhD RPh
Professor of Epidemiology & Affiliate
  Professor of Pharmacy
Northwest Center for Public Health
  Practice
University of Washington
Seattle, Washington
Chapter 14

Sean D Sullivan PhD
Professor of Pharmacy and Public Health
  and Community Medicine
Director
Pharmaceutical Outcomes Research and
  Policy Program
University of Washington
Seattle, Washington
Chapter 14

Simu K Thomas PhD
Manager
Health Economics and Outcomes
  Research
Novartis Pharmaceuticals Corporation
East Hanover, New Jersey
Chapter 10

Raymond J Townsend PharmD FCCP FAPRS
President
Wasatch Health Outcomes
Park City, Utah
Chapters 1, 11

John E Ware Jr PhD
Chief Executive Officer
Chief Science Officer
Chairman of the Board
QualityMetric Incorporated
Lincoln, Rhode Island
Chapter 7

Introduction to Pharmacoeconomics

CHAPTER 1

J Lyle Bootman,
Raymond J Townsend,
and William F McGhan

Health expenditures in the United States have been increasing as a percentage of the nation's gross domestic product (GDP).[1] Although the proportion of GDP spent on total health care has climbed steadily, the percentage spent on outpatient prescriptions has remained relatively constant over the past 30 years. Even though private health insurance and government programs cover a growing portion of drug expenditures, a sizable amount of drug costs is still paid directly by consumers. The cost of pharmaceuticals and pharmacy services have, therefore, become an important issue to patients, third-party payers, and governments alike. Today, and in the future, it is necessary to scientifically value the costs and consequences of drug therapy.

The basic value of drug therapy to prescribers and patients in the United States is evidenced by the increased therapeutic use of prescriptions. Community pharmacists dispense Approximately three billion prescriptions annually.[3] The number of prescriptions dispensed per person per year in the United States has increased dramatically over the past 50 years. The nation's hospitals provide billions of dollars worth of drugs and drug products to hospitalized patients.[4] Drugs available over the counter also serve an important role in the country's health care. Sales of nonprescription drugs have increased from $700 million in the 1950s to well into the billions of dollars.[5] These figures may be indicative of the value and perceived benefit that society attributes to medications. Most economists would acknowledge that a crude, lower-bound estimate of the value and benefits of drugs to consumers is the amount they spend on these products.

Pharmaceuticals and other therapeutic interventions have contributed to the important progress being made in the health status of the United States population. Corresponding to the introduction of new drug entities during the past several decades, the mortality rates for a number of diseases have declined substantially.[6] Drugs account for only a small proportion of the expenditures in hospital budgets, but drug therapy plays a crucial role in the efficient treatment of hospitalized patients. An average hospitalized patient receives six to eight different drugs on a typical day. Effective drug therapy helps to partially explain why the mean length of stay in hospitals has decreased over the years.[4]

Despite the general evidence supporting the use of pharmaceuticals, few data exist regarding the actual costs and benefits attributed to specific drug therapies. A primary reason is the lack of defined methodologies to evaluate medical interventions. Perhaps the current focus on reducing expenditures of pharmaceuticals and pharmacy services to save costs to the total healthcare system is inappropriate. One purpose of this book is to present economic and humanistic measurement methodologies that may be used not only to evaluate the outcomes of drug therapy, but also put them in perspective with other related healthcare expenditures.

Outcomes

The term "outcomes" is increasingly being used to describe the results and value of healthcare intervention. However, depending on perspective, the outcomes of health care are multidimensional. The clinician has traditionally been most concerned with clinical outcomes of treatments. More recently, healthcare payers and administrators have focused on the resource use or economic outcome of healthcare decisions. Patients, on the other hand, are becoming increasingly knowledgable and involved in decisions regarding their own health care and are seeking more information regarding the humanistic outcomes of therapy. Patients want to know how their quality of life will be affected or how satisfied other patients with their condition have been with various treatments.

As the healthcare marketplace is rapidly changing, there is a danger that the change will be driven primarily by the desire to contain cost. Clearly, cost-containment is an important objective. However, successful healthcare management as measured by the objectives of patients, physicians, and other healthcare providers, as well as by societal expectations, requires that the quality of care also be maintained. Outcomes measurement must take into account economic considerations while recognizing that acceptable clinical and humanistic outcomes are also important objectives. The true value of healthcare interventions, programs, and policy can be assessed only if all three dimensions of outcomes are measured and considered.

Definition of Pharmacoeconomics Research

Economics is about trade-offs and choices between wants, needs, and the scarcity of resources to fulfill these wants. When considering economics, most people think of the trade-offs between goods and services and money; however, the trade-off might also be expressed in humanistic terms. We are, therefore, careful to include both resource use and humanistic evaluations of drug therapy within pharmacoeconomic assessment.

Pharmacoeconomics has been defined as "the description and analysis of the costs of drug therapy to health care systems and society."[7] Pharmacoeconomic research identifies, measures, and compares the costs (ie, resources consumed) and consequences (ie, clinical, economic, humanistic) of pharmaceutical products and services. Within this framework are included the research methods related to cost-minimization, cost-effectiveness, cost–benefit, cost-of-illness, cost-utility, cost-consequences, and decision analysis, as well as quality-of-life and other humanistic assessments. In essence, pharmacoeconomic analysis uses tools for examining the impact (desirable, undesirable) of alternative drug therapies and other medical interventions.

Questions that pharmacoeconomics may help to address are as follows: What drugs should be included on the hospital formulary? What is the best drug for a particular patient? What is the best drug for a pharmaceutical manufacturer to develop? Which drug delivery system is the best for the hospital? How do two clinical pharmacy services compare? Which drugs should be included in a Medicaid formulary? What is the cost per quality-adjusted year of life extended by a drug? Will patient quality of life be improved by a particular drug therapy decision? What is the best drug for this particular disease? What are the patient outcomes of various treatment modalities?

In essence, pharmacoeconomic analysis uses important tools for examining the outcomes or impact of drug therapy and related healthcare interventions.

Historical Perspective

The emerging discipline of pharmacoeconomics has become a health science discipline by the pharmaceutical industry, academic pharmaceutical scientists, and pharmacy practitioners worldwide. As stated previously, it is generally defined as the description and analysis of the costs and consequences of pharmaceuticals and pharmaceutical services and their impact on individuals, healthcare systems, and society. The research methods used by scientists in this discipline (eg, cost-effectiveness, cost-utility, quality-of-life evaluations) are drawn from many areas: economics, epidemiology, medicine, pharmacy, and the social sciences. We believe that pharmacoeconomic analysis will have a significant impact on the delivery and financing of health care throughout the world. Furthermore, we believe that pharmacoeconomics may influence health care and the practice of pharmacy at a magnitude equivalent to the impact of clinical pharmacy and pharmacokinetics.

During the early 1960s, pharmacy began evolving as a clinical discipline within the healthcare system. It was during this time that the pharmaceutical science disciplines such as pharmaceutics, clinical pharmacy, drug information, and pharmacokinetics became a critical and integral part of pharmacy education and science. In the 1970s, pharmacoeconomics developed its roots. In 1978, McGhan, Rowland, and Bootman, from the University of Minnesota, introduced the concepts of cost–benefit and cost-effectiveness analyses.[8] Bootman et al.[9] also published an early pharmacy research article in 1979 in which cost–benefit analysis was used to evaluate the outcomes of individualizing aminoglycoside dosages in severely burned patients with gram-negative septicemia using sophisticated pharmacokinetic protocols. The actual term "pharmacoeconomics" did not appear in the literature until 1986 when the first of a two-part presentation by Townsend[10] was published describing the need to develop research activities in this evolving discipline. To date, many of the efforts in this discipline have been directed toward the refinement of the research methods and their application to evaluating pharmaceutical services and specific drug therapies.

Pharmacoeconomics continues to evolve similarly to another relatively new pharmaceutical science: pharmacokinetics. Pharmacokinetics surfaced in the 1950s in United States colleges of pharmacy and, in the 1970s, became an integral part of the pharmacy curriculum. Many of the theoretical models for pharmacokinetics are based on the physicochemical principles developed by physicists, chemists, and engineers. As a parallel, pharmacoeconomics has borrowed from the basic economic and social sciences for most of its theoretical models. McGhan, Rowland, and Bootman introduced course material related to pharmacoeconomics into the undergraduate and graduate pharmacy curricula as early as 1976 at the University of Minnesota. However, the educational content was emphasized at the graduate level—not at the undergraduate professional program levels. We are beginning to see much of this material incorporated at the PharmD education level alongside the discipline of pharmacotherapy.

Furthermore, upon examining the evolutionary path of pharmacokinetics, it is clear that its application in the clinical setting was a driving force that ensured its place in the professional pharmacy curriculum. We believe that pharmacoeconomics will obtain the same level of recognition when its application in the clinical setting is more complete. In other words, when pharmacy practitioners begin to apply the results of pharmacoeconomic research to therapeutic decision-making, thus positively influencing patient outcomes, the discipline will become an increasingly critical component of the pharmacy curriculum. Likewise, the successful implementation of "pharmaceutical care" will come about only with sufficient pharmacoeconomic research that adequately documents the degree to which the benefits of such care outweigh the costs associated with those services. In fact, the profession of pharmacy is unlikely to succeed in its role of providing pharmaceutical care without this critical body of knowledge. Pharmacists must become the key players in ensuring that drug therapy and related pharmacy services are not only safe and effective, but also provide real value in both economic and humanistic terms.

Overview of Pharmacoeconomic Methodologies

The purpose of this section is to acquaint the reader with the basic methodologic approaches regarding the economic evaluation of drug therapy. By definition, *pharmacoeconomic evaluations* include any study designed to assess the costs (ie, resources consumed) and consequences (clinical, humanistic) of alternative therapies. This includes such methodologies as cost–benefit, cost-utility, and cost-effectiveness (Table 1). Each of these methodologies is discussed in more depth in later chapters. Review articles that discuss the application of these techniques to healthcare evaluations also may assist readers in becoming more aware of the role of these tools.[8-30] The evaluation mechanisms delineated were often helpful in demonstrating the cost impact of innovative treatments, therefore granting them greater acceptance by healthcare providers, administrators, and the public.

Table 1. Pharmacoeconomic Methodologies

Methodology	Cost Measurement Unit	Outcome Unit
Cost–benefit	dollars	dollars
Cost-effectiveness	dollars	natural units (life-years gained, mg/dL blood glucose, mm Hg blood pressure)
Cost-minimization	dollars	assume to be equivalent in comparative groups
Cost-utility	dollars	quality-adjusted life-year or other utilities

COST-MINIMIZATION ANALYSIS

When two or more interventions are evaluated and demonstrated or assumed to be equivalent in terms of a given outcome or consequence, costs associated with each intervention may be evaluated and compared. This typical cost analysis is referred to as *cost-minimization analysis*. An example of this type of investigation regarding drug therapy may be the evaluation of two generically equivalent drugs in which the outcome has been proven to be equal, although the acquisition and administration costs may be significantly different.

COST-BENEFIT ANALYSIS

Cost-benefit analysis is a basic tool that can be used to improve the decision-making process in allocation of funds to healthcare programs. Although the general concept of cost-benefit analysis is not overly complicated, many technical considerations require a degree of explanation and interpretation to understand how it can be or has been applied.

Cost-benefit analysis consists of identifying all of the benefits that accrue from the program or intervention and converting them into dollars in the year in which they will occur. This stream of benefit dollars is then discounted to its equivalent present value at the selected interest rate. On the other side of the equation, all program costs are identified and allocated through a specific year and, again, the costs are discounted to their present value. Then, if all relevant factors remain constant, the program with the largest present value of benefits less costs is best in terms of its economic value.

Ideally, all benefits and costs resulting from the program should be included. This presents considerable difficulty, especially on the benefits side of the equation, as many benefits are either difficult to measure, difficult to convert to dollars, or both. For example, the benefits of improved patient quality of life, patient satisfaction with the healthcare system, and working conditions for the physician are not only difficult to measure, but are extremely difficult to assign a dollar value to. This problem has been addressed by many researchers in health economics, but has not been completely resolved. Generally, the analyst or researcher will convert as many benefits as possible into monetary units. The remaining variables are labeled as "intangible benefits" and left to decision-makers to include in their final deliberations. Cost-benefit analysis often has been used when comparing the value of dissimilar programs where the outcomes are in different units (eg, cost-benefit of having a neonatal care program vs a cardiac rehabilitation program).

COST-EFFECTIVENESS ANALYSIS

Cost-effectiveness analysis is a technique designed to assist a decision-maker in identifying a preferred choice among possible alternatives. Generally, cost-effectiveness is defined as a series of analytical and mathematical procedures that aid in the selection of a course of action from various alternative approaches. Cost-effectiveness analysis has been applied to health matters where the program's inputs can be readily measured in dollars, but the program's outputs are more appropriately stated in terms of health improvement created (eg, life-years extended, clinical cures).

An important point to be considered in both cost-benefit and cost-effectiveness analysis is that a program/treatment providing a high benefit (effectiveness)-to-cost ratio in terms of value to society may not be valued in the same way by all members of society. For example, drug therapy that reduced the number of patient-days in an acute care institution may be positive from a third-party payer's point of view, but not necessarily from the view of the institution's administrator who operated under a fixed level of revenue and depended on a fixed number of patient-days to meet expenses. What is viewed as cost-beneficial for society as a whole may be viewed differently by plan sponsors, administrators, health providers, governmental agencies, or even individual patients. One must consider whose interests are to be taken into account when using these analyses.

COST-UTILITY ANALYSIS

In examining Table 1, one can better appreciate the subtle differences between the techniques discussed to this point. *Cost-utility analysis* is an economic tool in which the intervention consequence is measured in terms of quantity and quality of life. It is much the same as cost-effectiveness analysis, with the added dimension of a particular point of view, most often that of the patient. Quite often the results of cost-utility analysis are expressed in the intervention cost per quality-adjusted life-year gained or changes in quality-of-life measurement for a given intervention cost. Although cost-utility analysis has been used somewhat successfully to aid in decisions regarding healthcare programs (eg, surgery vs chemotherapy), instruments that are reliable and sensitive enough to detect changes with drug treatments (eg, one antihypertensive agent vs another) are still needed.

COST-OF-ILLNESS EVALUATION

Cost-of-illness studies are important to pharmacoeconomic evaluations of new therapies. By evaluating the humanistic impact of disease and the resources used in treating a condition prior to discovery of a new intervention, the pharmacoeconomist can effectively establish a baseline for comparison. Although the value and methodologies of cost-of-illness studies have been debated, they remain prevalent in the pharmacoeconomic literature.[28,29] As with all pharmacoeconomic evaluation, when conducting or evaluating the cost-of-illness, it is important to carefully consider the design and intent of the study. There is value in having baseline information, but absolute conclusions regarding the value of an intervention versus an alternative can be made only after direct comparison.

COST-CONSEQUENCE ANALYSIS

A *cost-consequence analysis* has been defined as one "in which costs and effects are calculated but not aggregated into quality-adjusted life-years or cost-effectiveness ratios."[31] Simply, this type of analysis comprises a listing of all relevant costs and outcomes of drug therapy or healthcare intervention including direct medical costs, direct nonmedical costs, indirect costs, clinical outcomes, utility impacts, and quality-of-life impacts. Cost-consequence analysis provides the most comprehensive presentation of information describing the value of an intervention and has the advantage of being more readily understandable and more likely to be applied by healthcare decision-makers.[32] In this application, weighting of different costs and benefits is left to each decision-maker. Although this should lead to improvements in decision-maker welfare from an economic perspective, a possible drawback for disaggregated presentation of health outcomes is that decisions made at the individual decision-maker's level might not be made in the patient's or society's best interests. Another potential weakness of cost-consequence analysis is that all of the data are not always of comparable quality. Cost-consequence analyses in the literature often include a variety of data from clinical trials and other sources, since no single source is adequate to provide the breadth of information required.[33-37] Imputation and extrapolation are often necessary. Despite these considerations, cost-consequence analysis remains a useful approach to presenting relevant information for a wide range of healthcare concerns.

Pharmacoeconomics and Drug Development

The pharmaceutical industry spends billions of dollars annually for development of new drugs. As a percentage of pharmaceutical sales, these research and development (R & D) costs are certainly higher than those found in other industries.[2] The large number of compounds that must be evaluated to bring one drug to market contributes to the high R & D costs of drug development. This percentage is also higher than that found in other industries. It has been estimated that it takes $802 million and 14 years to bring a new drug to the market.[2] The process by which a drug is evaluated and developed for the marketplace is illustrated in Figure 1.

Because pharmacoeconomic data are becoming increasingly important to practitioners making drug formulary decisions, it is important to have these data as soon as possible after Food and Drug Administration approval. To do this, discussion and planning for pharmacoeconomic evaluation should begin during the early stages of drug development. A major question arises as to the ideal time to conduct pharmacoeconomic studies and the best process by which to do so. Pharmacoeconomic studies may be planned and conducted at the clinical development and Phase IV stages of postmarketing research. Basic research and development activities may be partially guided by preliminary pharmacoeconomic analyses. Therefore, studies may need to be

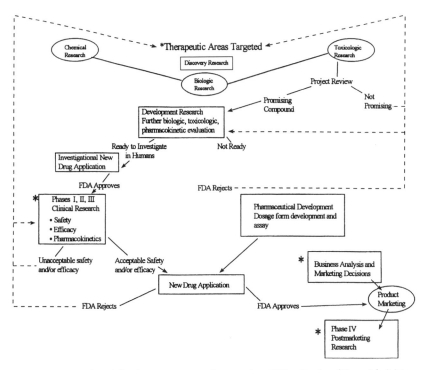

Figure 1. Research and development stages of a new drug. FDA = Food and Drug Administration. * = Pharmacoeconomic evaluations may be designed or conducted at these levels.

conducted at several stages of pharmaceutical research. The following is a summary of the research activity for each phase.

PHASE I TRIALS

The objective of the initial clinical trials, or Phase I, is to determine the toxicity profile of the drug in humans. The first Phase I trials usually consist of administration of single, conservative doses to a small number of healthy volunteers. The effects of increasing the size and number of daily doses are evaluated until toxic effects surface or the likely therapeutic dosage is substantially exceeded. It is during this stage that cost-of-illness studies should be accomplished to aid in deciding whether to further develop the drug and gather background data for future pharmacoeconomic evaluations. Cost-of-illness data may also aid in the development of preliminary models to assess the clinical benefits that must be achieved in order to have a marketable product.

PHASE II TRIALS

In Phase II trials, the drug is administered to a limited number of patients with the target disease. Patients without complicating, coexisting medical conditions are preferred for these trials. This reduces the number of variables that could confound analysis of the drug's activity and permits the potential therapeutic benefit of the new drug to be more clearly demonstrated.

Even in carefully selected patients, however, demonstrating the efficacy of a new drug is not easy or certain. To provide unequivocal evidence of the drug's therapeutic benefit, it is necessary to compare its effectiveness with that of standard medically accepted treatments or, where ethically appropriate, with a placebo. These comparisons also are used to establish the optimal dosage range for therapeutic activity of the new drug. During this phase, cost-of-illness studies can begin or continue, as can preliminary development of quality-of-life and resource utilization instruments. Models can be refined as more information is available about the clinical aspects of the drug.

PHASE III TRIALS

In Phase III trials, larger numbers of patients are given the new drug in the established dosage range and in the final dosage form. This larger sample size refines the knowledge gained during Phase II and helps identify patients who might have rare reactions to the drug. Patient selection is still closely supervised in Phase III, although some patients with coexisting medical problems are intentionally included to allow assessment of complication in the drug's use.

Discussion, planning, and implementation of pharmacoeconomic studies during this level of research are important. The prospective clinical study that has incorporated a pharmacoeconomic evaluation during the final stages of efficacy evaluation is close to the ideal situation. Critics of these studies claim that pharmacoeconomic evaluations will hinder the new drug application (NDA) process. Advocates of pharmacoeconomic evaluation correctly note that, unless a new drug treatment has no alternatives and is truly a breakthrough, the value of using it must be scientifically studied.

PHASE IV TRIALS

During the postmarketing phase, or Phase IV, retrospective and prospective pharmacoeconomic studies can be designed and conducted to gather data in support of the use of the drug. Postmarketing pharmacoeconomic studies are extremely important in that they allow evaluation of the costs and consequences of drug therapy without the altered interventions that occur in strictly controlled clinical trials. During tightly controlled clinical trials, pharmacoeconomics can only put value on efficacy; this only approximates the "real world." Once a product is on the market, cost-effectiveness can be determined. NOTE: *Efficacy* studies answer "can it work?" *Effectiveness* studies evaluate "does it work?"

As previously indicated, clinical trials are used to evaluate the efficacy and safety of therapies. The relationships between pharmacoeconomic evaluations and clinical trials are threefold.

1. The pharmacoeconomic evaluation may be a secondary objective of a trial designed primarily to study safety and efficacy.
2. The pharmacoeconomic evaluation may be the principal purpose of a clinical trial.
3. A pharmacoeconomic evaluation may be done retrospectively using clinical data obtained in previous trials.

Once a drug is marketed, either retrospective or additional prospective pharmacoeconomic studies may be designed and conducted.

Epidemiologic studies are frequently used to evaluate the effectiveness and safety of drugs. Epidemiologic data with regard to the disease and treatment under investigation can yield highly important information for economic evaluation of a specific drug therapy. Understanding the natural progression of the disease comorbidities and treatment enables estimation of the variables that may have pharmacoeconomic implications with regard to cost of illness and quality of life.

Epidemiology's role in pharmacoeconomic evaluations and considerations for conducting pharmacoeconomic research within clinical trials are the subject of Chapters 9 and 11, respectively.

Pharmacoeconomic Guidelines

Researchers and evaluators continue to develop and refine guidelines for pharmacoeconomic analysis. The uses and subject of the proposed guidelines are as follows:

1. Methodologic guidelines would guide researchers to appropriately design, conduct, analyze, and report economic and humanistic evaluations.
2. Reimbursement and pricing guidelines would outline the content, presentation, and evaluation of pharmacoeconomic data to determine or justify the price or reimbursement of a pharmaceutical product.
3. Approval guidelines would set the standards acceptable to a particular government to obtain approval to market a new product.
4. Promotional guidelines would set the criteria for the use of pharmacoeconomic data in support of pharmaceutical promotion to prescribers and consumers.

Although the intent of the call for guidelines is understandable, at present, the science of pharmacoeconomic research is still developing. It would not be desirable to implement guidelines that would limit the development of knowledge in this area. Suffice it to say that the substance of any guidelines involving research must be well grounded in appropriate methodology and sound scientific principles.

Challenges of Pharmacoeconomic Research

In the future, we will be routinely challenged to do pharmacoeconomic research, although merely performing the research will not solve all of the problems all of the time. To be useful, appropriate pharmacoeconomic evaluations must be tailored to the specific problem and decision at hand. Our challenge, therefore, begins with looking beyond the obvious and easy solutions.

Cost-minimization analysis is useful when comparing interventions with identical clinical and humanistic outcomes, but this can be the exception rather than the rule for many clinical applications outside of true generic substitution. Cost-benefit analysis would, at first glance, be the answer to more complex problems in that it would allow for evaluation of various interventions with multiple and dissimilar outcomes. Here, too, one must be careful to note the pitfalls and challenges associated with converting all of the benefits to monetary terms. (How do you place a monetary value on reduced blood pressure, insulin control, or improvement in quality of life?)

Allowing consequences to remain in natural and measurable terms means that cost-effectiveness analysis can be appropriate for many problems and help with many decisions when the outcomes of the interventions are measured in the same terms. But what about the patient and how the various treatments affect daily living and quality of life? Should decisions be made strictly on providing the best clinical outcome for the dollars spent? If so, perhaps cost-utility analysis, which takes into account patient preference and quality of life, should be the gold standard of pharmacoeconomic research. Alas, here too are the problems of measuring quality of life and preference in a changing world.

Present and future controversies surrounding pharmacoeconomic research also include arguments for methodologies of valuations and discounting. What is the most appropriate perspective to take when valuing costs and consequences: the patient, the third-party payer, or perhaps society? What of ethics? Will we be able to justify our decisions solely on the numbers obtained through scientific research?

One of the biggest challenges for pharmacoeconomic research lies in the education of those who are going to be evaluating the data derived from this research. Although the end users of pharmacoeconomic research data would like to have simple, clear-cut answers to their questions regarding the allocation of resources and the healthcare benefits derived from them, in actuality, the answers are quite complex. Pharmacoeconomics remains an art as well as a science. Even though the science may be perfectly clear, applying that science must be done artfully using professional judgment. Just as it is impossible to develop an algorithm for the treatment of a disease that is appropriate for all patients, it would be impossible to develop one for making pharmacoeconomic decisions. In the end, the user of pharmacoeconomic research data must be able to evaluate the scientific appropriateness and robustness of the research and make a decision regarding its usefulness in a particular situation. To do this, evaluators will need to understand the basic principles of pharmacoeconomic research.

The challenges of pharmacoeconomic research are inexhaustible; many are addressed within the chapters of this book. The real challenge, however, is not identifying the tools of pharmacoeconomic research, but rather discovering how and when to use them.

Summary

The overall costs of medical and pharmaceutical care continue to rise. The added value to society, individual healthcare institutions, and patients as weighed against cost has not been well established. The problem has become increasingly difficult to address because of the lack of understanding of methodologies for evaluation of new and existing drug therapy. The remaining chapters of this text provide in-depth information on specific methodologies often used in pharmacoeconomic investigations.

References

1. US Congress, Congressional Budget Office. Economic implications of rising health care costs. Washington, DC: Government Printing Office, 1992.
2. DiMasi JA, Hansen RW, Grabowski HG. The price of innovation: new estimates of drug development costs. J Health Econ 2003;22:151-85.
3. Flynn EA, Barker KN, Carnahan BJ. National observational study of prescription dispensing accuracy and safety in 50 pharmacies. J Am Pharm Assoc (Wash) 2003;43:191-200.
4. Scott L. Healthcare update. Mod Health 1994;24(June 20):18.
5. Cowley CT, Hager M. Some counter intelligence. Newsweek 1990;115(Mar 12):82-4.
6. Manasse HR. Medication use in an imperfect world: drug misadventuring as an issue of public policy. Am J Hosp Pharm 1988;46:929-44.
7. Townsend RJ. Postmarketing drug research and development. Drug Intell Clin Pharm 1987;21(1 pt 2):134-6.
8. McGhan W, Rowland C, Bootman JL. Cost–benefit and cost-effectiveness: methodologies for evaluating innovative pharmaceutical services. Am J Hosp Pharm 1978;35:133-40.
9. Bootman JL, Wertheimer A, Zaske D, Rowland C. Individualizing gentamicin dosage regimens on burn patients with gram-negative septicemia: a cost–benefit analysis. J Pharm Sci 1979;68:267-72.
10. Townsend RJ. Post marketing drug research and development: an industry clinical pharmacist's perspective. Am J Pharm Educ 1986;50:480-2.
11. Bootman JL, Rowland C, Wertheimer A. Cost–benefit-analysis: a research tool for evaluating innovative health programs. Eval Health Prof 1979;2: 129-54.
12. Bootman JL, Zaske D, Wertheimer AL, Rowland C. Individualization of aminoglycoside dosage regimens: a cost analysis. Am J Hosp Pharm 1979;36:368-70.
13. Stason WB, Weinstein M. Allocation of resources to manage hypertension. N Engl J Med 1977;296:732-9.

14. Weisbrod BA, Huston JH. Benefits and costs of human vaccines in developed countries: an evaluative survey. Washington, DC: Pharmaceutical Manufacturers Association, 1983.

15. Haaga JG. Cost-effectiveness and cost–benefit analysis of immunization programs in developing countries: a review of the literature. Washington, DC: Pharmaceutical Manufacturers Association, 1983.

16. Wagner JL. Economic evaluations of medicines: a review of the literature. Washington, DC: Pharmaceutical Manufacturers Association, 1983.

17. Dao TD. Cost–benefit and cost-effectiveness analysis of pharmaceutical intervention. Washington, DC: Pharmaceutical Manufacturers Association, 1983.

18. Vinokur A, Cannell CF, Eraker SA, Juster TF, Lepkowski JM, Mathiowetz N. The role of survey research in the assessment of health and quality-of-life outcomes of pharmaceutical interventions. Washington, DC: Pharmaceutical Manufacturers Association, 1983.

19. Little AD. Beta-blocker reduction of mortality and reinfarction rate in survivors of myocardial infarctions: a cost–benefit study. Washington, DC: Pharmaceutical Manufacturers Association, 1983.

20. Little AD. Use of beta blockers in the treatment of glaucoma: a cost–benefit study. Washington, DC: Pharmaceutical Manufacturers Association, 1983.

21. Little AD. Use of beta blockers in the treatment of angina: a cost–benefit study. Washington, DC: Pharmaceutical Manufacturers Association, 1983.

22. Dao TD. Cost–benefit and cost-effectiveness analyses of drug therapy. Am J Hosp Pharm 1985;42:791-802.

23. Drummond MF, Stoddart GL, Torrance GW. Methods for the economic evaluation of health care programmes. New York: Oxford University Press, 1987.

24. Klarman H. Application of cost/benefit analysis to health services and the special case of technological innovation. Int J Health Serv Res 1974;4:325-52.

25. Klarman H. Present status of cost–benefit analysis in the health field. Am J Public Health 1967;57:1948-58.

26. Rice DP. Measurement and application of illness costs. Public Health Rep 1969;84:95-101.

27. Crystal R, Brewster A. Cost–benefit and cost-effectiveness analysis in the health field: an introduction. Inquiry 1966;3:3-13.

28. Drummond M. Cost-of-illness studies. Pharmacoeconomics 1992;2:1-4.

29. Davey PJ, Leeder SR. The cost of migraine. More than just a headache? Pharmacoeconomics 1992;2:5-7.

30. MacKeigan LD, Bootman JL. A review of cost–benefit and cost-effectiveness analyses of clinical pharmacy services. J Pharm Marketing Manage 1988;2:63-84.

31. Russell LB, Gold MR, Siegel JE, Daniels N, Weinstein MC. The role of cost-effectiveness analysis in health and medicine. Panel on Cost-Effectiveness in Health and Medicine. JAMA 1996;276:1172-7.

32. Mauskopf JA, Paul JE, Grant DM, Stergachis A. The role of cost-consequence analysis in healthcare decision-making. Pharmacoeconomics 1998;13:277-88.

33. Aberg-Wistedt A, Cressell T, Lidberg Y, Liljenberg B, Osby U. Two-year outcome of team-based intensive case management for patients with schizophrenia. Psychiatr Serv 1995;46:1263-6.

34. Brooten D. Methodological issues linking costs and outcomes. Med Care 1997;35(suppl):NS87-NS95.

35. Lieu AT, Cochi SL, Black SB, Halloran ME, Shinefield HR, Holmes SJ, et al. Cost-effectiveness of a routine varicella vaccination program for US children. JAMA 1994;271:375-81.

36. Powe NR, Griffiths RI. The clinical-economic trial: promise, problems, and challenges. Controlled Clin Trials 1995;16:377.

37. Testa MA, Anderson RB, Nackley JF, Quality of Life Hypertension Study Group. Quality of life and antihypertensive therapy in men: a comparison of captopril with enalapril. N Engl J Med 1993;328:907-13.

Pharmacoeconomics: An International Perspective

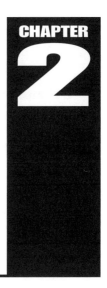

CHAPTER 2

Michael Dickson
and J Lyle Bootman

The application of economic analysis to pharmaceuticals is part of a larger global trend to maximize the value received for money spent on healthcare services. As discussed in Chapter 1, there has been an upward trend in healthcare expenditure as a percentage of gross domestic product in the United States as well as other countries. More to the point for payers, the per capita cost of healthcare services in general, and pharmaceuticals in particular, has risen steadily over at least the last 20 years (Figures 1 and 2). The trend is clearly upward for all countries shown, and the United States is well above the level of other countries. In general, European Union countries have lower per capita expenditures than non-European Union countries, with the exception of Australia, which has the lowest per capita expenditure for pharmaceuticals.[1] What accounts for this generally rising trend in pharmaceutical expenditure? Is it due to increased product quality, higher prices, increased utilization, or some combination of these causes?

In general, rising expenditure is due to a combination of the causes, thus inviting the question of how much increase in expenditure is contributed by each cause. If prices are increasing, can the increase be justified because better-quality products yield improvements in outcomes? If utilization is increasing, is this also contributing to better outcomes? To the extent that we can answer yes to these questions and price/utilization increases are commensurate with improvements in outcomes, increased expenditure could be justified. These are difficult relationships

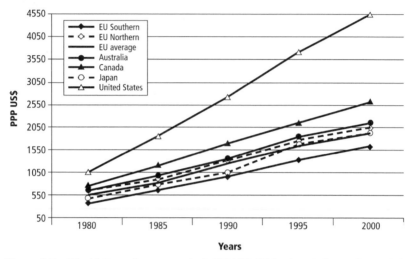

Figure 1. Total Health Expenditure per capita in PPP US$. EU Southern is France, Greece, Italy, Portugal, and Spain. Austria and Turkey are not included due to missing data. Data for 2000 are estimated. PPP = purchasing power party.

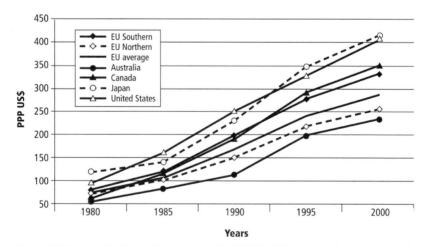

Figure 2. Pharmaceutical Expenditure per capita in PPP US$. EU Southern is France, Greece, Italy, Portugal, and Spain. Austria and Turkey are not included due to missing data. Data for 2000 are estimated. PPP = purchasing power party.

to assess. It is much easier to observe price and utilization changes than outcomes. Consequently, it is not surprising that much of the effort by payers to control pharmaceutical expenditure has focused on constraining prices and utilization. Payers are now interested in pharmacoeconomic analysis because the traditional controls have not arrested the trend in Figure 2. There is now an interest in assessing value received for money spent with the hope of moderating the pharmaceutical expenditure trend and establishing a reasonable relationship between expenditure and value received. Many payers are now focusing directly on value rather than its components.

Before examining pharmacoeconomic guidelines used by various countries, it is well to recall the simple relationship between price, quantity, expenditure, and value:

$$\text{Expenditure} = \text{price} \times \text{quantity}$$

$$\text{Value} = \text{expenditure/unit of outcome}$$

The price and quantity relationship is simple, but changes in value are more complex. Value is increased if expenditure decreases at a given level of outcome or outcome increases at a given level of expenditure. In a relative sense, value also will increase if outcome increases more rapidly or falls more slowly than expenditure. Thus, while pharmacoeconomic guidelines are usually expressed in terms of value, we should recognize that there are multiple pathways to improving value for money spent.

At the outset, it is important to understand that pharmacoeconomics does not answer the question of how much to spend on prescription drugs. The level of pharmaceutical expenditure is a political question that has multiple dimensions, of which economics is only one. How much to spend on prescription drugs also is influenced by social policies, public expectations, available resources, and competing needs. Pharmacoeconomics can be helpful in answering the question about value for money spent, but it is only one piece in the puzzle. This chapter is concerned only with the value question and how payers (usually governments) address the problem. Therefore, the objectives of this chapter are to:

1. describe the rationale for pharmacoeconomic guidelines and how they are used in selected countries,
2. demonstrate the relationships among pharmacoeconomic

guidelines and pharmaceutical reimbursement policies in these countries, and

3. discuss the implications of pharmacoeconomic guidelines for the availability of new chemical entities in the future.

The Pharmacoeconomic Guideline Concept

In most industrialized countries, with the notable exception of the United States, government is the primary payer for healthcare services, including prescription drugs. Many of these governments have a long history of using a variety of expenditure control mechanisms. Because these methods have not adequately reduced pharmaceutical expenditure (Figure 2), it is not surprising that payers have sought new methods. One of the more recently used approaches to expenditure control is the adoption of pharmacoeconomic guidelines. The concept of pharmacoeconomic guidelines, if not their application, is simple: applying economic analysis to determine the value of a prescription drug and using this information to help make drug pricing and reimbursement decisions. From the payers' perspective, the use of economic analysis is expected to reduce expenditure because they believe that high prices are the main contributor to expenditure. However, product manufacturers view economic analysis as a way to justify a product price.

As pharmacoeconomic data become more important in product marketing, payers have recognized the need for guidelines to ensure that the economic data presented to them are valid and organized in a format useful for their own decision-making. Thus, pharmacoeconomic guidelines are payer-specified standards for conducting and reporting economic analyses in support of a requested price or reimbursement for a product. These standards do not necessarily apply if an economic analysis is used to support product marketing rather than as part of a dossier submitted to a payer.

Pharmacoeconomic studies come from various sources, but the vast majority are either conducted or funded by pharmaceutical companies. From the payers' perspective, this introduces the possibility of bias, which is the rationale for specifying guidelines. The debate on the need for guidelines has three main themes. The payers' view is that guidelines are needed to ensure validity of the findings. An opposite view is that economic analysis of pharmaceuticals is in its infancy, and imposing guidelines now would only threaten future development. The third theme, a kind of middle ground, is that, if there are to be guidelines, they should be very general so as not to inhibit development of the discipline and to be broadly applicable.

Depending on the definition adopted, there are anywhere from a few to hundreds of pharmacoeconomic guidelines in use today by government and private payers. While the details of these guidelines may vary, there are some general themes by which guidelines can be classified for purposes of discussion. This chapter focuses on government payer guidelines used in three countries and private payer guidelines in the United States. The reader is cautioned that the number and shape of pharmacoeconomic guidelines change almost daily as countries implement or change methods. Therefore, this chapter can only provide a snapshot of pharmacoeconomic guidelines currently in use. The expectation is that these countries are representative of current conditions and indicative of trends.

The Regulatory Environment

In general, a new prescription drug is approved for marketing based on standards of safety, efficacy, and quality. After a product receives marketing approval, government payers will set a price or reimbursement level based on country-specific regulations. The product manufacturer will generally propose a price or reimbursement that becomes a basis for negotiations if negotiations are permitted. Because there is only one payer (the government), there is essentially no market for the new product until its price or reimbursement level is established. Therefore, the introduction of pharmacoeconomic guidelines in single-payer markets has been described by some as the fourth hurdle to marketing (the first three being safety, efficacy, and quality) because it introduces another review process. In markets where there are many payers, such as the United States, initial market access for new products is less constrained by pharmacoeconomic guidelines. In any pharmaceutical market, there are three ways in which pharmacoeconomic guidelines can be applied: during marketing approval, when setting product prices, and when fixing reimbursement levels for a product.

MARKETING APPROVAL

If pharmacoeconomic guidelines are applied as part of the marketing approval process, the rationale would be that new products should pass a threshold test for value. Such thresholds are difficult to express and more difficult to justify. There also exists the problem of what to do with products previously approved for marketing. In summary, it seems unlikely that pharmacoeconomic analysis will become a significant part of the marketing approval process, which has traditionally and universally been grounded in the principles of safety, efficacy, and quality.

PRICING DECISIONS

Countries that set product prices are the logical places to use pharmacoeconomic data. The manufacturer of a new product is typically asked to submit an economic dossier in support of a product price following the payer's pharmacoeconomic guidelines. The expectation is that products providing greater value can justify a higher price than lower-value products.

The seemingly scientific nature of this process weakens when attempting to establish a link between value and price. The conventional wisdom is that measuring value (cost/outcome) will yield the answer; however, there can be many assumptions in the definition of value (eg, costs to include, clinical endpoints to use, comparators). Theoretically, pharmacoeconomic guidelines will resolve many of these difficult issues, but both medical care and economics lack the quantitative properties necessary for definitive answers. The most we should expect from the application of pharmacoeconomic guidelines to pricing decisions is a better definition of issues separating the payer and the product producer.

REIMBURSEMENT STATUS

Rather than setting prices, some government payers create reimbursement schedules (consumer cost-sharing) for pharmaceuticals based on some scale such as price, therapeutic category, recipient income, and the like. Pharmacoeconomic regulations have been used to refine these scales or create another method for scaling consumer cost-sharing. Incorporating pharmacoeconomic data into reimbursement decisions has the advantage of rationalizing the consumer cost-sharing decision while avoiding the acrimony that accompanies pricing decisions; however, this is only a shift in focus. The fundamental problem remains: How should the cost of a prescription product be shared by the payer and the patient? Like the pricing situation above, setting a reimbursement level for a product is an explicit determination of value. Pharmacoeconomic data are useful in making this decision, but they are not the only factor to consider.

PRICING AND REIMBURSEMENT

These two decision points are sometimes used together (eg, in France) to provide more precise control over expenditure. Pharmacoeconomic data are especially useful for pricing and reimbursement if there is a significant private sector in addition to a large single payer. For example, a government payer might set a high product price and high reimbursement (eg, low consumer cost-sharing) for products with high value and in situations where it is important to limit the economic burden on users of the product. Conversely, low-value products might be given a low price, based on value, and low reimbursement (high consumer cost-sharing). This approach incorporates clinical and social parameters to create a value-based formulary.

Value and Price

A premise of pharmacoeconomic analysis is that the focus should be on value—this is sometimes interpreted as not focusing on price. However, another look at the earlier statement of value will show that price is an integral part of the value calculation. A more reasoned premise for pharmacoeconomic analysis is that value should not be viewed solely as a function of price, but considered more broadly in the context of economic, clinical, and humanistic outcomes.[2] Price is important, but should not be the only consideration in the determination of value. In practice, the price variable is often the only one that is manipulated by payers because they cannot control outcomes and often cannot constrain utilization.

Although the unease about expenditure trends (Figures 1 and 2) is general, prescription drugs present an unusual, if not unique, situation. For example, unlike a hospitalization, prescription drugs are viewed as products, not services. Furthermore, the same prescription drug is often available simultaneously in many countries, which clearly invites price and utilization comparisons. While a hospitalization may be seen as different across countries, few would see any difference in the same drug sold in different countries. Therefore, there is a tendency to focus on price differences among pharmaceutical products and dismiss all other aspects of pharmacotherapy; this leads to the conclusion that pharmaceutical prices alone determine value. The argument is made that a drug is the same everywhere and expenditure is rising because prices are too high. When price and reimbursement controls fail to achieve the desired result, payers attempt to control expenditure by restraining utilization through various means, including cost-sharing and limits on promotional expenditure.

Global Status of Pharmacoeconomic Regulation

Currently, only the governments of Australia, Canada, and the United Kingdom have operational pharmacoeconomic guidelines with explicit criteria for conducting and reporting the economic analysis of drug products. A few other Western countries have regulatory language suggesting that pharmaceuticals should give value, but these have not been standardized into explicit pharmacoeconomic guidelines. Canada is a bit unusual because the province of Ontario also has guidelines in addition to the federal guidelines. Nongovernmental pharmacoeconomic guidelines exist in the United States and are discussed here because they cover millions of insured lives and account for a substantial portion of United States drug expenditure.

Australian Guidelines

Australia was the first government to implement pharmacoeconomic guidelines. Because their approach has become a reference point, if not a model, for other countries, a discussion of the Australian guidelines is a logical departure point for understanding other guidelines.

The current Australian guidelines were preceded by a background paper in which the purpose, methods, and implications of economic analysis on pharmaceuticals for Australia were described.[3] In their conclusions, the authors acknowledged the complexity and difficulty of using economic analysis to make decisions about pharmaceuticals and suggested, "Staff training will be a priority; flexibility will be necessary during the development and introduction of formal requirements, and the pace of development must be controlled carefully."

About a year later, Drummond[4] observed that "...implementation of the guidelines will place considerable demands both on the industry and the Commonwealth itself." He expressed the belief that "...implemented sensibly they could form the basis for better decisions about the rational diffusion and use of medicines...if implemented inappropriately, the guidelines will be nothing more than an expensive way of slowing down the entry of new medicines." The initial Australian guidelines were published in 1992, became effective in 1993, were first revised in 1995, and most recently were updated with an interim document in April 2000.[5,6]

The guidelines were incorporated into the existing activities of the Pharmaceutical Benefits Advisory Committee (PBAC), which is responsible for making recommendations to the Minister of Health about drugs. As part of this responsibility, the PBAC also advises the Pharmaceutical Benefit Pricing Authority regarding "value for money" for drugs seeking admission to the Pharmaceutical Benefit Scheme (PBS). Although anyone may request that a drug product be added to the PBS, in practice, it is generally the product manufacturer that has the necessary data to support the request, especially in the case of new drugs. Admission to the PBS is critical to a product's success because only products on this list are subsidized by the government. In practice, the PBS regulates over 90% of the outpatient prescriptions dispensed in Australia.

The Australian guidelines specify two types of submissions (minor and major). No submission is required to list a generically equivalent product, and only a "minor submission" is necessary for clarifications and changes that do not affect pricing. The most extensive application of the guidelines is for preparation of a "major submission" that is required for a sponsor to[7]:

1. list a new drug on the PBS,
2. request a change in a current listing (eg, a new indication),
3. request a change in therapeutic relativity or price, or
4. list a new formulation of a currently listed drug for which a price premium is requested.

The report submitted by a product manufacturer in support of a listing and price for a new product must follow the guidelines. The complete submission contains clinical and economic information used by the PBAC to make its recommendation to the Minister of Health. Only the economic component of the guidelines is discussed below.

DETAILS OF THE PROPOSED DRUG AND ITS INDICATION FOR USE

The indication specified may be more narrow than what is specified in the marketing approval, but it may not go beyond what has been approved for the drug. The application also must specify the details of treatment (eg, daily dosage, the length of a course of therapy). A very important part of this section is a specification of the "main comparator," defined as "...the therapy most prescribers will replace in practice," which is often difficult to identify.[8] This is a key consideration, because establishing the economic value of a new product depends on the current cost of therapy for the main indication of the new product.

DATA FROM COMPARATIVE, RANDOMIZED TRIALS FOR THE MAIN INDICATION

The PBAC would like to have a head-to-head trial between the new drug and the main comparator; however, such a trial often is not available. In some cases, there may be different trials with both drugs against a common reference drug, but this also is not universally available. In some cases, such as for cancer drugs, the new medication may have been approved on evidence other than results of a randomized trial. Special rules apply in the latter case because, scientifically, it is difficult to establish the economic value of a product without randomized trials. The guidelines are quite specific that all randomized trial data should be provided and that an independent literature search will be conducted to verify the list provided. This rule is designed to ensure that product sponsors do not selectively present favorable trial results and exclude unfavorable results. The rules further specify that the report should include an economic evaluation of the data in the randomized trials with clear exposition of the strengths and weaknesses of aspects of the study that may introduce a bias.

If randomized trial data are not available, the product sponsor may submit appropriately analyzed literature using methods such as meta-analysis. The guidelines are specific about how data from nonrandomized trials should be analyzed and reported because these sources of information are scientifically weaker than randomized trial information.

MODELED ECONOMIC EVALUATION FOR THE MAIN INDICATION

Randomized trials conducted for the purpose of determining the safety and efficacy of a new drug often do not include economic data from which to estimate value. In addition, it is always necessary to estimate effectiveness of a new drug from efficacy data obtained in the trial. When it is not possible to estimate the economic value of a new drug using original data, the guidelines allow for economic modeling. Models require many assumptions, and there are specific requirements about how models should be prepared and reported. These requirements include reporting sources of information for estimating model parameters (eg, literature sources), populations on which the data are based (eg, 1,000 hypertensive males), the time horizon (eg, must be appropriate to the disease), the parameters of a sensitivity analysis (eg, which variables are used and why), and a justification of the outcome variable modeled.

ESTIMATED EXTENT OF USE AND FINANCIAL IMPLICATIONS

The previous specifications allow the PBAC to make a decision on whether to subsidize a new drug product based on its health benefits and value from a *societal perspective*. This section sets out requirements for estimating the financial impact of the new drug from the *perspective of the government health budget*. For example, a new drug may have excellent value but require additional expenditure from the health budget. Therefore, the product report is expected to estimate the volume of use and extent to which the new drug will be substituted for current therapy from which the financial implications for government health budgets can be determined. Obviously, the product sponsor must set a price for the product to conduct this analysis.

OTHER CONSIDERATIONS

Where discounting is appropriate (ie, benefits and costs extend beyond one year), the guidelines specify that a five percent discount rate should be used. All forms of economic analysis are acceptable if appropriate to the situation (eg, cost minimization, cost-effectiveness, cost-utility, cost-benefit); however, the use of cost-benefit analysis is discouraged because it often relies heavily on calculations of indirect costs and benefits. In general, the guidelines discourage inclusion of indirect costs and benefits because the perspective of the analysis is to be societal. For purposes of the Australian guidelines, the societal perspective does not include indirect costs because the Australian government view is that is sufficient unused capacity exits in the country to compensate for lost productivity due to illnesses. If inclusion of indirect benefits in the analysis can be justified, the report must include results with and without the indirect costs and benefits.

The guidelines suggest that, wherever possible, the outcomes of an economic analysis should be presented as the final outcome such as deaths prevented, life-years gained, or quality-adjusted life-years gained (eg, cost-effectiveness or cost-utility analysis). This is not always possible; surrogate measures are therefore acceptable but must be convincingly linked to the final outcome (eg, blood pressure as a surrogate outcome measure for an antihypertensive agent). The outcome must be specific to the main indication of the product and not include long-term consequences of a condition (eg, for an antihypertensive, the outcome should focus on blood pressure control and not end-stage renal disease). Regardless of the economic method used, the report must include an incremental analysis so that it is possible to determine the cost of each additional unit of outcome.

SUMMARY

The Australian guidelines are very specific on all the key elements of a standard economic analysis. Of special interest is the stipulation that product sponsors must provide an estimate of financial implications for the health budget. It is self-evident that a product must be both cost-effective (eg, provide value) and affordable to the government, which will pay most of the cost of the drug through its subsidy. Thus, the value of a new product is to be demonstrated at the societal level, but financial affordability is more narrowly defined.

If the PBAC decides not to recommend listing of a new product on the PBS, this presents the opportunity for negotiations between the PBAC and the product sponsor. Given the general character of economic analysis equations (cost per unit of outcome) and the fixed nature of the outcome (based on available clinical trial data or other evidence), this leaves price as the only variable to manipulate in an attempt to decrease the cost per unit of outcome. While there may be differences over the outcome assessment, it is clear that a price reduction from that specified by the product sponsor is likely to be necessary to achieve payer acceptance.

Another concern of the PBAC is the effect of diagnosis "creep" on the financial impact assessment provided in the economic analysis. Because the analysis estimates the financial consequences based on the main indication, there is the potential for increased expenditure if use of the new product creeps beyond this specific indication. The PBAC has the authority to restrict use of certain agents to guard against the problem of diagnosis creep.

Canadian Guidelines

The development of pharmacoeconomic guidelines in Canada began in 1991 with publication of draft guidelines by the Ontario Ministry of Health. The draft guidelines were revised in 1992 and became the basis for further development by an interprovincial working group.[9] After further revisions by the working group, this document was discussed at the the Collaborative Workshop on Pharmacoeconomics in June 1993.[10] The Ontario Ministry of Health, drawing on the Collaborative Workshop experience, revised and published their guidelines in November 1993.[11]

The Interprovincial Working Group proposed establishing a federal agency known as the Canadian Agency for Pharmaceutical Information Assessment (CAPIA) that would be responsible for developing national standards for comparative economic analysis of pharmaceuticals.[12] Although CAPIA was never established, the Canadian Coordinating Office for Health Technology Assessment (CCOHTA) effectively filled this role in 1994, and the guidelines were implemented.[13]

In the Canadian healthcare system, provinces are responsible for providing a set of healthcare services mandated by the federal government. Comprehensive health care is universally available and transferable among provinces. Unlike hospital and physician services, the federal government does not mandate a prescription drug benefit; however, all 10 provinces provide some type of government-subsidized drug program. In the absence of federal guidelines, it is not surprising to find considerable variability among provincial drug benefit programs. However, all provincial governments share a common desire to restrain pharmaceutical expenditure and therefore had an interest in fostering a national clearinghouse of pharmacoeconomic information.

At the federal level, price restraint on pharmaceuticals is exercised by the Patented Medicine Prices Review Board (PMPRB).[14] This board limits the launch price of new products and price increases on existing products. The board has authority over all patented products (both over-the-counter and prescription drugs), but not for unpatented products. It is not involved in the drug approval process. Pharmaceutical prices for any particular product can differ among provinces because of provincial initiatives to negotiate prices below the PMPRB-mandated ceilings.

As an example of a provincial drug benefit, Ontario subsidizes prescription drugs for the elderly (aged 65 and over), those receiving custodial or nursing home care, and those receiving certain types of public assistance payments.[15] Only products listed in the Ontario Drug Benefit Formulary/Comparative Drug Index are paid for by the Ontario Ministry of Health. Consumer cost-sharing is not required for prescriptions covered under the plan. Other provinces cover different groups and have different cost-sharing arrangements.

The Ontario guidelines are similar to those of Australia on the major features of economic analysis and reporting.[16] Ontario guidelines are less prescriptive on the type of economic analysis to be performed, but are more detailed with respect to the financial impact calculation. The latter is specified to be three years from product launch; the parameters of the estimate and sensitivity analysis are also specified. Product sponsors are not always required to provide an economic analysis, but it is clear that a premium price request must be supported with an economic justification. The Ontario guidelines also request that the data be summarized in a worksheet format, even though a complete report is attached.

Unlike the Ontario guidelines, the federal Canadian guidelines published by CCOHTA are not related to a specific government agency that will determine a price or reimbursement level for a product. Also, CCOHTA produces its own analysis rather than reviewing reports submitted by product sponsors. The CCOHTA guidelines were revised in 1997, and the most recent revisions are available on the CCOHTA Web site, which also provides a brief statement of its mission: "...encourage the appropriate use of health technology by influencing decision makers through the collection, analysis, creation and dissemination of information concerning the effectiveness and cost of technology and its impact on health."[17,18]

All of the major elements covered in the Australian and Ontario guidelines are included in the CCOHTA guidelines. Also included in these guidelines is explicit language about the decision-maker, which is somewhat separate from the concept of perspective. On this issue, the text indicates: "The primary audience (decision-maker) for the study should be identified. Secondary target audiences can also be listed."[17]

Later, under the heading of "perspective," the view is expressed that "All studies should report from a comprehensive societal perspective. That perspective should be transparently broken down into those of other relevant viewpoints, including that of the primary decision maker."[17] This level of detail regarding transparency and disaggregation of the data is found throughout the CCOHTA guidelines. In summary, the CCOHTA guidelines are similar to those for Ontario and Australia, but are more detailed.

United Kingdom Guidelines

Although these guidelines are often referenced as United Kingdom, they apply only to England and Wales. Scotland has a similar program known as the Scottish Intercollegiate Guidelines Network (SIGN). which develops clinical guidelines for Scotland.[19] Both the National Institute for Clinical Excellence (NICE),[20] the United Kingdom guideline agency, and SIGN are members of the Appraisal of Guidelines, Research and Evaluation collaboration (AGREE), an international network of guidelines programs.[21]

NICE is a special health authority within the National Health Service of the United Kingdom with the purpose of providing patients, health professionals, and the public with "...authoritative and reliable guidance on current best practice."[20] NICE issues technology appraisals and clinical guidelines. Pharmaceuticals are covered as part of the technology appraisal process, which also includes medical devices, diagnostic technologies, and surgical interventions. For technology assessments, NICE is charged to "appraise the clinical benefits and costs of those interventions notified by the Secretary of State and the National Assembly for Wales and to make recommendations." NICE also creates clinical guidelines that may refer to drugs in the context of clinical management. The NICE guideline approach is more like that of CCOHTA than Australia. Like CCOHTA, NICE does not set prices, nor does it establish reimbursement levels. NICE guidance does not override professional responsibility of health practitioners, but as participants in the National Health Service, health professionals are expected to "...take the guidance fully into account when exercising their clinical judgment."[20]

NICE is also like CCOHTA in that it does its own analysis internally rather than making an assessment submitted by a product sponsor. This means that both CCOHTA and NICE set their own agendas. In the case of NICE, the topics to investigate are referred by the Secretary for Health (in England) and the Welsh Assembly Government. The public and health professionals also have input through these two government bodies.

NICE guidelines are produced by one of several National Collaborating Centers following a standard set of guidelines that are monitored by another Collaborating Center. During development of a guideline, the group responsible for the assessment must consider both clinical effectiveness and cost-effectiveness. The process includes an extensive literature review and consultation with stakeholders before producing a draft guideline that is circulated for comment. The final report is submitted from the Collaborating Center to NICE, which issues the final guideline.

SUMMARY

NICE guidelines are issued following an internal development process that uses literature sources, as well as information provided by stakeholders that includes the manufacturer of a product that is the subject of analysis. NICE does not directly set prices, but rather a negative guidance suggesting that, on balance, a product is not cost-effective strongly implies that this is due to the price. There is somewhat of a disconnect between NICE guidance and its ultimate effect on use of a drug. While health professionals are not obliged to follow the guidance, there are clear indications that not following the guidance would at least need to be justified. If NICE is expected to positively influence value for money, it will require compliance with the issued guidelines.

Overview of Private and Public Sector Guidelines in the United States

Because the United States pharmaceutical market is split between a private sector and various government programs, the United States is not considered a single-payer market. There is no national drug benefit program that covers any segment of the population (Medicare provides health insurance for the elderly, but does not include an outpatient drug benefit); therefore, the absence of a single national pharmacoeconomic guideline is not surprising.

However, the Food and Drug Administration (FDA) has become involved in the issue of pharmacoeconomic assessments because it has jurisdiction over promotional claims for pharmaceutical products. Recently, product manufacturers have realized the advantages of making economic claims for their products and consequently have begun to generate pharmacoeconomic data with the intent of using it for marketing. The FDA has reviewed these claims prior to product launch and made decisions on a case-by-case basis rather than publishing a specific standard.[22] In the absence of separate standards for demonstrating an economic benefit, the FDA has set the same standard for economic claims that it uses for safety and efficacy claims (eg, two well-controlled randomized trials). Most manufacturers have found it difficult and expensive for their product to meet this threshold, which probably accounts for the absence of economic claims in marketing. An appreciation for pharmacoeconomic guideline activity in the United States requires consideration of both the private and public sectors.

FEDERAL GOVERNMENT ACTIVITY

At this time, there is no general United States government requirement to provide pharmacoeconomic data for the purpose of listing or reimbursing a product, and price setting is not a government function. However, two federal government entities (Veterans Affairs, the Department of Defense) do make economic assessments of pharmaceuticals. Both of these agencies have only recently begun pharmacoeconomic assessments.

The Veterans Affairs Pharmacy Benefits Management Strategic Health Care Group (VAPBM) publishes treatment guidelines and drug class reviews.[23] Each of these may contain opinions on the cost of therapy or, in the case of drug class reviews, recommendations on whether to admit a product to a formulary. However, the VAPBM has not published a set of guidelines used in their internally generated economic assessments.

The Department of Defense (DoD) Pharmacoeconomics Center (PEC) was founded to "improve the clinical, economic, and humanistic outcomes of drug therapy in support of the readiness and managed healthcare missions of the Military Health System (MHS)."[24] Activities of the DoD PEC include pharmacoeconomic analysis to support DoD formulary management, contracting activities, and clinical practice guideline development. These analyses are internally generated at the PEC. The PEC does not publish guidelines used for its assessments.

PRIVATE SECTOR ACTIVITY

The United States market for healthcare services is characterized by a large private sector dominated by insurers and managed care providers. Large insurers and managed care organizations have begun to employ some forms of economic analysis of pharmaceuticals to assist them with their formulary decisions. Because this is a problem shared by many insurers, the Academy of Managed Care Pharmacy (AMCP) has recently published guidelines for conducting formulary assessments that include an economic assessment. At this writing, the *AMCP Format for Formulary Submissions* was in use by managed care organizations covering in excess of 100 million lives.[25] Although not an official standard, the extent of coverage lends importance to the guidelines. The AMCP guidelines are intended to be a "...template for pharmaceutical and medical device manufacturers to use to construct a fomulary submission dossier designed to make the product evaluation process in formulary development more rational."[26] While the format covers all aspects of formulary decision-making, the discussion here is limited to the economic component.

The AMCP views the dossier format as a means for pharmaceutical manufacturers to justify the price of a new drug in terms of its value to the health plan. Methods of economic evaluation used by the product sponsor are not specified by the guidelines, but the methods chosen by the product sponsor are expected to be appropriate for demonstrating value. The guidelines do specify that the orientation of analysis should be disease based and not clinical trial oriented. The guidelines permit a variety of analytic approaches including prospective studies piggybacked onto pivotal clinical trials, naturalistic comparative studies, retrospective studies, and modeling studies. The data provided must be broadly applicable for the health plan to which the dossier is submitted, and it must be sufficient for the health plan to judge the merit of the individual studies submitted in support of the request for formulary listing.

The guidelines anticipate that economic models will be provided. When offered as support for the product, they must evaluate the impact of the new product on costs as well as clinical and humanistic outcomes for the plan's population. As mentioned above, the model must be disease based and consider all relevant treatment pathways. Results from the model are expected to provide either cost/consequences tables or cost-effectiveness ratios. The comparator is expected to be appropriate, the clinical endpoints must be relevant, and there must be a sensitivity analysis of the pivotal estimates and assumptions. While the model is disease based, the clinical and economic data are expected to be taken from clinical trials and modified to be realistic for the plan's population.

The *AMCP Format for Formulary Submissions* is very similar to the guidelines developed by Australia and CCOHTA, but there does appear to be more latitude on the selection of an economic evaluation method and the costs to include in the analysis. The guidelines recognize this by observing that major pharmaceutical manufacturers are already submitting outcomes modeling data as part of their submissions to national formularies for "...Australia, Canada, and other countries."[26]

OTHER GUIDELINES AND RECENT TRENDS

The guidelines reviewed above are those with the most longevity, but do not include the entire scope of activity. For example, New Zealand created guidelines in 1999,[27] and Norway now requires the submission of economic data for manufacturers seeking listing of a new product.[28] British Columbia, Canada, requires economic evidence from product sponsors seeking admission to their formulary. Pharmacare, the British Columbia drug benefit program, requires that product sponsors follow the CCOHTA guidelines when submitting dossiers.[29] Other countries, such as Denmark and Portugal,[21] have "voluntary" pharmacoeconomic data requirements, and Poland has proposed guidelines.[30]

Regardless of the development of guidelines, there has been an increasing number of pharmacoeconomic studies beginning in the 1990s. For example, in 1993, Drummond and colleagues[31] identified more than 60 economic evaluations of pharmaceuticals in 11 European countries reviewed. Pritchard[32] also noted the increased volume of economic studies ranging from about 1,000 in 1991 to over 2,000 in the year 2000. Founding of the International Society for Pharmacoeconomics and Outcomes Research (ISPOR) in the early 1990s fostered growth in economic evaluations of pharmaceuticals and serves as testimony to the interest in this area.

Perhaps because of the rising level of research activity, there have been many calls for standardization of the methods used to conduct economic evaluations of pharmaceuticals. Although governments established pharmacoeconomic guidelines to set standards for their own use, a need for further standardization has been consistently reported in the literature. Jacobs and colleagues[33] noted the divergence of published guidelines from accepted accounting standards, and ISPOR held a national conference to identify issues and suggest remedies.[34] Central to many of the issues are the problems of credibility and methodologic rigor. In the United States, a national panel was convened to make recommendations on standards for economic evaluations of healthcare technologies (including pharmaceuticals).[35,36] Drummond[37] has noted that there needs to be "...much more clarity of purpose in government guidelines, and methodological standards for economic analysis need to be refined." More recently, Pang[38] reviewed several multinational economic evaluations and assessed the factors that could create variations in cost-effectiveness between healthcare settings. He regards current guidelines as too limited to cope with the multinational scope of clinical trials and suggests alternatives that should be included in future guidelines. There continues to be disagreement over the usefulness of pharmacoeconomic guidelines, especially in a multinational context.

In the midst of all this diversity, there have been calls for a pan-European Union effort to standardize national pharmacoeconomic guidelines that would facilitate studies by manufacturers. The argument states that studies are both costly and time consuming, which ultimately increases the cost of drugs and delays their availability to the public. Furthermore, the same data should serve all decision-makers equally well. The counter position is that vast differences in national health policies, the structure of national healthcare systems, and varying levels of healthcare cost make harmonization difficult—if not impossible—at this time. However, a review of North American, European, and Australian guidelines suggests that much comparability already exists among national guidelines.[39] This study reviewed and compared 25 guidelines that were categorized as "formal," "informal," or "guidelines for health economic methods." When 15 important methodologic aspects were compared, the authors judged the guidelines comparable (within categories) on 40 percent to 100 percent of criteria for formal guidelines. Between-category comparability was rated as 75 percent. The most common disagreements among guidelines were on perspective, resources and costs to include in the analysis (probably a function of differences in perspective), and methods of evaluating resources used. While these are important areas of disagreement, it is somewhat surprising to find such a high degree of comparability. From a distance, it appears there is a continued movement toward development of national guidelines but little progress in harmonization across guidelines. However, there is some evidence that national guidelines are somewhat similar on their major dimensions.

It is difficult to know whether the call for standardization is the result of diverse research methodologies, the rising number of national guidelines, or some convergence of these trends. The consequence is clearly a greater emphasis on adopting standards for conducting and reporting pharmacoeconomic research.

This movement is being driven, at least in part, by payers who desire comparability, accuracy, and ease of use in the data they receive and use for decision-making. Their main concern is that much of the economic evaluation of pharmaceuticals is either funded or conducted by the product sponsor, which presents the potential for bias. This concern has given rise to at least two attempts to increase the transparency of the research process to reduce the perception of bias.

One such effort was that of the *New England Journal of Medicine*, which published an editorial policy on cost-effectiveness studies.[40] Concern over the potential for bias caused the editors to enunciate a policy on publication of cost-effectiveness analysis. Their concerns fall into three areas:

1. the relationship between industry funding and the investigators,
2. written assurance of the authors' independence regarding conduct of the research and publication of its results, and
3. complete disclosure of all data used in the analysis, all assumptions, and any model used in the analysis.

Subsequent letters to the editor show much disagreement with this policy.[41,42] Correspondents generally fault the policy for focusing on the source of funding rather than the quality of the work. These and other actions by the private sector in the United States have created an environment for economic evaluation that is similar to that of other countries where study criteria are mandated by the government.

The second United States effort to make pharmaceutical industry economic evaluations of pharmaceuticals more transparent is in the form of a set of ethical principles published by an independent academic group not affiliated with the pharmaceutical industry.[43] The academic group argues that competitive markets create pressure for bias that therefore requires adoption of standards to ensure integrity of scientific information. The authors stated that "Identifying studies that have followed protocols designed to reduce bias would allow readers to recognize the likelihood of bias in studies not so designated. As a result, competitive pressures would be channeled toward less biased, more useful research. Adherence to these standards would generate a seal of approval that could in itself be valuable in selling pharmaceuticals in an increasingly skeptical and competitive marketplace."[43] The six standards of practice presented by the authors are similar to those found in the Australian, Canadian, and Ontario guidelines. They include:

1. establishment of written agreements between companies and institutions (not individuals),
2. proper selection of comparators based on the situation,
3. transparency of the company–investigator relationship,
4. provisions on the control of data in stepwise funded projects,
5. preference for conservative assumptions, and
6. commitment to publish valid results regardless of their promotional value.

Implications

There are three undeniable global trends regarding pharmacoeconomic guidelines. First, the number of guidelines is increasing. Second, there is a movement to improve the credibility of pharmacoeconomic research. Third, there are frequent calls for harmonization of the various guidelines into some consolidated guidance. Of the many consequences that may result from any or all of these trends, only three are discussed here.

DRUG BENEFIT PROGRAMS

The rising trend of per capita pharmaceutical expenditure has been presented (Figure 2). This trend has persisted regardless of the methods used to constrain expenditure, and reasons for the rise have been discussed. It was noted that pharmacoeconomic guidelines were the most recent attempt to restrain expenditure by tying price or reimbursement to the value of a drug. Drummond,[37] for one, has noted that this may be an inefficient means of cost control if that is the objective. If value for money is the true objective, then it is possible that drug expenditure will rise even faster. Government payers will be reluctant to allow this, and the irresistable temptation will be to limit expenditure regardless of a product's estimated value. In this scenario, pharmacoeconomic guidelines become an expensive means of cost control. Payers are likely to disagree with this characterization of their intentions and would counter that pharmacoeconomic guidelines not only reward value, but also make clear to pharmaceutical companies which therapeutic markets hold the greatest potential for value. For example, producing one more β-blocker will not be as valuable as developing a new therapy for under-served conditions such as Alzheimer's disease and schizophrenia. Furthermore, the rationale is that a drug benefit that pays for products regardless of their value encourages marketing of un-needed products, therefore wasting scarce research resources.

If manufacturers respond to the value incentive, it is likely to result in a greater share of health expenditures devoted to phar-maceuticals through increasing government subsidies and ris-ing patient out-of-pocket costs. This will be due, in part, to the changing prevalence of disease in the industrialized world, as well as to the demand for pharmaceutical therapies. An aging population will use more chronic medications for longer periods of time, and much of the progress in medical interventions continues to be for less invasive forms of treatment, such as drugs. Whether pharmacoeconomic guidelines can encourage pharmaceutical manufacturers to develop more needed therapies is unknown, but the use of guidelines to constrain expenditure seems obvious.

CLINICAL MANAGEMENT

A clear objective in many pharmacoeconomic guidelines is to incorporate cost-effectiveness with clinical effectiveness in the decision to use a drug product. This position is implicit in many drug benefit programs regardless of their use of guidelines. For example, this is the principle in step-care and prior authoriza-tion programs. In step-care, a patient must demonstrate that less expensive therapies are not effective before gaining access to more expensive drugs. Prior authorization attempts to ensure that expensive therapies are used appropriately, but screens users before allowing access. Can a patient use a traditional an-tihistamine, or is a more expensive nonsedating antihistamine required? Will an H_2-antagonist produce the same outcome as the more expensive proton-pump inhibitor for a particular pa-tient? This is not a new philosophy, but it has applicability in the use of pharmacoeconomic guidelines because products that cannot demonstrate value may not be admitted to a formulary or given a subsidy. This practice brings with it some risk of mak-ing a product unavailable on the basis of economic criteria. While this is an issue of how to apply pharmacoeconomic guidelines, the content of a guideline could influence the trade-off between clinical effectiveness and cost-effectiveness.

APPLICABILITY TO PHARMACOGENOMIC PRODUCTS

From our current vantage point, we can get a glimpse of future drug therapy based on the principles of pharmacogenomics. While products based on pharmacogenomics may not be the norm for drug treatment, they are important in the context of pharmacoeconomic guidelines that purport to reward value (see Chapter 10). These products will be used to treat previously untreatable or poorly treated conditions which, by the definition of value for money embodied in pharmacoeconomic guidelines, will have high value. Treatment with pharmacogenomic products will be expensive because it will require diagnostic testing to identify patients who will benefit from treatment, the drugs will be expensive, and follow-up monitoring will be necessary. By definition, a pharmacogenomic drug will be specific to a very limited population.[44] Often, the conditions treated will be life-threatening or severely debilitating; this adds an emotional dimension and will encourage aggressive treatment even when the probability of success is low. We can observe this now for cancer, multiple sclerosis, and other serious conditions. The only difference is that pharmacogenomic drug treatment will be more costly and apply to a smaller pool of patients. Will the application of pharmacoeconomics be applicable to pharmacogenomic drugs? Will value be rewarded?

Summary

For the foreseeable future, a role for pharmacoeconomic guidelines seems assured, and it is evident that the main purpose of guidelines will be to limit pharmaceutical expenditure. It is not clear whether there will be standardization of methods used to conduct pharmacoeconomic studies, but the desires of payers using the information are likely to be sufficient to ensure that some form of standards are created. Manufacturers also have an interest in standards if they can increase the credibility of the data. Finally, harmonization of national standards seems a distant possibility given the many cultural, structural, and economic differences among countries even within the confines of the relatively homogeneous European Union. However, there continues to be interest in harmonization to improve the efficiency, if not the comparability, of data.

Besides the technical aspects of improving pharmacoeconomic guidelines, important differences remain between product sponsors and payers on the appropriate use of guidelines in policy decisions such as prices, reimbursements, and formulary listings. These differences are likely to remain given the divergent goals of producers and payers.

The applicability of pharmacoeconomic guidelines to future pharmaceutical markets is an open question. Development of pharmacogenomic drugs could substantially alter how guidelines are applied. The other area of uncertainty is the use of pharmacoeconomic data to make product claims for marketing purposes. Unless the credibility problems outlined above can be resolved, it seems unlikely that pharmacoeconomic data will be used more aggressively in marketing.

References

1. OECD Health Database (CD-ROM). OECD, producers. Paris: OECD, 2001.
2. Kozma CM, Reeder CE, Schulz RM. Economic, clinical, and humanistic outcomes: a planning model for pharmacoeconomic research. Clin Ther 1993;15:1121-32.
3. Evans D, et al. The use of economic analysis as a basis for inclusion of pharmaceutical products on the pharmaceutical benefits scheme. An unpublished background paper dated December 1989 and submitted to the PBAC. www.health.gov.au/pbs (accessed 2002 Apr 30).
4. Drummond M. Australian guidelines for cost-effectiveness studies of pharmaceuticals: the thin end of the boomerang? Pharmacoeconomics 1991;13 (suppl 1):61-9.
5. Guidelines for the pharmaceutical industry on preparation of submissions to the Pharmaceutical Benefits Advisory Committee (including submissions involving economic analysis). Canberra, Australia: Commonwealth Department of Health, Housing and Community Services, August 1992.
6. The 1995 guidelines, interim document. Australian Ministry of Health. www.health.gov.au (accessed 2002 Apr 30).
7. Guidelines for the pharmaceutical industry on preparation of submissions to the PBAC: part II. www.health.gov.au/pbs/pubs/pharmpac/part2.htm (accessed 2002 Apr 30).
8. Guidelines for the pharmaceutical industry on preparation of submissions to the PBAC: part III. www.health.gov.au/pbs/pubs/pharmpac/part3.htm (accessed 2002 Apr 30).

9. Detsky A. Guidelines for economic analysis of pharmaceutical products: a draft document for Ontario and Canada. Pharmacoeconomics 1993;15:354-61.
10. Schubert F, ed. Proceedings of the Canadian Collaborative Workshop on Pharmacoeconomics. Amsterdam: Excerpta Medica, November 1993.
11. Ontario guidelines for economic analysis of pharmaceutical products. Toronto: Ontario Ministry of Health, November 22, 1993.
12. Brogan T. Pharmacoeconomics: the Canadian experience. Scrip Magazine 1993;19(Nov):18.
13. Canadian Coordination Office of Health technology Assessment (CCOHTA). Guidelines for economic evaluation of pharmaceuticals: Ottawa, Canada: CCOHTA, 1st ed. November 1994.
14. Patient Medicines Price Review Board. www.pmprb-cepmb.gc.ca (accessed 2004 Apr 16).
15. Ontario drug benefit formulary comparative drug index no. 33. Toronto: Ontario Ministry of Health, 1993:viii.
16. Ontario guidelines for economic analysis of pharmaceutical products. Toronto: Ontario Ministry of Health, 1994. www.gov.ca/health (accessed 2002 Apr 30).
17. Guidelines for economic evaluation of pharmaceuticals: Ottawa, Canada: CCOHTA, 2nd ed. November 1997.
18. Canadian Coordinating Office for Health Technology Assessment guidelines. www.ccohta.ca (accessed 2004 Apr 16).
19. Scottish Intercollegiate Guidelines Network. www.sign.ac.uk (accessed 2004 Apr 16).
20. National Institute for Clinical Excellence. www.nice.org.uk (accessed 2004 Apr 16.
21. Appraisal of Guidelines, Research, and Evaluation. www.agreecollaboration.org (accessed 2004 Apr 16).
22. Bonastia CJ. What is the FDA's position on pharmacoeconomic data in promotion? Outcomes Measure Manage 1994;5(6):1-2.
23. Veterans Affairs Pharmacy Benefits Management. www.vapbm.org/PBM/menu.asp (accessed 2004 Apr 16).
24. Department of Defense Pharmacoeconomics Center. www.pec.ha.osd.mil (accessed 2004 Apr 16).
25. Neumann PJ. Evidence-based and value-based formulary guidelines. Health AFF 2004;23:124-34.
26. Academy of Managed Care Pharmacy. www.amcp.org (accessed 2002 Apr 30).
27. The Pharmac formulary management program. www.pharmac.govt.nz (accessed 2002 Apr 30).
28. Norwegian guidelines for phaarmacoeconomis analysis in connection with applications for reimbursement. www.legemiddelverket.no/eng/reg/ (accessed 2004 Apr 16).
29. Pharmacare and British Columbia pharmacoeconomic requirements. www. hlth.gov.bc.ca/pharme (accessed 2004 Apr 16).
28. Appraisal Guidelines Research Evaluation. www.agreecollaboration.org (accessed 2004 Apr 16).

30. Orlewska E, Mierzejewski P. Farmako Ekonomika Polish guidelines for condusting pharmacoeconomic evaluations (project). Farmako Ekonomika 2000;(suppl 1):12-20.
31. Drummond M, Ruttin F, Bienna A, Pinto CG, Horisberger B, Jönsson B, et al. Economic evaluation of pharmaceuticals. Pharmacoeconomics 1993;15: 173-86.
32. Pritchard C. Pharmacoeconomic guidelines around the world. Waltham, MA: Decision Resources, June 22, 2001:5-1–5-12.
33. Jacobs P, Bachynsky J, Baladi JF. A comparative review of pharmacoeconomic guidelines. Pharmacoeconomics 1995;8:182-9.
34. Advisory Panel Reports from the ISPOR conference on Pharmacoeconomics: identifying the issues. www.ispor.org/workpaper/adpanel/apr.pdf (accessed 2002 Apr 30).
35. Weinstein MC, Siegel JE, Gold MR, Kamlet MS, Russell LB. Recommendations of the Panel on Cost-Effectiveness in Health and Medicine. JAMA 1996;276:1253-8.
36. Siegel JE, Weinstein MC, Russell LB, Gold MR. Recommendations for reporting cost-effectiveness analyses. JAMA 1996;276:1339-41.
37. Drummond M. The emerging government requirement for economic evaluation of pharmaceuticals. Pharmacoeconomics 1994;6(suppl 1):42-50.
38. Pang F. Design, analysis and presentation of multinational economic studies. Pharmacoeconomics 2002;20:75-90.
39. Hjelmgren J, Berggren F, Andersson F. Health economic guidelines, differences and some implications. Value Health 2001;4:225-50.
40. The Journal's policy on cost-effectiveness analyses. N Engl J Med 1994; 331:669-70.
41. Powe NR. Cost-effectiveness analyses. N Engl J Med 1995;332:123-4. Author reply 124-5.
42. Steinberg EP. Cost-effectiveness analyses. N Engl J Med 1995;332:123-4. Author reply 124-5.
43. Hillman AL, Eisenberg JM, Pauly MV, Bloom BS, Glick H, Kinosian B, et al. Avoiding bias in the conduct and reporting of cost-effectiveness research sponsored by pharmaceutical companies. N Engl J Med 1991; 324:1362-5.
44. Dickson M, Reeder CE. Economics of cancer drug development. Oncol Spectrums 2001;2:542-9.

Cost Determination and Analysis

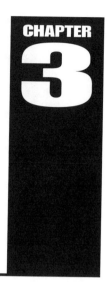

Lon N Larson

The price of a drug product is not the same as the cost of drug therapy. One objective of this chapter is to clarify this difference by defining and describing the concept of cost. A second is to describe how the cost of a therapy or service is determined. Unlike price, which is usually quite easily obtained, cost is more difficult to measure. The ultimate purpose of this chapter is to enable the reader to quantify the cost of a given program or service; in other words, to identify the resources used in a therapy and to assign monetary values to those resources.

The chapter begins with a brief description of production in the healthcare system and the definitions of cost-related terminology. This is followed by a description of the elements in the cost of illness and cost of therapy. The third section of the chapter provides a five-step approach to determining the cost of a therapy or service. The fourth section discusses issues in valuing resources in pharmacoeconomic analyses.

The concept of cost deals with the resources that are used or consumed in the production of a good or service. Production in the healthcare system is a two-step process. The ultimate products of the healthcare system are therapies that cure, prevent, or alleviate disease, thereby affecting health status. In producing these therapies, several services may be used: prescription drugs, laboratory tests, hospital stays, physician visits, and surgical procedures. Stated differently, these services are the inputs in a production process that produces therapies as its outputs. These services, in turn, require basic resources such as personnel, equipment, facilities, and supplies. In other words, healthcare services can be viewed as intermediate goods—they consume basic resources and, in turn, they are consumed in the production of therapies. In some pharmacoeconomic analyses, determining the basic inputs is important. For instance, to determine the cost of once-daily dosing, the basic inputs of labor and equipment should be specified. In contrast, to calculate the cost of treating an illness with drug therapy, determining the services used (ie, intermediate rather than basic inputs) is appropriate.

Several cost-related terms need to be understood. These include cost, direct and indirect cost, fixed and variable cost, average and marginal cost, and opportunity cost. *Cost* is defined as the magnitude of resources consumed.[1] The cost of a product or service is the monetary value of resources consumed in its production or delivery. Resources include labor, plant, equipment, and supplies.

A *direct cost* involves a transfer of money. If money is exchanged for the use of a resource, this is a direct cost. An *indirect cost*, in contrast, is an unpaid resource commitment.[1] No money is exchanged. Lost time from work is an indirect cost because output is lost due to the absence. Note that the economist and the accountant have different definitions of the term "indirect cost." The economic view is presented here. In accounting, indirect cost refers to overhead or shared expenses that are used in the production of several products. The allocation of shared costs, or the accountant's indirect cost, is discussed on page 55.

Resource use may or may not be affected by the volume of output. A *fixed cost* does not change with an increase or decrease in output. In contrast, a *variable cost* does vary or change with a change in the volume of output.[2] To illustrate, an employee's salary is a fixed cost, but a sales commission is a variable cost. Similarly, depreciation of plant and equipment is fixed, whereas cost of goods sold (drug products in the case of a pharmacy) is variable.

Average cost is the resources consumed per unit of output. It is derived by dividing total cost by volume or quantity of output. *Marginal cost* is the change in total cost of producing one additional (or one less) unit of output.[2] Because fixed cost remains unchanged as output increases, marginal cost may be viewed as the average variable cost. Thus, if a program involves principally variable costs, its average and marginal costs are similar. If, however, a program has a large amount of fixed costs (relative to variable costs), its marginal cost is less than its average cost.

Opportunity cost is defined as the amount that a resource could earn in its highest valued alternative use; it is the value of the alternative that must be foregone when something is produced.[1] Opportunity cost is the best measure of the value of a resource.[3] In a competitive marketplace, the price of a good or service—set through the interaction of supply and demand—is its opportunity cost. However, some healthcare services are relatively immune from price competition, and using price as a proxy for opportunity cost is hazardous. Inpatient hospital care, which is discussed in more detail on page 60, is an example. Other resources have no market prices—volunteer help, unpaid family assistance at home. Their opportunity cost is estimated by calculating potential earnings from another endeavor.

What are some of the implications of these definitions? First, cost should not be confused with charge or price.[4] Cost is the magnitude of resources consumed in producing a good or service. Price is what the customer is asked to pay for the good or service. A hospital is a good example, in which the charge for a service may not reflect resources consumed because of cross-subsidization between departments (eg, the very expensive aspirin). Second, cost is not the same as out-of-pocket payment. Often, the cost of a service is viewed as what the patient must pay out of pocket. This assumes that any third-party payment or charity care is without cost, and that is not the case. Third, cost should not be confused with flow of money. To illustrate, assume that a new program is started and staffed with existing personnel. Even though the personnel budget is unchanged, there is still a labor cost, or resource commitment, to the program. The personnel resource is consumed. The assumption is made that the time spent on this program could have been spent in another productive venture (ie, the opportunity cost of a foregone alternative).

Cost of Illness and Cost of Therapy

An illness consumes resources; thus, it has a cost.[4] The cost of an illness is the sum of three components: medical resources, nonmedical resources, and lost productivity or indirect costs. Medical resources are the services used to treat the illness, and they include hospital care, professional services, drugs, and supplies. The second category, nonmedical resources, can be classified as two types.[3,5] Personal costs consist of the patient's out-of-pocket expenses for goods and services outside the medical care sector. Transportation to the site of treatment and hiring a person to help with homemaker services are examples of personal nonmedical costs. The second type of nonmedical cost consists of resources consumed in other sectors because of the illness. For instance, an illness may cause resources to be consumed in the criminal justice system, and another may require special education programs. These are direct costs because money is exchanged. Even though they are nonmedical in nature, they are considered part of the cost of the illness because their use is caused by the illness. The illness also may be associated with productivity costs—economic losses that arise because of temporary or permanent disability. This is the third component of the cost of illness—also referred to as indirect costs. Productivity costs are sometimes classified as two types: morbidity costs (the time lost from work due to illness or disability) and mortality costs, arising from premature death.[6]

A medical therapy is intended to cure, prevent, or reduce the severity of an illness. As it does, the cost of the illness is reduced, and this reduction in the cost of the illness is the economic benefit of the therapy. However, a therapy uses or consumes resources. As with the cost of illness, the cost of a treatment also may be classified as medical, direct nonmedical (including personal and other sector), and indirect (or productivity). The net cost of therapy is the sum of the resources used by and saved by the therapy in those three categories. To illustrate with simplified examples, chronic renal dialysis may be performed at a clinic or at home. The medical resources used in clinic dialysis include equipment, facilities, and medical personnel. In addition, travel expense to the facility is a direct nonmedical expense. Finally, if the patient must miss work, the lost productivity is an indirect cost of the treatment. In comparison, home dialysis also includes equipment and supplies (medical costs), but facility fees and transportation costs are absent. However, home dialysis requires a trained helper. The helper's time (whether paid or not) is a cost of treatment. All of these items should be included in a comparison of the cost of the dialysis alternatives. Another example is providing intravenous medications at home rather than in a hospital. Medical costs (primarily in the form of hospital room and board) are saved with the former, but home care may involve more nonmedical resources, both personal (housemaker services) and other sector (Meals-on-Wheels).

Many pharmacoeconomic applications focus exclusively on medical costs. Excluding nonmedical costs is appropriate if the scope of the analysis is limited to the healthcare system or if the alternatives do not differ with respect to their effect on nonmedical resources. Including indirect or productivity costs is quite controversial, in part because wages may overstate the value of the decreased productivity associated with missed work. If indirect costs are included, the analysis should also be done without them so that their effect on the results can be seen.[7]

The total costs of a therapy—the complete picture of its impact on resource consumption—extend beyond the resources used in producing that therapy. In addition, the consequences of the therapy also affect the use of resources by consuming as well as saving them.[5] The consequences that affect the use of resources, and thus are included in the costs of a therapy, are of four types. One is the adverse effects of therapy. The resources used to treat them are considered part of the cost of therapy because those resources would not have been consumed in the absence of the therapy. A second consequence with resource implications is preventing or alleviating an illness. As an illness is prevented or reduced in severity, medical services are "saved." These are included in the cost of therapy as a savings (or negative cost). For instance, as hypertension therapy reduces the incidence of strokes, the savings of not having to treat the strokes that have been prevented are included in the net cost of hypertension therapy. Third, an intervention may provide information that causes resources to be used or saved. For instance, if a pharmacist's services increase the use of prescription medications by improving adherence or detecting untreated conditions, the costs of these medications are considered as part of the cost of the service. Fourth, and most controversial, a therapy may extend life, and medical care resources are consumed during those added life-years that would not have been consumed without the therapy. Whether these medical costs should be considered as part of the cost of the therapy is debatable.[7,8]

To summarize this section, the cost of an illness includes (1) the medical resources used to treat it, (2) nonmedical resources (personal and other sector), and (3) indirect costs (productivity losses). The net cost of a therapy (ie, the numerator of a cost-effectiveness ratio) from a societal perspective includes the first two of these categories: direct medical and nonmedical costs; whether indirect costs should be included is controversial. The total cost of a therapy includes (1) resources used in producing the therapy, (2) resources used in treating adverse effects, (3) resources saved if an illness is prevented or its severity reduced, (4) resources used (or saved) based on information acquired from the therapy, and arguably, (5) the medical resources used during the added life-years if death is postponed.

A Framework for Determining Costs

The framework for determining the cost of a therapy or service encompasses five steps: (1) specifying the ingredients or inputs, (2) counting the units of each resource or input, (3) assigning dollar values to the ingredients so that values approximate opportunity cost, (4) adjusting for differences in timing, and (5) allowing for uncertainty.

SPECIFYING THE RESOURCES

The initial step in determining the cost of a therapy or program is to identify the resources consumed by the program; that is, the ingredients used to produce the therapy or service. The goal is to develop a comprehensive list of the inputs that are used in producing it. In the case of a therapy, what medical services are used: Hospital care? Physician visits? Prescription drugs? What nonmedical services or indirect costs are involved? For a service, what types of personnel are required? What equipment and supplies?

A key point is that, to be meaningful, an economic evaluation must include all relevant resources, not just the ones that are obvious and/or easy to identify and measure. Identifying the inputs separately from assigning a dollar value to them reduces the likelihood of overlooking relevant items. Some resources may be found to be insignificant and possibly dropped from the analysis. However, this should be a conscious decision, made only after the resource has been identified and assessed.

In determining the relevance of resources, the analyst must specify the scope or perspective of the analysis. Economic evaluations may assume the viewpoint of a single provider, insurer, the healthcare system, or society. An example will help clarify this point. Consider a Medicare patient as she moves through the various levels of care from hospital to extended-care facility to home. From the hospital's perspective, its relevant costs are those incurred during the hospital stay. For instance, the hospital welcomes drug therapy that can reduce the length of stay and/or other services during the stay. An earlier discharge, however, may mean that more intensive and more costly nursing home care is required. This is relevant from the perspectives of the healthcare system and Medicare; it is irrelevant to the hospital. Finally, assume that the patient is discharged home and a family member assumes the role of caregiver. From society's perspective, the caregiver's time is a cost; however, the cost is outside the realm of the healthcare system and is not covered by Medicare. Thus, the cost of a healthcare program depends on one's perspective.

COUNTING UNITS

For each resource, a unit of use or unit of consumption should be specified. The magnitude of resource consumption is measured or counted in that unit. For instance, the use of a drug product may be measured in doses, physician services may be measured in procedures, and inpatient services may be measured in days. It is helpful to count and to report units separately from assigning monetary values because monetary values can vary. If units are counted and reported separately, the impact of a different monetary value can be easily estimated. Knowing the total monetary amount spent on a resource is less revealing than knowing the units consumed and the value assigned to each unit.

ASSIGNING DOLLAR VALUES

Once the resources used in a program have been identified and counted, they are assigned a monetary value. This is often quite complex. As a general rule, the time and effort spent in assigning a monetary value should be proportional to the importance of that resource. Major resources or cost items should receive more attention than minor items.

Several factors enter into this valuation process. In general, the best measure of a resource's value is its opportunity cost. One issue is the relationship between opportunity cost and market price. A second issue is the relationship between opportunity cost and average cost. A third issue is that some resources may be shared among several activities or programs and, therefore, must be allocated.

Opportunity Cost and Market Price

Although opportunity cost is the true cost of consuming a resource, market prices are probably the best indicator of value and should be used if available.[3] Market prices are appropriate for prices that are established through price competition. For some health services, however, there is little competition, and market prices may not be appropriate. Hospital charges, for instance, can be misleading because they may bear little (if any) relationship to resources consumed. If market price is not appropriate, a value must be derived from financial records or cost-accounting data. Similarly, for resources that have no price (eg, volunteers, unpaid assistance from a family member, lost homemaker productivity), the opportunity cost must be estimated.

Opportunity Cost and Average Cost

As mentioned earlier, marginal cost is the change in total cost that results from producing one additional unit of output. In general, marginal cost is a better indicator of opportunity cost than is average cost. Marginal cost also is a better indicator of resource value than average cost because the fixed expenses, which are included in the average cost, are consumed even in the absence of the additional unit. Likewise, when a unit of output is not produced (eg, a shortened hospital stay), the resources saved are equal to the marginal cost of the avoided output rather than its average cost. The problem is that, unlike average cost, the marginal cost is almost never known; it is not reported in nor easily derived from accounting reports.

Allocating Shared Resources

If a resource is consumed exclusively in the production of a single product or service, it is referred to as a direct cost in accounting. However, a resource also may be shared among several programs or departments; that is, it is not exclusively associated with one product or service. Cost allocation systems are designed to distribute these shared expenses appropriately among product lines or revenue departments (ie, the final outputs).[3]

Although the details of allocation systems are beyond the scope of this chapter, one fundamental issue is the basis by which an overhead expense is to be allocated. Costs can be allocated in numerous ways, including on the basis of square feet, time spent, and revenue generated. For example, in determining the cost of space for a program that does not have its own separate facility, housing expenses (eg, rent, utilities) are tied to area and are logically allocated on the basis of square feet. If personnel are shared among multiple products, the cost associated with each of the products may be allocated on the basis of time spent on each one. In allocating administrative expenses (eg, pharmacy director/manager) shared by many products, payroll expense or revenue generated may be used as a basis for allocation.

The key point is that, if a resource is used by multiple programs or services, the cost of that resource should be allocated among the programs. The cost should not be attributed to only one program, nor should it be omitted from others. If a pharmacist begins a new service, the personnel cost is not zero simply because the pharmacist was already on the payroll.

ADJUSTING FOR DIFFERENCES IN THE TIMING OF COSTS

A time preference is associated with money. We prefer to receive dollars now rather than later because they can generate benefits or returns in the interim. For the same reason, we prefer to pay out dollars later rather than now. In other words, a dollar today is worth more than a dollar tomorrow. As a simple example, suppose a lottery winner had the choice of receiving $1 million today or $1 million spread over 20 years; in all likelihood, the total sum would be taken today, so as to allow more time to enjoy and/or invest the winnings.

Because current and future dollars are not valued the same, future costs must be discounted to reflect their current value when a program extends over multiple years.[3] The present value (PV) can be calculated by multiplying the future cost (FC) by the discount factor (DF). The DF is dependent on two variables: the number of years into the future that the expense is incurred (n) and the discount rate (r).

For example, the DFs associated with discount rates of 3 percent and 6 percent for the next five years are

Year	3%	6%
1	0.971	0.943
2	0.943	0.890
3	0.915	0.840
4	0.889	0.792
5	0.863	0.747

The PV of $1,000 received a year from now is $971 if a discount rate of 3 percent is used and $943 with a rate of 6 percent.

The PV of a multiyear cost stream is the sum of the PV of the costs for each year. As an example, let's assume that a hypothetical treatment regimen has costs as follows: $3,000 in the first year, $2,000 in the second year, and $1,000 each year thereafter. Over three years, the unadjusted cost is $6,000. With a discount rate of 6 percent, the PV of the costs is $5,449 (which is the sum of each year's cost multiplied by the DF for that year).

The effects of two assumptions should be noted. In this calculation, we assumed that the expenses were incurred at the end of each period; therefore, the first-year costs (12 months in the future) were discounted using the factor for year 1, the costs for the second year (24 months out) were discounted by the factor for year 2, and so on. An equally acceptable assumption is that the expenses are incurred at the beginning of each year. Thus, the first-year costs are current—not future—and do not need to be discounted. The second-year costs (12 months in the future) are discounted with the factor of year 1; for the third year (24 months out), the factor of year 2 is used. In this case, the cost stream would be valued at $5,776.

The second assumption relates to the discount rate. As seen above, using a higher discount rate reduces the PV of future dollars. For instance, with a 3 percent discount rate, the three-year stream of costs (assuming they are incurred at the end of the year) is $5,714 (compared with $5,449 using a 6 percent discount rate).

A key issue is which discount rate to use. There is no set rule as to the best discount rate to use in economic evaluations. Theoretically, the discount rate should reflect the social rate of time preference. This is society's collective time preference, as measured by the real interest rate (interest rate minus rate of inflation) on long-term government securities. In practice, sensitivity analysis is frequently used, in which a range of rates is used in the calculations. The recommended discount rate is 3 percent, with rates of 5 percent and others between 0 percent and 7 percent used in sensitivity analysis.[8]

The relationship between discounting and inflation should be clarified. They are different concepts. As mentioned above, discounting is based on the time preference for money. Discounting is appropriate whenever a program or therapy extends over multiple years, even if the inflation rate is zero. Inflation is changes in prices. If data are collected in different time periods, the prices need to be adjusted to a uniform price to account for inflation. This is not discounting. Discounting is appropriate when the analysis is longitudinal, following the same subjects for more than one year. When projecting or estimating the cost in future years from current prices, no estimate is made for inflation. For example, the current price of long-term drug therapy is used in estimating future cost and then discounted by the real interest rate.

ALLOWING FOR UNCERTAINTY

Oftentimes, cost or resource consumption is not known with certainty; assumptions are made and estimated figures are derived. A method to compensate for this uncertainty is *sensitivity analysis.* In a sensitivity analysis, the economic evaluation is reworked using different assumptions or estimates of the uncertain costs.

Sensitivity analysis can be viewed as a "what if" analysis: What if a price increase (decrease) for a drug product is assumed? What if a different hospital per diem is used? What if different manpower requirements are assumed? Again, sensitivity analysis is essential for any cost that is not known with certainty. To assume that assumptions and estimates are factual can lead to erroneous conclusions.

Pharmacoeconomic Applications

This part of the chapter is devoted to exploring methods of determining the costs of various services of importance in pharmaceutical-related evaluations: personnel time, drug product costs, physician services, and hospital costs.

PERSONNEL TIME

Some economic evaluations, notably those dealing with a service, require the time spent on specific activities. For instance, the time devoted to dosage preparation and administration may be needed in assessing drugs with different dosing schedules or in evaluating drug distribution systems. Similarly, an evaluation of a clinical service requires the amount of personnel time needed to perform the service.

Work measurement techniques can be used to acquire this information. Two techniques are of relevance in cost determination: work sampling and stopwatch time study.[9] In work sampling, momentary observations are made at preselected times. After sufficient observations, the percentage of time devoted to each activity (including idle time) can be determined (ie, the number of observations for an activity divided by the total number of observations). Work sampling is especially useful with nonrepetitive tasks that are not entirely uniform from occurrence to occurrence.

Stopwatch time studies, on the other hand, are useful with repetitive tasks that are of short duration. This method directly measures the time required to complete a task or activity, such as processing a prescription or mixing a solution. Again, several observations of several persons are required to derive an average time for an average worker. After the time has been determined using one of these two techniques, the appropriate wage rates can be applied to derive the final labor costs.

One cautionary note is in order pertaining to opportunity cost; specifically, the opportunity cost of labor may not be reflected in the payroll. For example, if a hospital implements a new service without adding any personnel, this does not mean that the labor cost of the service is zero. Rather, the labor devoted to the program has an opportunity cost because it could have been devoted to other activities. Thus, the market value of the labor devoted to the program is rightfully considered a cost of the program. Similarly, a program may free up personnel time, but not affect the payroll. A notable example is switching from a drug requiring three-times-a-day dosing to one that requires once-daily dosing; obviously, nursing time is reduced. In this case, the payroll may be unaffected, but the nursing time saved can be devoted to other activities.

DRUG PRODUCTS

Drug products may have multiple prices. Buying groups, contractual agreements, quantity discounts, and competitive bidding have resulted in several prices for the same drug. Thus, drug products highlight the advantage of separating units from prices in measuring and reporting the cost of a therapy. If the number of doses is known, the appropriate price for a particular setting or institution can be applied. This cannot be done if only the monetary value of the drug product is reported.

A commonly used price for drug products in pharmacoeconomic analyses is average wholesale price (AWP). AWPs enable more realistic comparisons between products of different manufacturers. Even though the AWP is oftentimes higher than the actual acquisition cost, it is a standard price that is available to all purchasers. However, the AWP may be quite far removed from the actual purchase price. In some cases, most notable for generic products, the retail price paid by patients may be less than the product's AWP. In sum, the AWP should be used with caution.

PHYSICIAN SERVICES

For physician services (office visits, surgical procedures, outpatient laboratory and radiology services), two alternatives are frequently used in economic evaluations. One is to use the amount charged; in essence, this is the market price for the service. The second is to use the allowable charge (or usual and customary charge) of a third-party payer. It is important that the third-party fee schedule be reflective of cost and not be artificially low or discounted.

HOSPITAL SERVICES

Assigning value to hospital services is among the most difficult tasks in pharmacoeconomic evaluations; it also is often one of the most critical. An error in valuing hospital services, given their magnitude relative to other medical services, can easily overwhelm other costs and result in misleading conclusions. Again, a cardinal rule is: the more important (larger) a cost item, the more time and effort its valuation deserves. Thus, hospital services—the most expensive of all healthcare services—deserve special attention in pharmacoeconomic analyses.

The distinction between cost and charges was noted earlier. The amount charged is the price of a service, whereas the cost is the magnitude of the resources consumed in producing it. A few factors can cause the charge for a service to be potentially quite different from its cost. One is cost-shifting between departments. Some services in hospitals are priced much higher than their cost (eg, drugs), while others may be priced lower than their cost (eg, room and board). A second is the difference between average and marginal cost for hospital services.

Charges can be converted to costs using cost-to-charge ratios. These ratios vary from hospital to hospital. (These ratios typically use allocated costs rather than direct costs and, consequently, include overhead expenses.) A ratio is determined for each department or revenue center within the hospital. This ratio, multiplied by the charge figure from a given department, gives the underlying cost.

In a pharmacoeconomic analysis, the specific method of valuing hospital services will depend on the nature of the study and on the data available.[3] Again, the analyst seeks to determine which resources have been used (saved) and what is their opportunity cost. Three options will be considered here: an overall per diem encompassing all hospital services, utilization and cost of specific services, and payment rates by diagnosis-related group (DRG).

An overall per diem cost may be deceiving. The per diem figure is simply the average daily cost; that is, the sum of all costs (routine as well as ancillary services) divided by the number of patient days. There are two problems with using per diem costs. One is that it is an average of all fixed and variable costs. It is not equivalent to the marginal cost. As a hospital experiences one additional (or one less) patient day, the resources consumed (saved) are equal to the marginal cost and not the average cost. Two, a per diem cost assumes that all days are equal in terms of resource consumption. In actuality, the initial days of a stay are almost always more intensive in the use of ancillary services than are the latter days. Let us assume that one treatment alternative is associated with an average length of stay that is one day less than an alternative treatment. To use the per diem cost of the hospital (or one of its units) as the value of that day saved will likely overstate the resources actually saved.

A second, more refined option is to separate routine services from ancillary (or medical) services. Routine services are those that are relatively standard across all patient days (eg, room, dietary, laundry, administration). For these services, the average daily cost applies to each day. (It is not equal to marginal cost, and sensitivity analysis to account for this is appropriate.) Ancillary or medical services, such as pharmacy, laboratory, and radiology, vary by patient. Therefore, it is appropriate for the use of each of these services to be measured or estimated separately. In the example above, the savings of a one-day reduction in length of stay would consist of two components: the reduced need for routine services and the reduced use of each ancillary service.

A third valuation is the payment rate for DRGs. This can be useful if it is indicative of actual costs and not artificially low because of political or noneconomic factors. This global payment rate is useful in valuing admissions avoided or incurred. However, when comparing two treatment alternatives for a given DRG, the global payment rate is not very useful. For instance, if a treatment can be performed on an outpatient basis, the DRG payment rate may be a useful measure of the inpatient resources saved. When comparing two inpatient treatments for the same DRG, however, the payment rate is meaningless (although a cost system based on DRGs could be revealing).

In sum, one must be cautious in valuing the resources consumed (saved) in hospital services. Sensitivity analysis, using various assumptions, is certainly appropriate, if not essential.

Summary

This chapter has provided an overview of the major issues involved in determining and analyzing the cost of a service or therapy. Measuring and placing a monetary value on the resources consumed by a service or therapy are a central part of an economic evaluation. Determining and analyzing the cost of a service or therapy involves five steps: (1) specifying the ingredients (identifying the resources consumed), (2) counting units, (3) assigning monetary values, (4) adjusting for time, and (5) sensitivity analysis. Whether performing a study or critiquing one, careful attention should be given to the following question. What is the cost—the magnitude of resources consumed—by the alternatives being compared? In other words, what resources are consumed and at what cost?

The following are questions to consider when evaluating costs within an analysis:

1. What resources were included? Were they the appropriate ones? Were any resources omitted that should have been included?
2. What were the source(s) of estimates of resource use (quantities)? Were resources measured ("counted") appropriately in physical units?
3. What were the source(s) of per-unit cost (price) data? Were resources valued credibly?
4. Was discounting necessary? If so, was it done appropriately?
5. Were sensitivity analyses performed? Were they credible?
6. Was an incremental cost analysis performed (ie, was the cost of one alternative compared with the cost of another)?

References

1. Jacobs P, Rapoport J. Economic dimensions of the healthcare system. In: The economics of health and medical care. 5th ed. Gaithersburg, MD: Aspen, 2002:44-7.

Chapter 3: Cost Determination and Analysis ■ 63

2. Jacobs P, Rapoport J. Behavior of healthcare costs. In: The economics of health and medical care. 5th ed. Gaithersburg, MD: Aspen, 2002:129-31.

3. Drummond MF, O'Brien B, Stoddart GL, Torrance GW. Cost analysis. In: Methods for the economic evaluation of health care programmes. 2nd ed. New York: Oxford University Press, 1997:52-91.

4. Haddix AC, Shaffer PA. Cost-effectiveness analysis. In: Haddix AC, Teutsch SM, Shaffer PA, Duet DO, eds. Prevention effectiveness: a guide to decision analysis and economic evaluation. New York: Oxford University Press, 1996:103-29.

5. Weinstein MC. Principles of cost-effective resource allocation in health care organizations. Int J Technol Assess Health Care 1990;6:93-103.

6. Luce BR, Manning WG, Siegel JE, Lipscomb J. Estimating costs in cost-effective analysis. In: Gold MR, Siegel JE, Russell LB, Weinstein MC, eds. Cost-effectiveness in health and medicine. New York: Oxford University Press, 1996:176-213.

7. Drummond MF, O'Brien B, Stoddart GL, Torrance GW. Cost-effectiveness analysis. In: Methods for the economic evaluation of health care programmes. 2nd ed. New York: Oxford University Press, 1997:103-7.

8. Weinstein MC, Siegel JE, Gold ME, Kamlet MS, Russell LB. Recommendations of the Panel on Cost-effectiveness in Health and Medicine. JAMA 1996;276:1253-8.

9. Roberts MJ. Work measurement. In: Brown TR, Smith MC, eds. Handbook of institutional pharmacy practice. 2nd ed. Baltimore: Williams & Wilkins, 1986:90-110.

Cost-Benefit Analysis

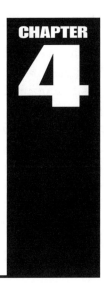

CHAPTER 4

William F McGhan
and Deborah S Kitz

C *ost-benefit analysis* (CBA) is a method for comparing the value of all resources consumed (costs) in providing a program or intervention with the value of the outcome (benefits) from that program or intervention.[1-5] In essence, CBA may be thought of as the monetary "yield" of an "investment." Will the benefits of a program exceed the cost of implementing it? Which program will produce the greatest net benefit?

The use of CBA is not a new concept in evaluating health programs. CBA is a basic tool that can be utilized to improve the decision-making process in the allocation of funds to healthcare and other programs.[6-11] While the overall concept of CBA is simple, many of the methodologic considerations require a certain degree of technical understanding to apply CBA appropriately.

CBA requires that both costs and benefits be valued in the same monetary units, for example, United States dollars. If a particular pharmaceutical regimen decreases the need for serum concentration monitoring, the dollar value of the eliminated tests is the benefit. Similarly, if the benefit is lives saved, a dollar value can be assigned to those lives (see Chapter 3 for a discussion of the human capital and willingness-to-pay methods for assigning a monetary value to a life).

Questions Cost-Benefit Analysis Can Answer

Single or multiple interventions may be assessed via CBA. For a single intervention, CBA may be used to determine whether a positive or predetermined minimum return will result from the intervention or to assess the intervention's ratio in comparison with the ratio(s) for other known treatment(s).

Multiple programs with similar or unrelated outcomes may be examined with CBA. Patrick and Woolley,[12] for example, conducted a CBA of three approaches to a pneumococcal vaccine program provided by a health maintenance organization (HMO): vaccinating no one, vaccinating all enrollees, or vaccinating all enrollees determined to be at high risk. For each approach, they determined the probability of disease, probability of adverse effects from the vaccine, cost of treating each of these events, and other costs for the HMO and the patients. The CBA indicated that a program of vaccinating only patients considered to be at high risk was most appropriate, even when the HMO's costs for identifying high-risk patients were included.

CBA of programs with unrelated outcomes is useful when funds are limited and only one program may be implemented. Should a hospital develop a cephalosporin surveillance program or a cholesterol-lowering program for employees? Which will generate the greatest benefit relative to the cost of implementing each program? Should a city government invest in a prenatal nutrition program, an AIDS awareness program, or three new community health centers?

CBA evolved from the need to ascertain estimates of the costs and benefits of public investment projects, such as bridges and dams. Expenditures for health care should produce net social benefits for the public. CBA techniques can be applied to make such resource allocation decisions in the healthcare field. Economists have reminded us that medical care is both an investment good and a consumption good. When considered as an investment good, medical care is an investment in human capital.[7,8,13,14] In economic terms, for example, the present value of a person's lifetime productivity (earnings) could be considered a measure of the potential benefit from any investment in "human capital."[15]

A major function in any planning process is formulating alternative ways to achieve desired objectives and choosing among those alternatives. Many times, decisions are made on the basis of intuition and personal judgment. CBA provides a more solid, rational basis for decision-making by requiring one to state precise definitions and objectives, identify criteria for judging results, quantify the results of each alternative, and examine the effects of assumptions and uncertainties.

Ideally, all benefits and costs caused by the program should be included. This presents considerable difficulty—especially on the benefits side of the equation—since many of the benefits are difficult to measure, difficult to convert into dollars, or both. For example, benefits such as patient comfort, patient satisfaction with the healthcare system, and working conditions for the physician are not only difficult to measure but are extremely difficult to convert into dollars. Although it may not be easy to conduct a full economic evaluation, an important advantage of CBA is that it forces those responsible to quantify inputs (costs) and outputs (benefits) as thoroughly as possible, rather than rest content with vague qualitative judgments or personal hunches.

Measuring Benefits

The economic benefits of a health program are defined as the reduction in costs realized because of the implementation of that program. The conventional classification of these benefits is threefold: direct, indirect, and intangible.

DIRECT BENEFITS

Direct benefits are defined as that portion of averted costs currently borne that are associated with spending for health services; they represent potential savings in the use of health resources. In other words, direct benefits are estimations of savings or direct costs. Direct costs include costs incurred prior to diagnosis and hospitalization, during hospitalization, during convalescent care, and during continued medical surveillance. These costs generally include expenditures for prevention, detection, treatment, rehabilitation, research, training, and capital investments in medical facilities, as well as professional services, drugs, medical supplies, and nonpersonal health services. Most often, direct benefits can be calculated with relatively less difficulty than indirect benefits.

INDIRECT BENEFITS

Indirect benefits represent the potential savings on indirect costs. Despite extensive treatment in the literature, indirect benefits are difficult to measure. They are the result of the avoidance of earnings and productivity losses that would have been borne without the health program in question. Rice[16] provided a systematic method of measuring indirect benefits. Her estimates include wage and productivity losses resulting from illness, disability, and death based on age and sex for major causal categories of morbidity and mortality.

INTANGIBLE BENEFITS

Intangible costs of ill health are difficult, if not impossible, to measure. These costs may be described as the psychic costs of disease such as those incurred from pain, suffering, and grief.[16]

The measurement of such intangible benefits poses an almost insuperable task. However, many economists emphasize that an attempt should be made to account for the extremely valuable "spillover" effects if possible. These effects have been evaluated in environmental and health programs.[7]

Discount Rates

CBA consists of identifying all of the societal benefits that will accrue from a health program and converting them into equivalent dollars in the year in which they will occur. This stream of benefit dollars is then discounted to its equivalent present value at the selected interest rate. Then, other things being equal, the program with the largest present value of benefits minus costs is the best in terms of its economic value. As a simple example, with a 10 percent inflation rate, $100 invested in a program today should be worth $110 in one year and $121 in the second year. We usually hope that programs will produce an even better return on the investment.

A challenge in CBA is how one determines the proper interest rate for discounting future benefits and costs. Prest and Turvey[17] recommended that the selection of a rate be based on similar projects, followed by sensitivity analysis of the problem to determine the effect of a range of discount rates as the final solution.

All benefits and costs that occur at different times must be adjusted to reflect comparable values. This is accomplished by converting dollar amounts into present values through the use of an interest rate referred to as the *discount rate* (Table 1). Although most economists agree that discounting should be emphasized, there is much discussion as to the appropriate rate for a given situation. The consequences of choosing a high or low discount rate are clear: a low rate favors projects with benefits accruing in the distant future, while a high rate favors projects with costs in the distant future. One commonly used rate is the current yield rate on long-term government bonds. This seems practical since it represents a riskless long-term alternative use of funds by a tax-free institution and, therefore, appears valid for use by hospitals in evaluating long-term investment proposals. Theoretical support can be found in the literature for practically any figure between the pure time-reference (riskless) rate as low as 4 percent and the corporate return on capital, approximately 20 percent.[10,18]

Steps in Conducting a Cost-Benefit Analysis

STEP 1

The first step in conducting a CBA is to clearly identify the intervention(s), program(s), therapeutic regimen(s), and research

Table 1. Effect of Discount Rates

	Cost of Therapies ($)	
Year	**Drug A**	**Drug B**
1	10,000	20,000
2	10,000	4,000
3	10,000	5,000
TOTAL	30,000	29,000
PV =	25,771	25,917

PV = present value.
Formula: $PV = FV [1/(1+i)^n]$
Note: Drug A unadjusted costs $1,000 more than Drug B, but if i = 8%, PV of Drug A is less. With time value of money, Drug A < Drug B.

questions to be evaluated. Patrick and Woolley[12] included identifying high-risk patients and treating adverse effects from the vaccine as part of the pneumococcal vaccine evaluation. The program went beyond administering vaccines and treating disease. For a cephalosporin surveillance program, it is not adequate to simply state that a program will reduce drug costs. What impact might the program have outside the drug budget? Will all patients receiving a cephalosporin have to be screened, or would it be more cost beneficial to do selective screening? Can the program reduce home-care costs? Will the patient be able to return to work sooner? What are the specific resources needed for the program?

STEP 2

The second step is to identify and value all of the resources consumed or costs of providing each intervention, program, or regimen. Different types of resources should be recognized. In their CBA of an outpatient parenteral antibiotic program, Poretz et al.[19] included expenses for training patients to self-administer drugs, physician visits, and supplies.

A hospital pharmacy would include expenses for personnel time (salaries, employee benefits), office space, computer hardware and software, additional telephone lines, and general supplies in a CBA of a cephalosporin surveillance program. A comprehensive comparison of two pharmaceutical therapy regimens would include costs for purchasing each drug, supplies consumed in administering each agent, salary and employee benefit expenses for personnel time (eg, pharmacists, nurses, physicians) consumed in preparing and delivering the drug, and hospital resources used to treat untoward effects of each regimen. Shapiro et al.[20] conducted this type of CBA of placebo versus cefazolin prophylaxis in women undergoing vaginal or abdominal hysterectomy and included expenses for hospital days, bacterial cultures, and antimicrobial agents.

STEP 3

Benefits are identified and valued in the third step. Benefits of the cephalosporin surveillance program might include decreased use of third-generation cephalosporins (ie, attempting to lower the drug purchasing budget with equally efficacious drugs), a lower incidence of drug interactions, and associated decreased use of resources to treat untoward patient events. For the hospital, the value of these benefits is their true cost savings. For the comparison of two pharmaceutical regimens, the benefits for the hospital of the regimen requiring a shorter duration of treatment would include cost savings from the decreased length of stay (assuming the hospital is only reimbursed for a fixed amount, as in diagnosis-related groups). Under a fee-for-service situation, a shorter length of stay benefits society but may actually decrease revenue for the hospital.

Recall that, if the benefit of an intervention is lives saved, a monetary value must be assigned to those lives. Similarly, if the benefit is fewer days of work missed, actual or estimated patient salary information may be used to assign a dollar value to these days.

STEP 4

The fourth step in CBA is to sum the value of all costs and then sum all the benefits of each program, intervention, or regimen. Total costs then may be subtracted from total benefits to determine net benefits:

$$\text{Net Benefits} = \text{Total Benefits} - \text{Total Costs}$$

Some investigators prefer to compute a cost-to-benefit ratio, while others prefer to calculate a benefit-to-cost ratio. Although the analytic approach is commonly called cost-benefit analysis, calculating a benefit-to-cost ratio frequently is appropriate because one usually expects the total benefits to exceed total costs, producing a ratio greater than 1:1.

$$\text{Cost-Benefit Ratio} = \frac{\text{Total Benefits}}{\text{Total Costs}}$$

If initial estimates of the benefit (yield) of an investment in a program (cost) must exceed a minimum dollar value before it is approved for implementation, net benefits would be calculated. A hospital pharmacy may determine that the net benefit of a biotechnology surveillance program must be at least $50,000 annually. In this case, net benefits should be calculated. Alternatively, a benefit-to-cost ratio should be computed if a criterion for implementing a program is that the benefits must be at least twice as great as the costs (ie, 2:1 benefit-to-cost ratio) regardless

of the absolute value of the benefits and costs. By comparing benefit-to-cost ratios of multiple programs, one can identify the program that produces the greatest "slide for the run," or yield, relative to the investment. In some ways, hospital budget allocation
decisions between expanding an outpatient pharmacy service versus a walk-in clinic versus a trauma program, for example, implicitly could compare the benefit-to-cost ratio for each program.

$$\text{Cost-Benefit Ratio} = \frac{\Sigma^n_{t=1}[B_t/(1+r)^t]}{\Sigma^n_{t=1}[C_t/(1+r)^t]}$$

where B_t = total benefits for time period t, C_t = total costs for
time period t, r = discount rate, and n = number of time periods.
The decision criterion is as follows:

> If B/C > 1, then benefits exceed costs and
> the program is socially valuable.
> If B/C = 1, then benefits equal costs.
> If B/C < 1, then benefits are less than
> costs; therefore, the program is not socially
> beneficial.

The major problem with selecting this method is in choosing "r,"
the discount rate (see page 68).

Another formula used in CBA relates to the logical concept of
net present value (NPV).[3]

$$\text{Benefit} - \text{Costs} = \text{NPV} = \Sigma^n_{t=1}[(B_t - C_t)/(1+r)^t]$$

Table 2 presents a simplified example of the type of data utilized in cost-benefit calculations. One can see that it is important on the costs side to include items beyond simply the acquisition cost of a drug, such as administration costs and the cost of
adverse drug reactions. On the benefits side, days back at work
and extra months or years of life are converted into dollars.

Table 3 illustrates that the cost-benefit mathematical formulas can be misleading depending on the potential differences in
the magnitude of dollars and time involved when comparing the
costs and benefits of competing programs. Table 2 presents simplified versions of the different cost-benefit mathematical approaches to illustrate how the decision factors can vary. From
these options, practitioners must select which formula is most
appropriate at their institution or perhaps all three formulas
should be presented in the proposal.

In the example provided below, Program A might represent a proposal for a medium-sized computer in the pharmacy, while Program B might represent a large computer system with multiple decentralized terminals. Although Program B has a higher cost-benefit ratio and rate of return, it is an expensive system and the pharmacy may not want to commit such a substantial amount of funds. Numerous other examples could be considered here that change the results from the various formulas and make it more difficult to select between programs.

It should be emphasized that, for the limited investment streams presented in this example, the calculations have been greatly simplified. The calculations and comparisons become more complex as benefits are accrued at different increments of time and as costs and benefits are properly discounted with the more complete formulas presented earlier.

Perspective of the Analysis

An important consideration in conducting a CBA and other types of clinical economic evaluations is the perspective of the

Table 2. Example of Simplified Cost-Benefit Analysis Applied to Drug Therapy

	Cost of Therapies ($)	
Parameter	Drug A	Drug B
Costs		
Acquisition	300	400
Administration	50	0
Monitoring	50	0
Adverse effects	100	0
Subtotal	500	400
Benefits		
Days at work	1,000	1,000
Extra months of life	2,000	3,000
Subtotal	3,000	4,000
Benefit-to-cost ratio	3,000/500 = 6:1	4,000/400 = 10:1
Net Benefit	2,500	3,600

analysis. For whom are the costs and benefits being assessed? The patient? Department manager? Third-party payer? Practitioner? Society?

Different resources are considered costs and benefits, and the dollar value of each may vary depending on the perspective from which the analysis is conducted. A hospital pharmacy department may include expenses for a portable computer as part of their costs for an outpatient parenteral therapy program. However, these costs are not relevant to the patient. Similarly, a patient who is able to return to work considers this a benefit of the outpatient program, but this is not a benefit to a hospital. Patients may incur out-of-pocket expenses for transportation to outpatient follow-up visits. These costs do not have any direct impact on the third-party payer, hospital, pharmacy department, or clinician.

McGhan[2,3] has also pointed out that a factor considered to be a benefit from one perspective may be a cost from another perspective. For example, a hospital may view decreased inpatient days as a benefit (under fixed price payment such as diagnosis-related groups) of having an outpatient parenteral therapy program. However, a patient covered by health insurance that includes a higher copayment for outpatient care and 100 percent coverage for inpatient care would view the decreased inpatient days as a cost. Although insurers would consider the change from inpatient surgical care to outpatient lithotripsy for renal stones a benefit, urologists may consider this to be a cost, particularly if the payment for lithotripter services is lower than for surgical care. In the same way, outpatient drugs to dissolve gall-

Table 3. Example of Sample Comparisons Using Different Cost-Benefit Approaches

Program	Costs (t_0)	Benefits (t_1)	Cost-Benefit Ratio (B/C)	Net Present Value (B-C)	Internal Rate of Return (B-C)/C
A	$10,000	$15,000	1.5:1	$5,000	50%
B	$100,000	$180,000	1.8:1	$80,000	80%

stones may be a savings to society but a cost (loss) to hospitals.

Koplan and Preblud[21] included costs from different perspectives in their clinical economic evaluation of the mumps vaccine. For children with mumps, they included estimates of wages lost by parents staying home with the children, expenses for transportation to office visits, cost of the vaccine, and acute care costs. Although they did not place a dollar value on the ability to return to work, Rosenfeldt et al.[22] and Nevitt et al.[23] did include the ability to return to work as a benefit of coronary bypass surgery and total hip arthroplasty, respectively.

Under fixed-payment schemes for hospital care, the importance of specifying the perspective from which the analysis is being conducted is magnified. These payment schemes mean that high patient-care expenses generated by the hospital no longer increase third-party payer payments. Extensive and unnecessary use of technology or biotechnology, for example, may generate high patient-care costs for the hospital, but do not affect third-party payments. On the other hand, pharmaceutical therapy that shortens the length of stay or eliminates the need for serum concentration monitoring may generate savings for the hospital. From the insurer's perspective, however, no savings will accrue; the payment is fixed. Insurers' costs may increase, however, if a patient receives inpatient care when ambulatory or home care is more feasible and effective.

Fixed-price payment also imposes a relatively new requirement on cost-benefit and other clinical economic analyses performed from the perspective of the hospital: true costs must be assessed. *True costs* are the value of the resources used in providing a service. Charges, which bear no consistent relationship to costs and often are set to maximize revenue, are irrelevant in assessing hospital expenses or savings under fixed-price payment.

Determining the hospital's cost for a service usually is not a trivial task. Determining the cost of different modes of intravenous antibiotic therapy, for example, may involve time and motion studies of personnel time (and assigning salaries and employee benefits) devoted to reconstituting and administering the agent and hospital expenses for supplies used in each mode. Although determining hospital costs may be a time-consuming, detailed process, it is a critical element of any clinical economics analysis performed from the perspective of the hospital.

Consider the perspective from which the analyses will be conducted in the initial design. More than one perspective should be included in the analysis. However, attention should be devoted to distinguishing the value of costs and value of benefits from each perspective.

Making Assumptions

Frequently, investigators find it necessary to use secondary data sources to make assumptions or projections about the value of one or more variables in a clinical economic evaluation. This occurs most often when the clinical economic analysis is not being performed in conjunction with the clinical evaluation or when no acceptable retrospective data are available. In the example of the outpatient parenteral therapy program, a hospital may have to estimate annual mileage for a supply delivery van. Information about the hospital's catchment area and experience of other hospitals may guide the estimates. Nevertheless, the investigator needs to be confident that the value of this variable will not influence the conclusions of the evaluation.

Sensitivity analysis is a method of determining whether the conclusion of an economic evaluation changes when the value of one variable is varied while other variables are held constant. Will the benefit-to-cost ratio fall below 1 if expenses for computers are higher than estimated? If personnel expenses for the cephalosporin surveillance program are actually 25 percent higher than projected, will the net benefits of the program become negative? In other words, sensitivity analysis allows one to determine whether the original conclusions are upheld through the range of variation in the value of the variable in question. Does the benefit-to-cost ratio remain above 1 through the range of variation (regardless of changes in the value of the ratio)? Do the net benefits remain positive? If the conclusions are upheld, there is a higher degree of validity in the assumptions. However, if the conclusions change, efforts should be made to determine the true value of the variable or to state explicitly that the conclusions are sensitive to the value of that single variable.

For example, Koplan and Preblud[21] varied the incidence of disease, discount rate, and costs per vaccine dose. Under all reasonable ranges of each variable, they found that the benefit-to-cost ratio of mumps vaccine remained above 1. Thus, they felt confident of the general findings about the economic aspects of *mumps vaccine.*

Eisenberg and Kitz[24] included sensitivity analysis in their economic evaluation of outpatient antibiotic treatment for osteomyelitis. Initially, they used information from a previous report indicating that 50 percent of patients could return to their normal routines (eg, work, school) during outpatient parenteral antibiotic therapy. To determine whether the general conclusions were sensitive to the value of the variable, they reanalyzed the data with 0 and 100 percent "return to routine" rates. The original conclusions were upheld under these two values of this variable: benefits would accrue to patients from an outpatient program.

Patrick and Woolley[12] included sensitivity analysis in their CBA of three approaches to pneumococcal pneumonia vaccine for an HMO population. Their overall conclusions about identifying and immunizing high-risk patients did not change when they varied the cost of the vaccine, duration of the program, likelihood of adverse effects, cost of illness, and several other factors.

One approach to sensitivity analysis is to increase and decrease the assumed value of the variable by a significant percent (eg, 50 or 100 percent). Another approach is to select the mean (eg, for salaries) for the initial analysis and then repeat the analysis with the lowest and highest value of the variable.

Cost-Benefit or Cost-Effectiveness Analysis

Cost-benefit and cost-effectiveness analyses are useful tools for assessing the clinical economic impact of medical care programs or interventions. There are, however, several important distinctions between the two approaches.

First, CBA may be applied to single or multiple programs, while cost-effectiveness analysis is applied to multiple programs. Second, CBA may be used to compare programs with disparate outcomes. In contrast, cost-effectiveness analysis is a method for identifying the least costly approach to achieving a single outcome. A third distinction is that CBA requires that all the outcomes or benefits be assigned a dollar value. The outcome or effect is not valued in cost-effectiveness analysis. Some investigators find it distasteful to place a monetary value on a benefit such as lives saved and thus prefer cost-effectiveness analysis.

Which approach should you use in the pharmacy arena? It depends. A general guideline is that cost-effectiveness analysis is most appropriate when a single effect or outcome can be defined. An effect might be providing antibiotic prophylaxis for patients undergoing surgery for nonperforated appendicitis or providing postsurgical analgesic therapy. CBA is usually most appropriate when a single program is to be evaluated or when funds are limited and budget allocation decisions must be made among programs with unrelated outcomes.

McGhan et al.[3] were one of the first pharmacy researchers to suggest that CBA is an important technique for justifying clinical pharmacy services. Are the costs of implementing a service offset by savings (benefits) from the service? These types of questions will be asked with increasing frequency as hospital administrators and departmental managers respond to cost-containment pressures created by fixed-price payment.

Cost-Benefit Analysis in the Literature

As noted throughout this chapter, many of the CBA reports in the clinical pharmacy arena have focused on the use of antibiotics. Poretz et al.[19] conducted a CBA of an outpatient parenteral therapy program with ceftriaxone for patients with serious infections. They conducted a telephone survey to determine expenses for training sessions, supplies, physician visits, and transportation to follow-up visits. Income information and days of work missed by patients and companions were used to assess productivity losses. Data also were collected regarding third-party payer coverage for components of care. The benefit-to-cost ratio of this outpatient therapy program was about 3.7:1; average total weighted benefits were approximately $6,600 and costs were about $1,800. The authors noted that insurance coverage was less comprehensive for outpatient care than for inpatient care, suggesting that analysis of these types of programs from the patient's perspective should consider out-of-pocket expenditures for direct medical care routinely covered when provided to inpatients.

A type of CBA of another outpatient parenteral therapy program was conducted by Kunkle and Iannini.[25] Their analysis was limited to an estimate of per diem hospital costs (exclusive of ancillary services), a conservative estimate of daily patient wages, and an estimate of nursing time consumed in delivering intravenous antibiotics.

Shapiro et al.[20] incorporated a CBA in a clinical trial of antibiotic prophylaxis for hysterectomy. This approach to conducting an economic evaluation is attractive because data regarding untoward effects, treatment failures, and other clinical parameters are collected concurrently with economic data. A danger of this approach, however, is that a particular aspect of therapy, such as serum concentration monitoring, may occur simply because of the clinical trial. Such monitoring would not be part of standard clinical practice and inadvertently will be included in the economic assessment. It is necessary to exclude from the cost and benefit calculations the clinical trial–related expenses that would not occur in normal practice. Identifying these factors may be difficult, particularly if little information is available about routine practice with a new drug.

The CBA performed by Shapiro el al.[20] included expenses for operative site or urinary tract infections or febrile morbidity that occurred while the subjects were inpatients and within six weeks of discharge following abdominal or vaginal hysterectomy. Although the authors used charge rather than cost data to assess expenses for hospital days, cultures, and antibiotic agents, the results indicated that the net benefit of prophylaxis versus placebo was about $100 per patient for abdominal hysterectomy and nearly $500 for vaginal hysterectomy.

Vaccination programs also have been evaluated through CBA. In addition to Patrick and Woolley's[12] evaluation of pneumococcal pneumonia vaccines, Koplan and Preblud[21] conducted a CBA of mumps vaccine for children in the United States. They included data on disease incidence, vaccine efficacy, mumps, encephalitis, hearing loss, and death and found a benefit-to-cost ratio of at least 7.4:1. Results of clinical economic evaluations of vaccines have been summarized by other authors who pointed out that issues regarding target populations for the vaccines, vaccine efficacy, and expenses for administering the vaccines are important and should be examined periodically to reassess the findings of earlier economic evaluations.

For further examples of CBA studies, the National Institute on Drug Abuse has information on several CBA and cost-effectiveness analysis studies related to drug abuse prevention and treatment.[26] In addition, Table 4 compares three studies that have examined the costs and consequences of various vaccine interventions. This table illustrates that different types of interventions and different target populations provide a range of results that need to be compared and considered in designing cost-beneficial programs.[27-29]

Summary

CBA is an approach to clinical economic assessment. It requires that the costs and benefits both be measured in the same units, usually dollars. A single intervention may be evaluated or multiple interventions with different outcomes may be compared with CBA. Net benefits or benefit-to-cost ratio may be computed to determine the yield of an investment in a diagnostic, therapeutic, or screening intervention.

References

1. McGhan WF, Lewis NJ. Guidelines for pharmacoeconomic studies. Clin Ther 1992;3:486-94.
2. McGhan WF. Dilemmas in evaluating health care and clinical programs. Drug Intell Clin Pharm 1981;15:684-7.
3. McGhan W, Rowland C, Bootman JL. Cost-benefit and cost-effectiveness: methodologies for evaluating innovative pharmaceutical services. Am J Hosp Pharm 1978;35:133-40.
4. Bootman JL, McGhan WF, Schondelmeyer SW. Application of cost- benefit and cost-effectiveness analysis to clinical practice. Drug Intell Clin Pharm 1982;16:235-43.
5. Bootman JL, Wertheimer AL, Zaske D, Rowland C. Individualizing gentamicin dosage regimens in burn patients with gram-negative septicemia: a cost-benefit analysis. J Pharm Sci 1979;68:267-72.
6. Crystal R, Brewster A. Cost-benefit and cost-effectiveness analysis in the health field: an introduction. Inquiry 3 (1966):3-13.
7. Mishan EJ. Cost-benefit analysis. 4th ed. London: Routledge Press, 1988.
8. Drummond MF, O'Brien B, Stoddart GL, Torrence GW. Methods for the economic evaluation of health care programs. Oxford: Oxford University Press, 1997.
9. Weinstein MC, Stason B. Foundations and cost/effectiveness analysis for health and medical practitioners. N Engl J Med 1977;296:716-21.

Table 4. Comparing the Results of Three Vaccine Studies

Reference	Patient Group	Results	Cost Savings/ Benefit
Nichol et al.[27]	healthy, working adults	43% decrease in absenteeism due to URI 36% decrease in absenteeism due to all illness 44% decrease in physician office visits for URI	$46.85 per person vaccinated direct benefit to employers who saw a healthier workforce with the use of the influenza vaccine
Nichol et al.[28]	elderly (≥65 years of age)	decrease in hospitalization rates for influenza, pneumonia, and acute and chronic respiratory diseases 37% decrease in hospitalization rates for CHF	$117 per person vaccinated improved health not only by preventing influenza illness, but also by preventing other medical conditions
Neuzil et al.[29]	healthy and at-risk women <65 years of age	substantial morbidity and mortality from acute cardiopulmonary events during the influenza season excess hospitalizations and deaths most pronounced in women at risk, but women not at risk also had significantly increased rates of cardiopulmonary hospitalizations during the influenza season	influenza vaccine beneficial in high-risk populations and the general population by reducing morbidity, mortality, and healthcare costs

CHF = congestive heart failure; URI = upper respiratory tract infection.

10. Gold MR, Siegel JE, Russel LB, Weinstein MC. Cost-effectiveness in health and medicine. New York: Oxford University Press, 1996.

11. Klarman H. Application of cost/benefit analysis to health services and the special case of technological innovation. Int J Health Serv Res 1974;4: 325-52.

12. Patrick KM, Woolley FR. A cost-benefit analysis of immunization for pneumococcal pneumonia. JAMA 1981;245:473-7.

13. Klarman H. Present status of cost-benefit analysis in the health field. Am J Public Health 1967;57:1948-58.

14. Rice DP. Cost-of-illness studies: fact or fiction? Lancet 1994;344:1519-20.

15. Mishan EJ. Evaluation of life and limb: a theoretical approach. In: Harberger A, et al., eds. Benefit/Cost Analysis. Chicago: Aldine-Atherton, 1971:103-23.

16. Rice DP. Measurement and application of illness costs. Public Health Rep 1969;84:91-101.

17. Prest AR, Turvey R. Cost-benefits analysis: a survey. Econ J 1965;75:683-735.

18. Marglin SA. The social rate of discount at the optimal rate of investment. J Econ 1963;77:95-111.

19. Poretz DM, Woolard D, Eron LJ, Goldenberg RI, Rising J, Sparks S. Outpatient use of ceftriaxone: a cost-benefit analysis. Am J Med 1984;77(4C)77-83.

20. Shapiro M, Schoenbaum SC, Tager IB, Muñoz A, Polk BF. Benefit-cost analysis of antimicrobial prophylaxis in abdominal and vaginal hysterectomy. JAMA 1983;249:1290-4.

21. Koplan JP, Preblud SR. A benefit-cost analysis of mumps vaccine. Am J Dis Child 1982;136:362-4.

22. Rosenfeldt FL, Lambert R, Burrows K, Stirling GR. Hospital costs and return to work after coronary bypass surgery. Med J Aust 1983;1:260-3.

23. Nevitt MC, Epstein WV, Masem M, Murray WR. Work disability before and after total hip arthroplasty: assessment of effectiveness in reducing disability. Arthritis Rheum 1984;27:410-21.

24. Eisenberg JM, Kitz DS. Savings from outpatient antibiotic therapy for osteomyelitis: economic analysis of a therapeutic strategy. JAMA 1986;255: 1584-8.

25. Kunkle MJ, Iannini PB. Cefonicid in a once-daily regimen for treatment of osteomyelitis in an ambulatory setting. Rev Infect Dis 1984;6:S865-9.

26. National Institute on Drug Abuse. Measuring and improving costs, cost-effectiveness, and cost-benefit for substance abuse treatment programs. www.nida.nih.gov/impcost/impcostindex.html (accessed 2004 Mar 10).

27. Nichol KL, Lind A, Margolis KL, Murdoch M, McFadden R, Hauge M, et al. The effectiveness of vaccination against influenza in healthy, working adults. N Engl J Med 1995;333:889-93.

28. Nichol KL, Margolis KL, Wuorenma J, von Sternberg T. The efficacy and cost effectiveness of vaccination against influenza among elderly persons living in the community. N Engl J Med 1994;331:778-84.

29. Neuzil KM, Reed GW, Mitchel EF Jr, Griffin MR. Influenza-associated morbidity and mortality in young and middle-aged women. JAMA 1999;281:901-7.

Cost-Effectiveness Analysis

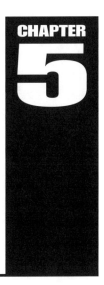

CHAPTER 5

Grant H Skrepnek

The use of economic assessments in health care has rapidly increased as a result of demands to achieve efficiency under conditions of heightened resource scarcity and constraint. Unlimited wants and finite resources characterize the market for healthcare technology, ultimately requiring those who allocate or consume products and services to engage in an investment or capital budgeting process. Under such conditions, optimal gains are sought through the most efficient allocation of time, people, money, goods, and services. Within this, various healthcare treatment options must be considered in addition to the perspectives of numerous economic agents. Although a variety of methods exists in aiding decision-making in this context, cost-effectiveness analysis (CEA) has emerged as a pragmatic and powerful methodology for assessing potential benefits of new technology, such as those involving innovative pharmaceuticals. In particular, the growing number of pharmaceutical therapies from which to choose, rising healthcare costs, and the response to the consumer's question "Are we receiving the greatest benefit from our healthcare dollar?" are important facets surrounding the adoption of pharmacoeconomic methods. Pharmacoeconomics can assist in generating the maximum benefit in terms of patient outcomes for an overall population and can supplement decisions made strictly from a clinical stance. The methodology can also offer insight in assessing the value of pharmaceutical products and services and in affording optimal balances between cost and quality in health care. Overall, economic evaluations are intended to improve efficiency by attempting to achieve maximum outcomes for the resources consumed.

Although cost-containment pressures are an important consideration in the utilization of CEA, public policy decisions warrant a broader viewpoint to assess an optimal investment that maximizes gains from healthcare spending. Thus, focusing only upon decreasing costs relating to specific cost centers (eg, pharmaceutical budgets) may not necessarily provide an overall benefit to society or to the healthcare system.[1,2] Specific to therapeutics, establishing a decision strategy to utilize products with only the lowest acquisition cost may offer misleading results, as issues pertaining to clinical effectiveness, monitoring, required concomitant therapies, or treatment of adverse effects are essentially negated under the premise. As such, both individual patient care and overall social welfare may be compromised if comprehensive analyses are ignored. Analysts considering only resource consumption, without including outcomes related to therapeutic interventions, would be engaging in only a partial form of economic evaluation.[3]

Cost-Effectiveness Analysis Defined

Within the discipline of pharmacoeconomics, the CEA exists as a comprehensive form of economic analysis that seeks to define, assess, and compare resource consumption (inputs) with consequences of care (outputs) between two or more alternatives.[3] Pharmacoeconomics can be used to determine whether products or services provide sufficient value to the market to allow for reimbursement or adoption and guide appropriate use, and can be extended to be used during pipeline research and development of pharmaceutical products.[4-7]

Consistent with other pharmacoeconomic designs, inputs in CEAs are measured in physical units and valued in monetary units; these costs are contingent upon the established perspective of the study (eg, managed care organization, government, patient, third-party payer, society). The CEA design is differentiated from other pharmacoeconomic assessments in that non-monetary, natural unit terms of health improvement are employed as outcome measures (eg, clinical laboratory values, years of life saved, or prevention of an event).[8,9] Outcomes expressed in physical terms have intuitive appeal to those working within healthcare settings, as clinical effects of therapies or services are often the primary consequence of interest, such as low-density lipoprotein cholesterol (LDL-C), forced expiratory volume in 1 second (FEV_1), millimeters of mercury (mm Hg), years of life saved, or number of symptom-free days. Although some scholars view the CEA as being a less comprehensive investigation relative to a cost-benefit analysis, utilizing natural unit outcomes may be supported for numerous reasons.[10-12] Foremost, clinicians and healthcare decision-makers often have greater familiarity and comfort with clinical outcome measures, as these indicators are regularly used in practice settings. CEA does not explicitly warrant that the value of a human life be determined as is required in a cost-benefit analysis. Importantly, a limitation of CEA is that the methodology often does not adequately address broad issues of social welfare that can be addressed by the cost-benefit analysis.

CEA is a framework for guiding and augmenting decisions and should not necessarily be considered a complete substitute for other forms of assessment or clinical expertise. Consistent with other types of economic analyses, assumptions may be required regarding issues that are not easily quantified, thus rendering conclusions that may be somewhat speculative. Furthermore, issues of broad public policy and those involving ethics, morals, or value judgments may not be adequately addressed by the economic calculus.[13]

Advantages and disadvantages of the cost-effectiveness methodology must be considered either when employing the design or in assessing the studies that utilize it. Aside from those previously mentioned, additional advantages of CEA are that researchers do not have to place a dollar value on clinical outcomes and that treatments can be compared when it is impossible or inappropriate to use monetary outcomes (eg, What is the dollar value of an LDL-C level?). Furthermore, different treatments that have the same treatment goal may also be evaluated. Principally because nonmonetary outcomes are measured, the methodology can only compare options with the same type of outcome, and only one outcome can be measured at a time. For example, two treatments with two distinctly different outcomes (ie, years of life saved vs disability days avoided) cannot necessarily be assessed in unison with CEA. In certain instances, this may be considered a substantial limitation, especially if treatments do not have similar measurable intermediate outcomes (ie, outcomes that are established or thought to be related to a final event of clinical importance). Given that many pharmaceutical products are not necessarily considered perfect substitutes that can be compared via a single unit of effectiveness, multiple effects of individual products are poorly integrated within the CEA methodology. A new technology may offer no substantial cost-effective improvement relative to a specific clinical outcome, such as a lipid profile or blood pressure, but may offer improvements in mortality plus a side effect profile that substantially improves quality of life relative to comparators.

CEA is often utilized as a dynamic methodology that is frequently combined with other pharmacoeconomic study designs. Elements of a cost-benefit analysis may be incorporated that include the monetary benefits related to the treatment of the disease state. Although a given CEA may focus upon aspects of reduced morbidity (eg, avoided complications of therapy), extensions may attempt to quantify monetary consequences associated with complications that are avoided. Other investigators have viewed the cost-utility analysis as a form of CEA, making an assumption that a quality-adjusted life-year is defined as a natural unit outcome.[14] Currently, the explicit distinction between CEA and cost-utility analysis is often made by numerous scholars.[3] Generally, comprehensive evaluations of the described nature often fall under the rubric of CEA in scientific journals.

PROPER USE OF THE TERM "COST-EFFECTIVE"

A common misconception in the use of the term *cost-effective* is that only the least expensive alternatives should be sought or that the most effective alternatives are relevant; cost-effective does not necessarily indicate simply the cheapest or most effective option. From an economic viewpoint, these interpretations are rather naïve because resource consumption and consequences are considered only in isolation.

Doubilet et al.[15] recognized that a comprehensive definition of cost-effectiveness includes multiple dimensions. Overall, a therapy or other technology may be deemed a cost-effective strategy when the outcome is worth the cost relative to competing alternatives (ie, there is value being offered to the market for the money and resources needed to acquire and utilize the good or service). An intervention can be considered cost-effective when it is found to be: (1) less expensive and at least as effective as alternatives, (2) more expensive and more effective than alternative therapies (with the additional benefit worth the additional cost), or (3) less expensive and less effective (in instances where the extra benefit provided by the competing therapy is not worth the extra expense). Figure 1 presents the cost-effectiveness grid, indicating areas that are considered cost-effective versus strategies which are cost-ineffective. *Dominant* strategies are defined as offering both lower cost and higher effectiveness compared with an alternative, while a *dominated* strategy is one that costs more than the comparator and is less effective. Options requiring a trade-off include technologies that present a higher cost with higher effectiveness or lower cost with lower effectiveness relative to comparators.

		Cost of Alternative A Relative to Alternative B		
		LOWER	**EQUAL**	**HIGHER**
Effectiveness of Alternative A Relative to Alternative B	**HIGHER**	+ (Dominant)	+	+/− (Trade-off)
	EQUAL	+	Arbitrary	−
	LOWER	+/− (Trade-off)	−	− (Dominated)

Figure 1. The cost-effectiveness grid.[3]

Principles of a Cost-Effectiveness Analysis

The general steps in conducting a CEA that are applicable to all settings have been outlined by Warner and Luce[16] and Dao[17] and are summarized in Figure 2. Although other approaches may be relevant, the steps that appear may be considered a rational and beneficial starting point in conducting CEAs.[18]

More specific aspects of these general steps in conducting a pharmacoeconomic investigation include the following:

1. establishing the perspective;
2. specifying alternatives;
3. specifying possible outcomes;

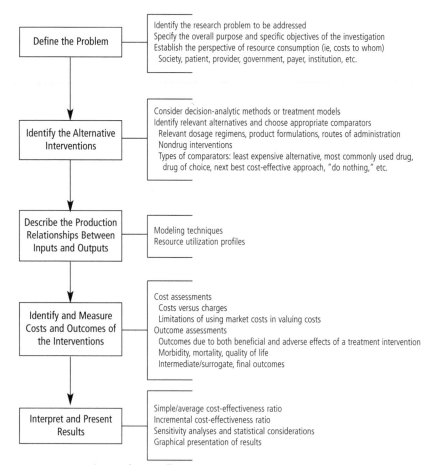

Figure 2. General steps of a cost-effectiveness analysis.[16,17]

4. specifying and monitoring healthcare resources consumed;
5. assigning dollar values to resources consumed;
6. specifying and monitoring non–healthcare resources;
7. specifying the outcomes and unit of effectiveness;
8. specifying other aspects of the alternatives that may be important in addition to the identified outcomes;
9. analyzing the data; and
10. conducting a sensitivity analysis on key or uncertain assumptions and variables.

STEP ONE: DEFINE THE PROBLEM

Conducting an appropriate CEA begins by understanding the research problem in light of the alternatives that exist and the perspective desired within the investigation. A clear and precise research purpose should be drawn upon which specific objectives concerning the alternatives may be established to be investigated. Expert opinion and literature reviews must be utilized to assist in clarifying the focus of the study, potentially identifying other relevant outcomes, and ascertaining the limitations and generalizability of the endeavor.

Problem Identification

Relevant to a CEA, identifying the problem that needs to be solved involves two approaches: one focusing upon the disease state as the area of primary interest and another centering upon the technological advance itself. During the CEAs that characterized the emerging stages of pharmacoeconomics, studies generally began by identifying specific health problems (eg, morbidity, disability, mortality) associated with a certain disease. Analysts were then motivated to identify and compare a wide variety of preventive and therapeutic modalities with respect to relative cost-effectiveness. More recently, a specific intervention strategy (eg, a given drug, service, surgical procedure, or medical instrument or device) often serves as the starting point. The problem to be solved is whether the intervention in question (eg, Drug X) is cost-effective rather than to determine the most cost-effective alternative for reducing morbidity and/or mortality from a particular condition. As the analyst begins with a given treatment option, the specific regimens may then be investigated for single or multiple conditions.

Although both of the aforementioned problem orientations are legitimate and can arrive at identical CEAs, the latter may result in an inappropriate omission of key comparators.[16] For example, orientation toward comparative cost-effectiveness of cefaclor with amoxicillin for the treatment of acute otitis media may divert focus away from other treatments that should be investigated (eg, amoxicillin/clavulanate or trimethoprim/sulfamethoxazole). More generally, orientation toward comparative cost-effectiveness of a new pharmaceutical with other drugs in its therapeutic class may result in researchers overlooking the possibility that another drug, a nondrug treatment, a preventive approach, or no treatment whatsoever are reasonable alternatives that could be investigated simultaneously.

In conducting a CEA of drug therapy, the analyst must always contemplate the implications of the problem orientation. If the problem is formulated in terms of a specific drug or drug class, consideration should be given to documentation in the medical literature of the acceptability of alternatives to the drug or drugs in question. Regardless, it is quite proper to focus on drug–drug comparisons if the condition in question is known to require drug therapy.

Selection of Objectives

Following problem identification, specific objectives are developed for comparing the cost and effectiveness of alternative interventions. A research decision must be made concerning how the problem statement can be quantifiably incorporated into the study's methodology.

Selection of appropriate, measurable objectives is not always a simple or straightforward task. Careful attention must be directed toward the link between the health problem in question and the specific objective. Illustrating this, Warner and Luce[16] provided an example of morbidity and mortality resulting from myocardial infarction (MI) concerning the importance of this aspect of a CEA. Clearly, both morbidity and mortality resulting from MIs are important components of the health problem. Approaches to quantifying the problem would vary depending on which objective the analyst selects: decreasing the mortality rate of patients having an MI versus reducing the incidence of

MIs. The first would suggest a variety of emergency treatment alternatives, whereas the latter involves more preventive approaches. The selection of either does not allow consideration of intervention approaches suggested by the other. That is, preventive efforts would be expected to have little impact on the mortality rates of those who did experience an MI, and emergency treatment interventions would have little effect on the incidence of MIs. Building upon this, analysts have three choices when such incompatibilities exist between objectives: (1) select only one objective, thereby reducing the scope of the analysis; (2) include both objectives, realizing the resulting analysis may be inconclusive due to the lack of a common unit of measure; or (3) identify another objective that incorporates both facets. In the case of MIs, a reasonable solution might be to select the measurement of quality-adjusted life-years as an objective; both preventive and treatment approaches are consistent with this outcome.

An illustration of the difficulties involved in selecting objectives is fairly specific to drug formulary decisions.[19] In such situations, the pharmacy and therapeutics committee may typically consider the addition, deletion, or restricted use of a new technology. Thus, the problem orientation is intervention-based rather than health problem–based. Most pharmaceutical products are used for more than one indication, and each indication may have different relevant outcomes. Since a decision to add, delete, or restrict the use of a drug must consider all potential uses, the pharmacy and therapeutics committee does not have the option of selecting a single measure from several seemingly incompatible measures. Either multiple objectives or some composite objective must often be identified.

To ensure the appropriateness of the objectives developed for the study, the analyst should be confident that those chosen reflect the most important dimensions of the health problems and are relevant to the alternative interventions that will be compared. Furthermore, an outcome measure should be selected that is sensitive to the actual differences likely to be encountered between interventions. For example, if the percent of patients cured with comparative drug regimens is expected to be similar, but time to healing or symptom resolution or recurrence rates are expected to differ, an objective that reflects the latter measures may be recommended.

Perspective

The various economic agents and decision-makers within health care have legitimate differences in perspective that can affect which elements of resource consumption should be included in a pharmacoeconomic analysis. Perspective addresses the question, "Costs to whom?" The broadest viewpoint, that of society (ie, the aggregate of all society members, present and future), generally stipulates that all direct and indirect costs and benefits are addressed in addition to all intangible concerns. Perspectives that are more narrow than those of society, and potentially more useful for the specific decision-maker, include those of employers, governments, specific providers of care, managed care organizations, hospitals, insurers, or patients. Given that these viewpoints are less broad, it is logical that an individual perspective might not consider some costs and benefits important to society as a whole.

An illustration of the importance of establishing perspective is that patients are often only concerned with costs to the extent that they themselves are responsible for payment. The insured individual pays only when there are deductibles, coinsurance, and limits on coverage, which often represent only a small portion of the total costs. The patient, however, is extremely concerned with risks of productivity loss, morbidity, mortality, and quality of life. The acute care hospital, conversely, is concerned only with costs prior to discharge and the effects on patient productivity, and rehabilitation costs outside of the institution may typically not be included for this perspective. From the view of the insurer, only costs within the scope of coverage are relevant. By including different components of costs and outcomes for each viewpoint, conflicting decisions may arise from analyses with differing perspectives. As such, conducting a CEA from multiple perspectives may be warranted to offer information to numerous decision-makers in the marketplace.

Establishing the perspective in a CEA may be challenging for several reasons. Often, conventional economists advocate that a societal perspective be taken, as the goals of the cost-effectiveness or cost-benefit analysis have historically been to determine what society should do with regard to resource allocation. This approach, however, may not accurately reflect the primary concerns of a given patient, provider, or payer. A more pragmatic position is to accept that the proper perspective of a CEA should consider that of the individual or organization for whom the analysis is being conducted or for decision-makers requiring results of the investigation. This approach may also be too limited—regardless of the point of view of the decision-maker for whom the analysis is being conducted, it is likely that these individuals need to know how other economic agents will assess the research question.

Broad policy recommendations emanating from pharmacoeconomic assessments may have to be adopted, implemented, enforced, and perhaps withstand litigation by agencies, institutions, and individuals that have their own viewpoints. As addressed earlier, one solution is to offer numerous perspectives and include subanalyses that reflect the interests of the various parties.[17] Expanding upon this concept, it has been suggested that a method of weighting be considered concerning the various subanalyses, allowing the analyst the ability to offer predictions based upon the power distribution of the various economic agents.[20] Notwithstanding the approach taken, the choice regarding the explicit perspective (or multiple perspectives) must be taken prior to beginning the CEA.

STEP TWO: IDENTIFY THE ALTERNATIVE INTERVENTIONS

CEAs provide the most meaningful information to decision-makers when an attempt is made to relate a new technology to alternatives that exist in each specific marketplace. Rather than examining the cost-effectiveness of a new therapeutic agent alone (or drawing comparisons with placebo), a full economic assessment involves comparisons of resource consumption and outcomes with one or more alternatives.[3] Based upon the objectives of the investigation or specific regulatory requirements, researchers may choose comparators that include the least expensive alternative, a less expensive regimen relative to the new technology, the most commonly used drug within the therapeutic class, a preferred agent or drug of choice, a standard therapy from a given drug class, or a therapy that provides the next highest magnitude of cost-effectiveness.

Relating to the problem statement of the research endeavor and the specific objectives of the study, one would expect that the narrower the problem and objectives, the fewer relevant alternatives would be necessary to consider. However, the choice of comparators must also take into account the number of alternative therapies that exist for the given disease state. If an investigation seeks to address the consequences of gastrointestinal ulcers, all alternatives must be directed toward those outcomes. Thus, if the established objective is to increase healing rates of patients who present only with active ulcers, preventive alternatives might be excluded. Expanding this, comparators may be expected to vary according to clinical practice settings or guidelines as well as time. Differences in comparators would also be expected relative to each country, population, or institution, because the mix of available products and alternatives may not necessarily be equivalent. The choice of relevant, appropriate alternatives in a CEA is crucial, as it specifies the baseline from which cost-effectiveness ratios are computed. Furthermore, alternatives or treatment protocols should be described in sufficient detail that other researchers could replicate the investigation in their own treatment settings. Justification must also be offered for the choice of comparator relative to other therapies that exist.

In perhaps the simplest case, individual drugs may be compared with each other for a single condition. The pharmaceutical products would not necessarily be required to be from different drug classes, although differences do usually exist with respect to some relevant pharmacologic property. Interventions being compared may consider entirely different classes of drugs (eg, β-blockers versus thiazide diuretics for treatment of hypertension). When classes of drugs are compared, a single drug from each class is often selected as representative for the entire class. Interventions may also be investigated across multiple disease conditions, as is required for many formulary decisions.[19] For example, proton-pump inhibitors might be compared for both treatment of existing ulcers and prophylaxis of recurrent ulcers. Depending on the scope of the problem and specific objectives being addressed, it may be necessary to include nondrug therapy (eg, surgery) or even no therapy as alternative interventions.

STEP THREE: DESCRIBE THE PRODUCTION RELATIONSHIPS BETWEEN INPUTS AND OUTCOMES

Defining the research problem, objectives, perspective, and relevant alternatives establishes the initial, conceptual framework of a CEA. The next step in the analysis (ie, describing the relationship between resource consumption and outcomes) builds upon this foundation. Describing the production relationship ultimately results in the identification and measurement of resource use required to provide each intervention. It also provides the technical framework for the quantitative assessment and comparison of net costs with net effectiveness.

There are several methods for characterizing the production relationship; these approaches generally involve the development of a model that specifies how inputs are combined and how much output a given group of inputs will produce. The method required to assess the production relationships may be as simple as populating a table or flow chart wherein all inputs and their quantities are documented where they enter the production process. One technique that may be useful in identifying and measuring costs is to develop a resource utilization profile that parallels the structure of a decision-analytic model, wherein all healthcare resource consumption is delineated according to each step of the decision tree. The amount of resources consumed would subsequently be calculated based upon the defined cost drivers to dollar amounts; these values would then be used to estimate the costs of the intervention. Other techniques for modeling include Monte Carlo and Markov Chain methods, regression analysis, or life-table approaches.[21-26]

Production costs are those associated with providing an intervention and are determined by first itemizing the resources used to actually provide the intervention. For each event identified, health resource consumption must be identified (eg, services by physicians and other healthcare professionals, hospital services, diagnostic tests, drug therapy). This information must be specific, detailing the exact quantities and types of resources needed. For services conducted by professionals, the specific services and the type of professional providing them must be precise (eg, Is the service provided by a physician, nurse, or pharmacist, and how specialized are these professionals?). One particular service provided by nurses that is especially relevant to drug therapy CEAs is drug administration. For pharmacists, time involved in traditional dispensing services (eg, compounding, supervision of technicians) in addition to pharmaceutical care activities (eg, pharmacokinetic monitoring) that are components of the intervention should be itemized. The number of times each service is provided by each of these professionals and the time required per episode should also be included. For hospital services, the type of unit on which the services are provided should be recorded (eg, intensive care unit, burn unit, emergency department). Furthermore, the number of days or hours spent in each type of unit is needed. The type of diagnostic tests and the number of times each is used must be assessed. For drug therapy, the analyst must detail the specific drugs, doses, dosing interval, duration of therapy, and route of administration.

An important aspect in conducting economic assessments involves the evaluation of incremental inputs and outputs. In brief, the tendency of many analysts is to rely solely upon average inputs needed to produce a single unit of output (ie, the average cost to add one additional life-year). There are several problems with this approach, among which is the overestimation of opportunity costs of an intervention by inclusion of its associated fixed inputs. The appropriate course is to utilize an incremental analysis and pose the question: For each additional unit of output gained, how much additional input will be required? In addressing this, a subtle distinction exists between the terms *marginal* and *incremental* that deserves brief discussion. Within economics, marginal analyses are frequently conducted to assess the production of an additional unit of output. Given that real-world decision-making often requires the consideration of comparators plus output changes that are broader in scope, extensions to the classically defined marginal analyses are often more appropriate. Studies that involve changes in discrete quantities of output between alternatives are termed *incremental analyses*, which are essentially considered a practical application of a marginal analysis to include relevant comparators.

STEP FOUR: IDENTIFY AND MEASURE COSTS AND OUTCOMES OF THE INTER-VENTIONS

Cost Assessments

The basic purpose of cost analyses in pharmacoeconomics is to identify the centers of resource consumption required for the production of a good or service wherein monetary values would be assigned to these resources. These cost analyses follow proper understanding of the production relationships that were briefly addressed earlier. Concerning cost studies, however, distinctions must be firmly established between costs as defined by *accounting* versus *economic* costs. Whereas the accountant defines costs as historical monetary outlays or expenses used to prepare financial statements, economists are concerned with opportunity costs (ie, what must be foregone to produce a good or service, thus considering the revenue that may be generated by other uses of resources for projects of similar risk).[27,28] Opportunity costs are essentially those that are lost relative to the cost of comparable and forsaken alternatives; these can only arise in instances with scarcity given that a limited amount of resources exists to meet all wants or needs. From the position of corporate finance, investment decisions focus upon elements of economic costs rather than those involving accounting costs.[28] In identifying and measuring costs within pharmacoeconomic analyses, the explicit specification of the perspective of the study is required, as this perspective dictates what costs represent the opportunity costs to be assessed. Another important consideration in discussing costs is to note that costs may differ from both charges and price; actual costs would be expected in most instances to be lower than charges and market prices, as several aspects beyond the marginal cost of production are omitted in an actual cost. Finally, the resource consumption that is investigated within CEAs is contingent upon the perspective of the study and can differ substantially between economic agents. Caregiver time and lost productivity (ie, indirect costs) may be costly to the patient or to society, but not from the perspective of the provider or payer. Additionally, intangible costs (eg, pain and suffering) would often be expected to impact a patient to a greater extent than a payer.

An area of debate that has been addressed concerning the CEA surrounds the merits of including unrelated future health-care costs. Some scholars have stated that these costs, which include the costs of treating diseases that would not have occurred if the patient had not lived longer as a result of the original intervention, should be incorporated.[3,29] However, others contend that these costs should not be included, as incorporating such costs would overestimate the costs associated with life-saving interventions.[16,17,30,31] Furthermore, it seems inconsistent to include consumption of healthcare resources in added years without including productivity and other types of consumption that are associated with prolonged life.

Outcomes Assessment

Similar to clinical trial investigations, the precise description and definition of outcomes is required in cost-effectiveness studies. Intuitively, the outcomes should be clinically relevant and measured in an objective fashion. These outcomes should also follow standard measurement criteria such that the results are acceptable within the healthcare community. For example, oncologic investigations often assess response by measuring tumor area, whereas measuring the volume of the tumor itself may not necessarily be considered routine.

Within the design of the CEA, the effectiveness of an intervention is not valued in monetary units. Although health status is multidimensional, researchers and practitioners are often concerned with a single health measure and the most efficient means of reaching a preferred health status. For example, a question may be posed concerning which of two drugs would produce the greatest number of cures per dollar spent. Here, the number of cures can serve as the single measure of health effectiveness. Similarly, a single measure for mortality could be the number of lives saved (or lost) by each intervention.

The ECHO model (economic, clinical, and humanistic outcomes) is one method of classifying the various outcomes in pharmacoeconomic analyses.[32] Although all of these outcomes are considered relatively inseparable and realizing that no single outcome type is necessarily more important than another, clinical outcomes are typically of prime interest in the CEA due to the scope of the methodology. Clinical outcomes are often expressed in terms of morbidity and mortality rates or laboratory values associated with a disease or intervention. However, because many current interventions are directed toward alleviating disease conditions or relieving symptoms rather than saving lives, the ability to measure quality of life is often of consequence. Given the importance of quality of life as an outcome, the topic should at least be addressed in the presentation of the results, even if it is done so only in descriptive terms. In specific disease states warranting assessments of both the quality and quantity of life, quality-adjusted life-years may also be included in addition to a clinical outcome measure, thus incorporating elements of a cost-utility analysis.

Often, it is most desirable to analyze clinical endpoints that are considered a final outcome (eg, cure of acute conditions, control of chronic conditions, life-years saved, strokes avoided, survival/death) primarily because these have a direct relationship with a patient's morbidity or mortality. Although preferable, such measures are not always easily captured. Due to the time frames involved, collecting data on final outcomes is often impossible or impractical to undertake, thus advocating the utilization of intermediate outcomes within a study.

Intermediate versus Final Outcomes

An *intermediate outcome* (eg, mm Hg, FEV_1, CD4+ count) is a surrogate endpoint related to the final outcome of interest. The use of an intermediate measure is often established in feasibility: these endpoints are often more readily available and, given the extended time frame required to collect final outcomes, are more practical to focus upon within a research endeavor. When intermediate measures are used, a strong empirical relationship between the final outcome of importance must be established or the intermediate measure exists as a critical clinical measure in itself.[3] Using a surrogate outcome affords researchers shorter time frames of investigation, as intermediate events accumulate more rapidly than final events.

The choice of a reliable and valid intermediate outcome is an area of debate in many disease states and, although advanced methods exist to assess the association between the primary clinical outcome of interest and a surrogate endpoint, continued work is still required.[33,34] Overall, the findings based upon these surrogate measures are frequently generalized to the final outcome of clinical interest. Regardless of the empiric strength of association between the intermediate and final outcome, investigators should include discussion of how the surrogate extrapolates to the final outcome. For example, the association between a patient's serum cholesterol level and coronary heart disease or tumor response and survival in oncology addresses the potential disconnection between surrogate and final endpoints.

Randomized Clinical Trials: Efficacy versus Effectiveness

While cost estimates used in a CEA are often collected from either a clinical trial or secondary sources, outcome measures are commonly approximated by data obtained from randomized clinical trials (RCTs). Concerning data obtained from RCTs, a strong distinction should be drawn between the terms efficacy and effectiveness.[35] *Efficacy* data emanate from RCTs, wherein conditions are controlled, adherence is almost perfect, and the population investigated is relatively homogenous. Conversely, *effectiveness* data involve real-world, naturalistic settings; patient populations may be diverse, diagnoses may be incorrect, and medication adherence may be substantially less than ideal. Overall, efficacy focuses upon the question of "Can it work?," while effectiveness addresses the broader issue of "Will it work?" Given the aforementioned factors, the difference between efficacy and effectiveness can be substantial. In all, treatment regimens can be efficacious, but may not necessarily offer the same degree of effectiveness. Extending this, therapies may be effective, but may not necessarily provide value.

Efficacy data are considered easier to obtain than effectiveness data, primarily due to the regulatory requirements of pharmaceuticals to go through phase trials. However, the framework of the randomized, placebo-controlled clinical investigation may not necessarily be considered the most favorable for economic assessments.[36] Aside from the biased study design of RCTs, the comparator used within the experimental design of most clinical trials is defined as that of no treatment whatsoever, which is often an unrealistic comparator for real-world or economic decision-making. Results from RCTs regarding drug efficacy can be used and adjustments made to reflect expected conditions of actual use, such as inaccuracies in diagnosis and prescriber and patient nonadherence with recommended regimens.[3] These adjustments are often subjective, as few data are available for most drugs regarding the relationship between degree of adherence and drug effect. Although analysts are strongly cautioned to recognize the limitations of economic assessments based upon RCT study designs, measuring effectiveness also presents numerous challenges that must be considered.[37] In instances in which pharmacoeconomic analyses are conducted in parallel to RCTs where efficacy is the key outcome of interest, the description of the investigation is often defined as a *cost-efficacy analysis*.

Discounting Cost and Effectiveness Measures

Regardless of whether all cost variables within a CEA are adjusted for inflation or even if the inflation rate is zero, discounting of the monetary inputs is warranted if the time frame of the pharmacoeconomic investigation exceeds one year. Being a fundamental aspect of finance, that of the "time value of money," a time preference exists for capital because secured funds can be immediately allocated to generate interest or profits from risk-free investments (eg, Treasury bills). Additionally, individuals identify that there is also a bona fide time preference for capital, in that monies obtained immediately are free from financial uncertainties that may occur in the future. No debate exists in the discipline of finance concerning the importance and requirement of discounting; the only area of debate is which discount rate to employ. Typically, discount rates used in pharmacoeconomic analyses may be three or five percent domestically and may vary in international settings; a sensitivity analysis is advocated for any discount rate chosen.[38]

Although the need to discount cost variables is an accepted fact, controversy remains regarding nonmonetary health outcomes.[13] Given that the inputs of the cost-effectiveness ratio are discounted, some scholars have stated that omitting discounting from outcomes leads to unequal comparison; discounted effectiveness measures would thus be warranted on the grounds that these valuations are made relative to discounted costs.[29] Theoretically, the process of discounting outcomes has also been supported because people may have a time preference for additional life-years, preferring an additional year of life sooner rather than later. This argument is not entirely straighforward, as other scholars have illustrated that no trade-off or time preference could exist in possessing an extra year of life sooner rather than later: an individual simply cannot have extra years of life in the future if the years are not offered earlier.[16] Regardless of whether discounting outcomes is supported on theoretical grounds, the choice of discount rate to utilize is highly questionable and may become especially suspect if intermediate clinical outcomes are used (eg, LDL-C).

STEP 5: INTERPRET AND PRESENT RESULTS

Cost-Effectiveness Ratios

The basic decision criterion for cost-effectiveness establishes that innovations are adopted in the marketplace and that such innovations are allocated optimally in the market. That is, goods or services that provide increased value with respect to both costs and consequences relative to competitors are utilized. Decisionmakers seek to incorporate treatment options that maximize an outcome relative to resources consumed and ensure that the outcome is explicitly positive in nature. Although a cost-effectiveness ratio can offer information on the cost per life-year saved subsequent to an intervention, the methodology does not necessarily offer a robust mechanism for establishing the value of that additional life-year.

Results from a CEA are typically expressed as a cost-effectiveness (C/E) ratio; the numerator of the ratio reflects total costs, while the denominator is the expression of the outcome variable. Thus, as presented in terms of cost-to-effect, the findings from a CEA may be expressed as an average cost of $50 per one percent reduction in hemoglobin A_{1C} or an incremental cost of $5 per symptom-free day gained. In general, the lower the numerator and the higher the denominator of the C/E ratio, the greater the investment value offered from a technology, leading to what is implicitly considered a *preferred* strategy. Recalling the proper use of the term cost-effective, conditions do exist wherein more expensive therapies are worth the extra cost or cheaper alternatives are not worth the savings.

Two forms of the C/E ratio exist: (1) average, or simple, and (2) incremental (ICER). The average/simple C/E ratio is a straight-forward approach, defined as follows:

$$\text{average (simple) C/E ratio} = \frac{\text{cost}}{\text{effect}}$$

where cost represents the cumulative costs measured within the investigation for a given treatment alternative and effect is the natural unit outcome of interest. The average C/E ratio is calculated for each treatment alternative, and comparisons are drawn relative to the differences between the new therapy and the chosen comparator. Results are subsequently interpreted as the average cost per unit of effectiveness (eg, average cost per cure or average cost per percentage decrease in mm Hg).

Although average C/E ratios provide useful information for analysts, incremental analyses are considered a hallmark of CEA; incremental analyses should always be conducted within a CEA. The ICER is defined as a ratio of the difference in costs between two alternatives to the difference in effectiveness between the alternatives and is calculated according to the following equation:

$$\text{ICER} = \frac{\Delta \text{cost}}{\Delta \text{effect}} = \frac{\text{cost}_{\text{New Technology}} - \text{cost}_{\text{Comparator}}}{\text{effect}_{\text{New Technology}} - \text{effect}_{\text{Comparator}}}$$

where cost and effect are defined consistently with those used to compute the average C/E ratio; new technology can also be defined as other alternatives, and comparator reflects a baseline intervention. The interpretation of the ICER differs from the average C/E ratio—results denote the cost to produce or achieve a one-unit increase in an outcome relative to a chosen baseline rather than an average cost per outcome. For example, an incremental analysis may be used to determine the cost of obtaining one additional cure within the population for a new alternative relative to a chosen comparator as opposed to the average cost to treat the entire population for each alternative. Results emanating from the ICER may differ from the average C/E ratio; on occasion, the difference can be large, potentially changing the final recommendation that is offered to or made by the decision-maker.

An important caveat exists with the ICER in cases wherein a technology offers both decreased cost and increased effectiveness relative to a given baseline comparator; this caveat builds upon the concepts provided in the discussion of the cost-effectiveness grid in Figure 1.[3] Under the conditions described above, an explicit connotation of a *dominant* strategy exists and a negative ICER is subsequently observed—the new technology offers value in the marketplace with respect to both aspects of cost and effectiveness and should ultimately be accepted. Conversely, if an option is more expensive and less effective than an existing baseline comparator, the option is considered *dominated*, with the recommendation of rejecting this intervention; a negative ICER is also observed in this scenario. Caution has been recommended in interpreting negative ICERs beyond an assessment of the sign of the numerical value; that is, although information is present within the magnitude of the value, its interpretation differs than when the value is positive.[39] In cases where the cost of a new technology is higher than its comparator and its subsequent effect is also higher or if the cost of the new technology is lower and the effect is lower, a trade-off must be made: Is the increased cost of either the new technology or the comparator worth the added benefit?

In instances wherein a new treatment is both more effective and less expensive, the decision-maker's choice is relatively straightforward: to accept the new technology based on the merits of decreased resource consumption and improvement in outcomes. When no clear dominant strategy exists, however, the choice may become somewhat more challenging. In the latter instance, the ICER calculated may be compared relative to a *threshold value* (ie, the amount representing a decision-maker's willingness to pay to obtain for the incremental gain in outcomes). Decision-makers will most often choose to adopt a technology wherein the ICER is either equal to or less than the established (or subjective) threshold value. Debate currently exists and will likely continue surrounding the baseline ICER that is acceptable and what ICER above a threshold value is also acceptable.

Illustrating a separate form of dominance, the observation of *extended dominance* occurs when a particular option has a higher ICER than a subsequent and more effective alternative.[40] Given a scenario wherein one treatment yields three different options, Option A offers an ICER of $100 per additional unit of effectiveness relative to an established baseline, Option B yields an ICER of $200 per additional unit of effectiveness, and Option

C has an ICER of $125 per additional unit of effectiveness, extended dominance describes Option B among the choices. Within this example, Option B is dominated, and a decision-maker should observe which combinations of Options A and C offer optimal benefits when considering resources to be allocated.

To illustrate the differences between the simple/average and incremental C/E ratios, Example One presents two treatments as follows: Treatment One (a baseline comparator) costs $500 to treat 100 patients and Treatment Two (a new innovation) costs $750 to treat the same number of individuals. The effectiveness measure is a final outcome, cure rate, wherein 95 percent of the patients are cured with Treatment One and 97 percent of the patients are cured with Treatment Two. Calculating the average C/E ratio yields a relatively small difference between the average costs to treat the patient groups between the two alternatives, $246.88. However, an incremental analysis finds the cost of Treatment Two to be substantially higher, costing $12,500 to obtain one additional cure.

Sensitivity Analyses and Statistical Issues

Consistent with all types of scholarly research, care should be taken in the presentation and interpretation of results from the CEA. Discussion should clearly identify the critical uncertainties of the analysis with the likely impact of these uncertainties on the findings. Furthermore, methodologic limitations and external validity should be explicitly offered in addition to other relevant considerations that have not been addressed in the analysis. For example, if outcomes such as changes in quality of life were identified but not addressed in a quantifiable manner, discussion should be offered on the likely impact upon the analysis.

To account for potential aspects of uncertainty within pharmacoeconomic assessments, a sensitivity analysis is often incorporated to ascertain the robustness of the estimates that are obtained.[41] This approach systematically varies the critical parameters of variables to determine whether the overall decision criteria changes. To illustrate this, if a researcher chooses a discount rate of three percent, a sensitivity analysis may be conducted wherein the discount rate is varied between zero and 10 percent to observe whether the estimates or final decision criteria are robust. If the results of the sensitivity analysis change the final estimates to a small magnitude when the discount rate is altered, confidence in the results is increased. Conversely, if the research findings change substantially, the analyst should be more concerned about the uncertainty of the particular estimate.

Beyond the discount rate, other variables that have potentially high levels of uncertainty include efficacy rates (especially comparative efficacy of the alternative interventions), adverse reaction rates, event rates in untreated individuals, estimates of cost components, adherence rates, and variables wherein subjective assumptions are made. The limitation of sensitivity analyses generally surrounds a lack of consensus that exists on the specific variables and parameters to vary, the range of the values to be varied, and the challenges in interpreting results, particularly concerning more advanced methods.[42,43]

Example One
Calculating Average/Simple and Incremental Cost-Effectiveness (C/E) Ratios

Given:

Treatment One
   total cost to treat 100 patients = $500
   effectiveness = 95% cure rate

Treatment Two
   total cost to treat 100 patients = $750
   effectiveness = 97% cure rate

Computations:
1. What is the average/simple C/E ratio for each therapy?
2. What is the incremental C/E ratio comparing Treatment One versus Treatment Two?

Solution: Average/simple C/E ratio

Treatment One
   500/0.95 = $526.32 average cost per cure
Treatment Two   Difference = $246.88
   750/0.97 = $773.20 average cost per cure

Solution: Incremental C/E ratio

Treatment One vs Two
   (750–500)/(0.97–0.95) = $12,500 per additional cure to use Treatment Two

A useful approach to uncertainty in pharmacoeconomic assessments beyond sensitivity analyses involves reporting confidence intervals around the various estimates.[43,44] Many pharmacoeconomic investigations present a single point estimate for the ICER that is computed based upon average values for costs and effects. This brings about several statistical issues, given that both costs in the numerator and effects in the denominator represent separate distributions of data that encompass differing levels of uncertainty. For example, given the degree of skew, a median or mean value (or potentially transformed figure) may be most appropriate for analysis. Furthermore, point estimates may not be considered to be reflective of the amount of variance present within the distributions. Partially addressing the limitations of sensitivity analyses as well as the issues surrounding point estimates, confidence intervals are frequently used to better express the nature of the data that exist within C/E ratios. Approaches include the Box method, Fieller's theorem, nonparametric bootstrap, and Taylor's series.[44] Of these, research supports that Fieller's theorem and nonparametric bootstrap generally outperform other techniques.[45] Beyond confidence intervals, the application of Bayesian methods to capture probability distributions of the ICER offers another method of managing the uncertainty within CEAs.[46]

League Tables

The CEA is used to determine the value of new technology that will augment decision-making considering conditions of scarcity. The hallmark of the CEA in ascertaining potential gains from innovation is the incremental analysis and, although computing an economic metric such as the ICER is required, doing so does not necessarily address the issue of broad comparative assessments between therapies or investigations. One way that addresses this issue and may be employed to judge the relative valuation of a technology with others in the marketplace is through the use of league tables.[47]

A *league table* rank-orders interventions according to ICERs based upon an established outcome, such as a cost per year of life saved.[48] Some economists favor the defining outcome of the cost-utility analysis, the quality-adjusted life-year, to be the preferred denominator for broad comparative decision-making between programs.[49] Two uses of a league table exist: (1) allocating funds on a fixed budget, wherein therapies are included in a rank-ordered and listwise fashion until the entirety of the budget is allocated, and (2) comparing treatment approaches both between alternatives and relative to a threshold value.[50] A primary advantage of a league table is that it aids in establishing a broad summary to allow for a more sound valuation of options. In theory, although a league table may offer guidance, the information presented is contingent upon the findings of several studies that may differ substantially relative to methodologies utilized. Thus, it is recommended that these tables seek to represent information that reflects the diversity of findings that may exist, particularly relating to comparators used, subpopulations studied, and information concerning the ICER (eg, mean, variance, confidence intervals). The methodology used to determine outcomes may also be of importance.[50]

Graphical Depictions of Data

Mathematical presentations of C/E ratios are clearly required when representing the results of the investigation. Two approaches that may be used to supplement numerical depictions offer strength via graphical means: (1) cost-effectiveness plane and (2) economic efficiency frontier.

The *cost-effectiveness plane* is a method of depicting the incremental cost-effectiveness of a new treatment relative to a chosen comparator.[39] This technique places the difference in costs between two treatment options on the Y-axis versus the difference in effectiveness on the X-axis, thus establishing the baseline comparator at the origin. Building upon the cost-effectiveness grid presented earlier in Figure 1, a dominant strategy offering lower costs and increased effectiveness would appear in the bottom, right-hand region of Figure 3, labeled Quadrant II. If the new technology is more expensive and less effective, the dominated strategy would appear in the top, left-hand region of the graph labeled Quadrant IV. Trade-offs are required of decision-makers in both Quadrant I (ie, Is the increased cost of the new treatment worth the increase in effectiveness?) and Quadrant III (ie, Is the decrease in effectiveness worth the cost savings?). Importantly, the C/E ratio is represented as the slope of the line from the origin of the graph (ie, the comparator) to the point representing the new technology; a negative slope corresponds to a negative ICER, which indicates either a dominant or dominated strategy. Revisiting Example One, which compared two different treatment strategies, Treatment Two provides both increased cost and increased effectiveness; the results would be placed within Quadrant I, requiring a trade-off by the decision-maker.

The *economic efficiency frontier* is an additional method to graphically present results from a cost-effectiveness analysis, illustrated in Figure 4.[51] Defined as a set of points that represent preferable strategies, the efficiency frontier is comprised of the options that form a boundary nearest the region of dominant

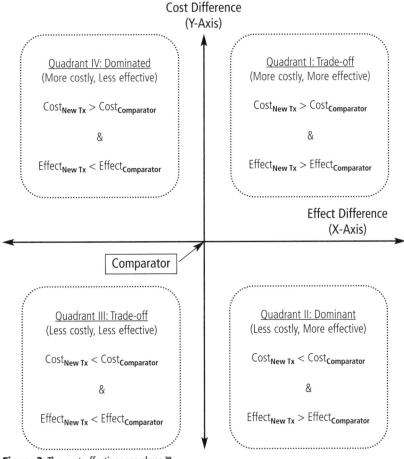

Figure 3. The cost-effectiveness plane.[39]

strategies (ie, the area in the graph represented at the bottom, right-hand corner: choices with lower cost and higher effectiveness). C/E ratios are represented within the graph as the slope of respective lines. The average/simple C/E ratio is reflected by the slope of a line from the origin of the graph to the option of interest; the ICER is reflected as the slope of a line drawn between two particular options.

In Example Two, two options are considered: a new technology versus usual medical care. Given that the new treatment offers both increased effectiveness and decreased costs, one may presume initially that it dominates usual medical care; a negative ICER is indeed observed. Placement of the new option versus the comparator appears in the bottom, right-hand region of the cost-effectiveness plane (ie, Quadrant II). Attention should be drawn toward the economic efficiency frontier concerning the slopes of the lines denoting average and incremental costs; the negative ICER is reflected with a negative slope function relative to the baseline comparator, usual medical care.

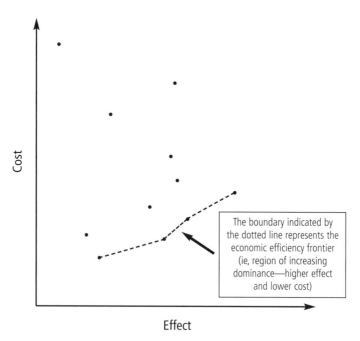

The boundary indicated by the dotted line represents the economic efficiency frontier (ie, region of increasing dominance—higher effect and lower cost)

Figure 4. The economic efficiency frontier.[51] The points within the graph illustrate various treatment options.

Summary

Throughout the scope of health care, choices have to be made concerning the allocation of scarce resources, as all wants and needs cannot be met under conditions of constraint. At its very essence, these circumstances require what is analogous to an investment or capital budgeting decision. The CEA provides powerful methodology by which the researcher can identify, measure, and compare both resource consumption and patient outcomes associated with innovative healthcare technologies. In conducting a pharmacoeconomic investigation, a well-defined problem statement and concrete objectives provide the foundation of a sound methodologic design. An explicitly stated perspective is required in a CEA, as the resources consumed are contingent upon specific viewpoints of the economic agents within health care. Appropriate treatment alternatives must be identified, and each must be critically evaluated in relation to other available options within the marketplace.

Overall, the specification of perspective, selection of comparators, and choice of outcome measures establish the means by which CEAs are utilized by decision-makers in real-world settings. The analyst's presentation and discussion of results is critical to appropriate interpretation by readers—the hallmark of the CEA is in computing the ICER between options. To account for uncertainty and establish confidence in estimates, sensitivity analysis of key variables, assumptions, and uncertainties should be conducted; the presentation of confidence intervals, relevant descriptive statistics, and diagnostics is also advocated. Consistent with all research, the limitations and generalizability of findings must also be addressed.

The barriers in utilizing CEAs parallel those that exist for all pharmacoeconomic investigations. Given that information required for decisions in clinical settings must be timely, studies must exist when a new chemical entity is approved and when other therapeutic agents enter the marketplace. Consideration of issues regarding changes in price, the epidemiology of disease, or insurance coverage are also of importance. Generalizability of studies is dependent upon the population investigated, as well as the perspective of the study itself. These issues may be of special concern with research conducted in multinational

<u>Example Two</u>
A Dominant Strategy

Given:
  New Treatment Option
    total cost of treatment   = $7,000
    percent of patients with no adverse events = 70%
  Usual Medical Care
    total cost of treatment   = $7,500
    percent of patients with no adverse events = 50%
Computations:
  1. What is the average/simple C/E Ratio for each option?
  2. What is the incremental C/E ratio comparing the new treatment versus usual
     medical care?
  3. Where would the new treatment be placed on the cost-effective plane?

Solution: Average/simple C/E ratio
  New Treatment Option
    7,000/0.70 = $10,000 average cost per successfully treated patient
  Usual Medical Care
    7,500/0.50 = $15,000 average cost per successfully treated patient
Solution: Incremental C/E ratio
  New Treatment Option vs Usual Medical Care
    (7,000–7500)/(0.70–0.50) = –$2,500
    {The new treatment option offers decreased cost and increased effectiveness
     (ie, dominant strategy), yielding a negative ICER}
Solution:

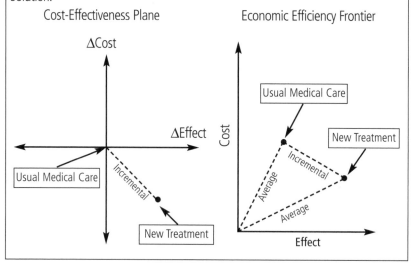

Cost-Effectiveness Plane   Economic Efficiency Frontier

venues or when extrapolating findings from one distinct health-care system to another. The methodologies and results from pharmacoeconomics can be complex and difficult to understand by actual decision-makers, and the methodologies themselves are continuing to evolve and increase in rigor. Although certain areas of consensus exist, the broad harmonization of principles and guidelines is not necessarily advocated by all scholars.[52]

The choice of utilizing a CEA versus other methods depends upon the specific questions identified by researchers, the types of alternatives investigated, and the information required by final decision-makers. Consideration of the various advantages, disadvantages, limitations, and generalizability must remain of paramount importance. When considering chronic conditions or cases wherein symptom control takes precedence over survival or cure, the CEA may simply not capture all dimensions of concern.

Despite potential drawbacks, pharmacoeconomic analyses are useful tools to augment decision-making for policymakers, providers, insurers, and other consumers in health care. In light of this, the term cost-effective is used to imply value for money rather than to merely identify the cheapest option. Managers of pharmaceutical programs must be constantly aware of the broad impact in adopting products and services with only the lowest acquisition costs, as other aspects within health care may worsen as a result. In addressing the welfare of society as a whole, the optimal balance of resource allocation with respect to outcomes affords all persons a maximum benefit with regard to the innovations and options in health care.

References

1. Pauly MV. The economics of growing health care expenditures. LDI Health Policy Res Quart 1991;1:1-21.
2. Neumann PJ, Johannesson M. From principle to public policy: using cost-effectiveness analysis. Health Affairs 1994;13:206-14.
3. Drummond MF, O'Brien B, Stoddart GL, Torrance GW. Methods for the economic evaluation of health care programmes. 2nd ed. New York: Oxford University Press, 1997.
4. DiMasi JA, Caglarcan E, Wood-Armany M. Emerging role of pharmacoeconomics in the research and development-making process. Pharmacoeconomics 2001;19:753-66.
5. Motheral BR, Grizzle AJ, Armstrong EP, Cox E, Fairman K. Role of phar-

macoeconomics in drug benefit decision-making: results of a survey. Formulary 2002;35:412-21.

6. Drummond M, Dubois D, Garattini L, Horisberger B, Jönsson B, Kristiansen S, et al. Current trends in the use of pharmacoeconomics and outcomes research in Europe. Value Health 1999;2:323-32.

7. Drummond MF, Jonsson B, Rutten FFH. The role of economic evaluation in the pricing and reimbursement of medicines. Health Policy 1997;40: 199-215.

8. McGhan WF. Pharmacoeconomics and the evaluation of drugs and services. Hosp Formulary 1993;28:365-78.

9. Bootman JL, Larson LN, McGhan WF, Townsend RJ. Pharmacoeconomic research and clinical trials: concepts and issues. DICP 1989;23:693-7.

10. Birch S, Gafni A. Cost-effectiveness/utility analyses: do current decision rules lead us to where we want to be? J Health Econ 1992;11:279-96.

11. Phelps C, Mushlin A. On the near equivalence of cost-effectiveness and cost-benefit analyses. Int J Technol Assess Health Care 1991;7:12-21.

12. Johannesson M, Jonsson B. Economic evaluation in health care: is there a role for cost-benefit analysis? Health Policy 1991;17:1-23.

13. Towse A. Health economics—a useful tool or a threat? Scrip 1994;May: 30-3.

14. Gold MR, Siegel JE, Russell LB, Weinstein MC, eds. Cost-effectiveness in health and medicine. New York: Oxford University Press, 1996.

15. Doubilet P, Weinstein MC, McNeil BJ. Use and misuse of the term "cost-effective" in medicine. N Engl J Med 1986;314:253-5.

16. Warner KE, Luce BR. Cost-benefit and cost-effectiveness analysis in health care: principles, practice, and potential. Ann Arbor, MI: Health Administration Press, 1982.

17. Dao TD. Cost-benefit and cost-effectiveness analysis of drug therapy. Am J Hosp Pharm 1985;42:791-802.

18. Warner KE, Hutton R. Cost-benefit and cost-effectiveness analysis in health care: growth and composition of the literature. Med Care 1980;18: 1069-84.

19. Gagnon JP, Osterhaus JT. Proposed drug–drug cost effectiveness methodology. Drug Intell Clin Pharm 1987;21:211-6.

20. Luft HS. Benefit cost analysis and public policy implementation: from normative to positive analysis. Public Policy 1976;24:437-61.

21. Beck JR, Pauker SG. The Markov process in medical prognosis. Med Decis Making 1983;3:419-58.

22. Detsky AS, Naglie G, Krahn MD, Naimark D, Redelmeier DA. Primer on medical decision analysis. Part 1—getting started. Med Decis Making 1997;2:123-5.

23. Detsky AS, Naglie G, Krahn MD, Naimark D, Redelmeier DA. Primer on medical decision analysis. Part 2—building a tree. Med Decis Making 1997;2:126-35.

24. Detsky AS, Naglie G, Krahn MD, Naimark D, Redelmeier DA. Primer on medical decision analysis. Part 3—estimating probabilities and utilities. Med Decis Making 1997;2:136-41.

25. Krahn MD, Naglie G, Naimark D, Redelmeier DA, Detsky AS. Primer on

medical decision analysis. Part 4—analyzing the model and interpreting the results. Med Decis Making 1997;2:142-51.

26. Sheldon TA. Problems of using modeling in the economic evaluation of health care. Health Econ 1996;5:1-11.

27. Sendi P, Gafni A, Birch S. Opportunity costs and uncertainty in the economic evaluation of health care interventions. Health Econ 2002;11:23-31.

28. Skrepnek GH. Accounting- versus economic-based rates of return: implications for profitability measures in the pharmaceutical industry. Clin Ther 2004;26:155-74.

29. Weinstein MC, Stason WB. Foundations of cost-effectiveness analysis for health and medical practices. N Engl J Med 1977;296:716-21.

30. Russell LB. Is prevention better than cure? Washington, DC: Brookings Institute, 1986.

31. Garber AM, Phelps CE. Economic foundations of cost-effectiveness analysis. Stanford, CA: National Bureau of Economic Research, 1995.

32. Kozma CM, Reeder CE, Schultz RM. Economic, clinical, and humanistic outcomes: a planning model for pharmacoeconomic research. Clin Ther 1993;15:1121-32.

33. De Gruttola VG, Clax P, DeMets DL, Downing GJ, Ellenberg SS, Friedman L, et al. Considerations in the evaluation of surrogate endpoints in clinical trials: summary of a National Institutes of Health workshop. Control Clin Trials 2001;22:485-502.

34. Freeman LS, Graubard BI, Schatzkin A. Statistical valuation of intermediate endpoints for chronic diseases. Stat Med 1992;11:167-78.

35. Sommer A, Zeger SL. On estimating efficacy from clinical trials. Stat Med 1991;10:45-52.

36. Drummond MF, Davies L. Economic analyses alongside clinical trials: revisiting the methodological issues. Int J Tech Assess Health Care 1991; 7:561-73.

37. D'Agostino RB, Kwan H. Measuring effectiveness: what to expect without a randomized control group. Med Care 1995;33(4 suppl):AS95-105.

38. Luce BR, Simpson K. Methods of cost-effectiveness analysis: areas of consensus and debate. Clin Ther 1995;17:109-25.

39. Black WC. The CE plane: a graphical representation of cost-effectiveness. Med Decis Making 1990;10:212-4.

40. Weinstein MC. Principles of cost-effective resource allocation in health organizations. Int J Technol Assess Health Care 1990;6:93-105.

41. Agro KE, Bradley CA, Mittman N, Iskedjian M, Ilersich AL, Einarson TR. Sensitivity analysis in health economic and pharmacoeconomic studies. An appraisal of the literature. Pharmacoeconomics 1997;11:75-88.

42. Doubilet P, Begg CB, Weinstein MC, Braun P, McNeil BJ. Probabilistic sensitivity analysis using Monte Carlo simulation. Med Decis Making 1985;5:157-77.

43. Willan AR, O'Brien BJ. Confidence intervals for cost-effectiveness ratios: an application of Fieller's Theorem. Health Econ 1996;5:297-305.

44. Bala M, Mauskopf JA. The estimation and use of confidence intervals in economic analysis. Drug Inf J 1999;33:841-8.

45. Polsky D, Glick HA, Willke R, Schukman K. Confidence intervals for cost-

effectiveness ratios: a comparison of four methods. Health Econ 1997; 6:229-42.

46. Box GEP, Tiao GC. Bayesian inference in statistical analysis. Hoboken, NJ: John Wiley & Sons, 1992.

47. Drummond MF, Torrance GW, Mason J. Cost-effectiveness league tables: more harm than good? Soc Sci Med 1993;37:33-40.

48. Mason J. Cost-per-QALY league tables: their role in pharmacoeconomic analysis. Pharmacoeconomics 1994;5:472-81.

49. Mason J, Drummond M, Torrance GW. Some guidelines on the use of cost effectiveness league tables. BMJ 1993;306:570-2.

50. Mauskopf JA, Rutten F, Schonfeld W. Cost-effectiveness league tables: valuable guidance for decision makers? Pharmacoeconomics 2003;21:991-1000.

51. Eisenberg JM. Clinical economics: a guide to the economic analysis of clinical practices. JAMA 1989;262:2879-86.

52. Luce BR. Working toward a common currency: is standardization of cost-effectiveness analysis possible? J Acquir Immune Defic Syndr Hum Retrovirol 1995;10(suppl 4):S19-22.

Cost-Utility Analysis

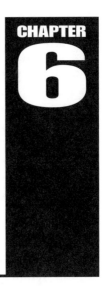

Stephen Joel Coons
and Robert M Kaplan

As observed by Neumann and Weinstein,[1] the American public has a love–hate relationship with medical technology. Medical technologies are lauded for saving lives and improving the quality of medical care while, at the same time, they are condemned as the primary cause of the unchecked growth of medical care costs.

Our society's ambivalence stems, in part, from the lack of critical information as to what value is received for the tremendous amount of resources expended on medical care. As Maynard[2] has stated, it is commonplace in health care "for policy to be designed and executed in a data-free environment!" Although the implicit objective of medical technology is to improve health outcomes, there is minimal evidence of the true effectiveness of many current healthcare practices.[3] In addition, measures of the overall quality of the United States healthcare system, such as access to primary health care, health indicators (eg, infant mortality, life expectancy), and public satisfaction in relation to costs, provide evidence that the United States trails other countries that spend significantly less on medical care.[4]

Earlier chapters have discussed the pressing need to maximize the net health benefit derived from the utilization of limited healthcare resources. Cost-effectiveness analysis and cost-benefit analysis have been presented as methods for assessing the costs and consequences of healthcare technologies, particularly pharmaceuticals. The purpose of this chapter is to discuss another method for evaluating the value obtained for the money spent: cost-utility analysis (CUA).

What Is Cost-Utility Analysis?

CUA is a formal economic technique for assessing the efficiency of healthcare interventions. It is considered by some to be a specific type of cost-effectiveness analysis in which the measure of effectiveness is a utility- or preference-adjusted outcome.[5,6] However, in this chapter, we will consider it as a separate and distinct economic technique.

CUA is one of the newest, and perhaps most controversial, types of economic evaluation. The controversy stems mainly from the measurement of utility. *Utility* is the value or worth placed on a level of health status, or improvement in health status, as measured by the preferences of individuals or society.[7] Measurement of health state utilities or preference values is necessary for calculation of the most commonly used outcome measure in this type of analysis: quality-adjusted life-years (QALYs) gained. There is no true consensus as to the most appropriate measurement approach. (The measurement of utility is discussed in greater depth starting on page 128.)

Nevertheless, CUA has some distinct advantages over cost-benefit analysis and cost-effectiveness analysis. Cost-benefit analysis suffers from the difficulty of translating all costs and consequences into monetary terms.[8] It is especially difficult to translate patient-reported outcomes (eg, quality of life) into dollars. In addition, cost-benefit analysis carries the potential for discrimination because it favors treatment for people who are working or those who are more wealthy. Cost-effectiveness analysis is limited by the inability to simultaneously incorporate multiple outcomes from the same intervention or to compare interventions with different outcomes. In cost-effectiveness analysis, although the outcome measure is in natural units (eg, life-years saved), no attempt is made to value the consequence or outcome in terms of quality or desirability. In contrast, CUA incorporates the quality of (or preference for) the health outcome achieved.[7] CUA, using QALYs gained as the outcome measure, is the most common approach to combining quantity and quality-of-life outcomes in economic evaluations.[9]

In addition, CUA is the approach to the economic evaluation of health care that was recommended by the Panel on Cost-Effectiveness in Health and Medicine.[10] The Panel was convened by the United States Public Health Service (USPHS) in 1993 to assess the state-of-the-science and to provide recommendations for conducting cost-effectiveness studies in order to improve the quality of the analyses and to enhance comparability. Concerns of the USPHS included the imprecise use of the term "cost-effective" in the healthcare evaluation literature and the unabating need for high-quality data to help inform healthcare resource allocation decisions. A primary outcome of the Panel's $2^{1}/_{2}$ years of research and deliberation was a standard set of methodologic practices to be followed when conducting and reporting CUAs, called a Reference Case. The specific guidelines for the Reference Case are provided in the Panel's summary report.

When Is Cost-Utility Analysis Appropriate?

Drummond et al.[7] enumerated several circumstances in which CUA may be the most appropriate analytic approach:

1. When health-related quality of life is *the* important outcome—for example, when comparing interventions that are not expected to have an impact on mortality, but a potential impact on patient function and well-being (eg, treatments for osteoarthritis).

2. When health-related quality of life is *an* important outcome—for example, evaluation of the outcomes associated with the treatment of acute myocardial infarction. Not only is lives saved an important outcome measure, but also the quality of the lives saved (eg, the impact of a treatment-induced stroke in a survivor).

3. When the intervention affects both morbidity and mortality and a combined unit of outcome is desired—for example, evaluation of a therapy, such as estrogen use by postmenopausal

women, that can improve quality of life, may reduce mortality from certain conditions (eg, heart disease), but may increase mortality from other conditions (eg, uterine cancer).

4. When the interventions being compared have a wide range of potential outcomes and there is a need to have a common unit of outcome for comparison. This is most commonly the case when a decision-maker must allocate limited resources among interventions that have different objectives and resultant benefits—for example, the choice between providing increased prenatal care or expanding a hypertension screening and treatment program.

5. When the objective is to compare an intervention with others that have already been evaluated in terms of cost per QALY (or equivalent) gained.

The identification, valuation, and measurement of costs is covered in Chapter 3. In addition, an extensive review of the critical issue of cost determination in the context of the published CUA literature from 1967 to 1997 has been provided by Stone et al.[11] Chapter 7 covers quality-of-life assessment. Health-related quality of life is an integral part of CUA; however, not all instruments measuring this component have outcome scores that can be incorporated into CUA. As stated by Hopkins,[12] quality-of-life measures:

...have proved successful in tracking the effects of medical and surgical interventions and reflecting apparently more realistically the outcomes of these interventions. However, the multidimensional nature of these scales is perceived by some as a disadvantage, as it is difficult to compare outcomes between patients and across procedures. How can there be a "trade-off," for example, between reduction in pain and depression of mood? There is therefore considerable interest in attempting to value a health state in terms of a single number. Such valuations can then be integrated with the dimension of time in that state to allow comparisons of values achieved by different interventions in different clinical disorders. The best known of these integrated indices is the quality-adjusted life-year....

QALYs integrate in a single summary score the net health improvement gains, in terms of both quantity and quality of life, experienced by a group of individuals. Although some economic evaluations reported in the literature have used disease-specific quality-of-life scales or general health profiles as outcome measures, most have incorporated valuations of health state preferences or utilities for the purpose of calculating QALYs.[9] This chapter focuses on assessing the health state utilities needed to calculate QALYs, the CUA ratio's most commonly used denominator.

However, before proceeding, we must clarify some terminology. The term *utilities* used in health state valuation literature does not correspond to the classical use of the same term by economists and philosophers of the 19th century. The current use of the term is derived from von Neumann and Morgenstern's[13] theory of rational decision-making. Torrance and Feeny[14] have suggested that, to avoid confusion, it would be preferable to call some of the valuations discussed in the following section health state "value preferences" rather than utilities. As described by Drummond et al.,[7] "preferences" is the broader term that subsumes both "utilities" and "values." Although we agree, in this chapter that distinction will not be made consistently and the terms health state utilities, preferences, and values will, at times, be used interchangeably. This will be discussed in greater detail below.

Need for Health State Utility Assessment

Health care has different objectives. The objective of the care provided by a diabetologist might be a reduction in diabetic complications. Oncologists strive to keep their patients alive and may be satisfied with a short increase in survival time, whereas primary care providers often focus on shortening the cycle of acute illnesses for which mortality is not an immediate concern. All of these providers are attempting to improve the health of their patients. However, they each measure health in a different way. Comparing the productivity of a diabetologist to that of an oncologist may be like comparing apples to oranges. In other words, there is usually no way to directly compare the productivity of different providers when the intended outcomes are different.

The diversity of objectives and resulting outcomes in health care has led many analysts to focus on the simplest common ground. Typically, that is mortality or life expectancy. When mortality is studied, those who are alive are statistically coded as 1.0 and those who are dead are statistically coded as 0.0. Mortality allows the comparison between different diseases. For example, we can compare the years of life lost from heart disease with the years of life lost from cancer. The difficulty is that everyone who remains alive is given the same score. A person with end-stage renal disease is given the same score as someone who is healthy. Utility assessment allows the quantification of levels of wellness on the continuum anchored by death and optimum health.

Conceptual Model

To evaluate health-related quality of life, we must consider all of the different ways that illness and its treatment affect outcomes. It can be said that there are only two central categories of outcomes: life duration and quality of life.[15] We are concerned about any illness or disability because it might make us live a shorter period of time. In addition, we are concerned about the impact of an illness or the effects of its treatment on quality of life. Assessment should consider three basic questions[16]: Does the illness or its treatment shorten life? Does the condition or its treatment make life less desirable and, if so, how much less desirable? What are the duration effects; that is, how much life is lost or how long is the period of diminished quality of life?

Life duration, or quantity of life, as affected by an illness or its treatment is the easier of the concepts to measure. Actuarial mortality data allow for the determination or estimation of the shortened quantity of life. However, the impact of an illness or its treatment on the quality of life is less obvious or objective.

Health-related quality of life is a multidimensional construct. Its general measurement can result in a single outcome score (ie, health index) or an array of scores for individual quality-of-life dimensions (ie, health profile). The index and the profile represent the two complementary approaches to quality-of-life assessment: the decision theory or utility approach and the psychometric approach, respectively.[17] Chapter 7 addresses quality-of-life assessment. This chapter's discussion of quality of life focuses on the incorporation of the utility approach in CUA.

Over the past three decades, there has been growing interest in using quality-of-life data to help evaluate the cost-effectiveness of healthcare programs. As touched upon earlier, CUA expresses the outcomes of health care in a common outcome unit, such as a QALY.[18] The same outcome has been described as well-years[15] or healthy years of life.[19] QALYs integrate mortality, morbidity, and preferences into a comprehensive index number. If a man died of a stroke at age 50 and we would have expected him to live to age 75, it might be concluded that the disease was associated with 25 lost life-years. If 100 men died at age 50 (and also had a life expectancy of 75 years), we might conclude that 2500 life-years (100 men × 25 years) had been lost.

Death is not the only outcome of concern in stroke. For many adults, the stroke results in disability over long periods of time. The quality-of-life loss can occur even when life expectancy is unaffected. Quality-of-life consequences of illnesses can be quantified and used to adjust length of life for its quality. For example, a disease that reduces quality of life by half will take away 0.5 QALYs over the course of one year. If it affects two people, it will take away 1.0 QALYs (2 × 0.5) over a one-year period. A medical treatment that improves quality of life by 0.2 for each of five individuals will result in the equivalent of 1.0 QALY if the benefit is maintained over one year. This system has the advantage of considering both benefits and adverse effects of interventions in terms of the common QALY units.

Concept of Relative Importance of Dimensions

Nearly all health-related quality-of-life measures have multiple dimensions. The specific dimensions vary from measure to measure. There is considerable debate about which dimensions need to be included in a comprehensive measure of health-related quality of life. The ones most commonly included are physical functioning, role/social functioning, and mental health/emotional well-being.

Different dimensions can be useful in assessing the impact of a disease as well as positive and negative treatment effects on quality of life. For example, a medication to control hypertension might be associated with low probabilities of dizziness, tiredness, impotence, and shortness of breath. The major challenge is in determining what it means when someone experiences an adverse effect. This requires the effect to be placed within the context of the total health outcome. For example, should a patient with insulin-dependent diabetes mellitus discontinue therapy because of skin irritation at the injection sites? Clearly, local irritation is an adverse effect of treatment. But, without treatment, the patient would die. Often the issue is not whether treatment causes adverse effects, but how these effects should be placed within the context of overall health. Ultimately, it must be determined whether treatment interventions produce a net benefit or a net deficit in health status.

Many measures of health-related quality of life simply tabulate frequencies for different symptoms or represent health status using profiles of outcomes. Figure 1 is a representation of one such profile.[16] The figure represents three hypothetical treatment profiles. It is common in the presentation of these profiles to connect the points even though increments on the x axis are not meaningful. T-scores (y axis) are standardized scores with a mean of 50 and a standard deviation of 10. Treatment 1 may produce benefits for physical functioning but decrements for role functioning. Treatment 2 may produce decrements for physical functioning but increments for role functioning. This information may be valuable for diagnostic purposes. However, ultimately, clinicians make some general interpretations of the profile by applying a weighting system. They might decide that they are more concerned about physical than role functioning, or vice versa. It must be recognized that judgment about the relative importance of dimensions is common. Physicians may ignore a particular test result or a particular symptom because another one is more important to them. Typically, however, it is done arbitrarily. We suggest that the process by which relative importance is evaluated can and should be studied explicitly.

There are a variety of conceptual and technical issues relevant to preference or utility assessment.[20-23] For example, different approaches to preference assessment can yield different results. However, these differences might be expected because the varying approaches are based on different underlying conceptual models. As a result, the preference assessment techniques ask different questions. The following sections attempt to elucidate some of these conflicts.

Concept of Quality-Adjusted Life-Years

The concept of QALYs has been discussed in the literature for over 30 years. Perhaps the first application was suggested by Fanshel and Bush.[24] Soon after, Torrance[25] introduced a conceptually similar model. Since then, a variety of applications have appeared. Although most of these models are conceptually alike, variations between the approaches have led to some inconsistent findings, some of which are highlighted later in the chapter.

Despite the differences in approach, some important assumptions are similar. For example, all of these approaches assume that one full healthy-year of life is scored as 1.0. Years of life in less than optimal health are scored as less than 1.0. The basic assumption is that two years scored as 0.5 add up to the equiva-

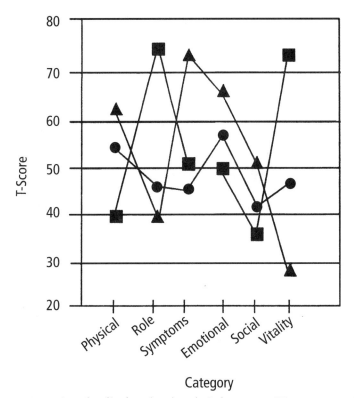

Category

Figure 1. Comparison of profiles from three hypothetical treatments.[13] T-scores are standardized scores with a mean of 50 and a standard deviation of 10. ▲ = treatment 1; ● = treatment 2; ■ = treatment 3.

lent of 1.0 year of complete wellness. Similarly, four years scored as 0.25 sum to the equivalent of 1.0 completely well–year of life. A treatment that moves a patient from 0.5 to 0.75 produces the equivalent of 0.25 QALYs if it is maintained for a year. If applied to four individuals, and the duration of the treatment effect is one year, the effect of the treatment would be equivalent to 1.0 completely well-year of life. The disagreement among most researchers is not usually over the QALY concept, but rather over how the preferences or utilities for health states between 0.0 and 1.0 are obtained.

However, that is not to say that there are no concerns about using QALYs in health policy decisions.[26-30] Mehrez and Gafni[31,32] have proposed that the healthy-year equivalent is a more appropriate outcome measure than the QALY. They assert that the healthy-year equivalent, like the QALY, combines both quality of life and quantity of life; however, healthy-year equivalents more fully represent individuals' preferences in the calculation of the trade-offs between quality and quantity of life. Nord[33] and Ubel et al.[34] contend that the promise of CUA as a tool to guide healthcare allocation decisions cannot be fulfilled until the current concept of QALYs is replaced by an outcome measure that incorporates societal values (eg, fairness, distributional equity). Although important, a discussion of these concerns is beyond the scope of this chapter.

History of the Utility Theory

The history of the utility theory and its applications to health outcomes assessment has been reviewed by Torrance and Feeny.[14] Health utility assessment has its roots in the work of von Neumann and Morgenstern,[13] who published their classic work more than a half century ago. Their mathematical decision theory characterized how a rational individual should make decisions when faced with uncertain outcomes. They outlined axioms of choice that have been formally evaluated and have become basic foundations of decision analysis in business, government, and health care. Their work has been expanded upon by Raiffa[35] and others.[36,37] Torrance and Feeny[14] emphasized that the use of the term *utility theory* by von Neumann and Morgenstern was unfortunate. Their reference to utility differs from the more common uses by economists that emphasize consumer satisfaction with commodities that are received with certainty. Nineteenth-century philosophers and economists assumed the existence of cardinal (or interval level) utilities for these functions. A characteristic of cardinal utilities is that they can be aggregated across individuals and used to inform social policy.

By the turn of the century, Pareto challenged the value of cardinal utilities and demonstrated that ordinal utilities could represent consumer choice.[38] In a classic essay, this work was extended by Arrow and Debreu.[39] Arrow[40] had previously argued that there are inconsistencies in individual preferences under certainty and that meaningful cardinal preferences cannot be measured and may not even exist. As a result, most economists maintain that averaged or aggregate preferences have little meaning.

There are several reasons why Arrow's work may not be applicable to the aggregation of utilities in the assessment of QALYs. First, utility expressions for QALYs are expressions of consumer preference under uncertainty. The traditional criticisms of microeconomists are directed toward decisions under certainty rather than uncertainty.[14] A second issue is that Arrow assumed that the metric underlying utility was neither meaningful nor standardized across individuals. Substantial psychometric evidence suggests that preferences can be measured using scales that have meaningful interval or ratio properties.[41,42] Utility scores must possess at least interval scale properties to be used in the calculation of QALYs.[43]

It is also important to recognize that different approaches to the calculations of QALYs are based on very different underlying assumptions. One approach considers the duration someone is in a particular health state as conceptually independent from the utility for the state.[15,18] The other approach merges duration and utility.[14] This distinction is central to the understanding of the difference in approaches and the required evidence for the validity of the utility assessment procedure.

In the approach advocated by Kaplan and Anderson[15] and Weinstein and Stason,[18] utilities for health states are obtained at a single point in time. For example, persons in a particular health state, such as confinement to a wheelchair, who performed no major social role are asked to assess the utility of that health state. Suppose that this state is assigned a value of 0.5. Patients in this state are then observed over time to empirically determine their transitions to other states of wellness. If they remain in that state for one year, then they would lose the equivalent of 0.5 well-years of life. The key to this approach is that the preferences only concern a single point in time and that the transition is determined through observation or expert judgment. The alternative approach emphasized by Torrance and Feeny[14] and Nord[44] obtains preference for both health state and duration. These approaches also consider the more complex problems of uncertainty. Thus, they are consistent with von Neumann and Morgenstern's[13] notion of decision under uncertainty in which probabilities and trade-offs are considered explicitly by the judge.

Methods for Assessing Utility

CUA requires an assessment of preferences for health states. A variety of different techniques have been used to assess these preferences. These techniques are summarized briefly. Then, comparisons between the techniques are considered. Some analysts do not measure preferences directly. Instead, they evaluate health outcome by simply assigning a reasonable value.[45] However, most current approaches have respondents assign values to different health states on a scale ranging from 0.0 (for dead) to 1.0 (for perfect health). The three most commonly used techniques for the direct elicitation of health state preferences are rating scales, standard gamble, and time trade-off. In addition, magnitude estimation and the person trade-off approach are sometimes used. Each of these methods is described briefly.

RATING SCALES

Rating scales require the respondent to assign a numeric value to objects. There are several methods for obtaining rating scale information. The category scale, exemplified by the familiar 10-point rating scale, is efficient, easy to use, and applicable in a large number of settings. Typically, the subjects read the description of a case and rate it on a 10-point scale ranging from 0 for dead to 10 for asymptomatic optimal function. The endpoints of the scale are typically well defined.

Another common rating scale method is the visual analog scale. The visual analog method shows a subject a line, typically 10 centimeters in length, with the endpoints well defined. The subject's task is to mark the line to indicate where their preference rests for one or more health states in relation to the two poles.

Appropriate applications of rating scales reflect contemporary developments in cognitive sciences. Judgment-decision theory has been dominated by the belief that human decisions follow principles of optimality and rationality. A considerable amount of research has challenged the normative models that have attempted to demonstrate rational choice. The development of cognitive theories, such as information integration theory,[46] provides better explanations of the cognitive process of judgment. Information integration theory includes two constructs: integration and valuation. A large body of evidence indicates that rating scales provide meaningful metrics for the expression of these subjective preferences. Although there have been some challenges to the use of rating scales, most biases can be overcome with the use of just a few simple precautions, such as clear definitions of the endpoints and preliminary practice with cases that make the endpoints salient.

MAGNITUDE ESTIMATION

Magnitude estimation is a common psychometric method that is believed by psychophysicists to yield ratio scale scores. In magnitude estimation, a specific case is selected as a standard and assigned a particular number. Then, other cases are rated in relation to the standard. Suppose, for example, the standard is assigned the number 10. If a case is regarded as half as desirable as the standard, it is given the number 5. If it is regarded as twice as desirable, it is given the number 20. Ratings across subjects are standardized to a common metric and aggregated using the geometric mean. Advocates for magnitude estimation argue that the method is meaningful because it provides a direct estimate of the subjective ratio. Thus, they believe, the magnitude estimate has the properties of a ratio scale. However, magnitude estimation has been challenged on several grounds. The method is not based on any specific theory of measurement and gains credibility only through face validity.[46] Further, the meaning of the scores has been challenged. For example, the values are not linked directly to any decision process. What does it mean if one case is rated as half as desirable as another? Does it mean that the respondent would be indifferent between a 50–50 chance of the higher valued outcome and a certainty of the alternative valued as half as desirable? These issues have not been systematically addressed in the health status literature.

STANDARD GAMBLE

Category rating and magnitude estimation are methods commonly used by psychometricians. Typically, the tasks emphasize wellness at a particular point in time and do not ask subjects to make trades or consider aspects of uncertainty. Several methods more explicitly consider decisions under uncertainty. The standard gamble offers a choice between two alternatives: choice A—living in health state i (a chronic health state between perfect health and death) with certainty, or choice B—taking a gamble on a new treatment for which the outcome is uncertain. Figure 2 shows this trade. The respondent is told that a hypothetical treatment will lead to perfect health with a probability of p or immediate death with a probability of 1–p. They can choose between remaining in state i that is intermediate between wellness and death or taking the gamble and trying the new treatment. The probability is varied until the subject is indifferent between choices A and B. For example, if a subject is indifferent between choices A and B when p = 0.65, the utility of state i is 0.65.

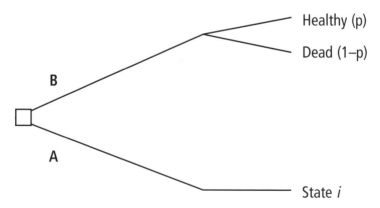

Figure 2. Standard gamble for a chronic health state. i = chronic health state; p = probability of achieving perfect health.

The standard gamble has been attractive because it is based on the axioms of utility theory. The choice between a certain outcome and a gamble conforms to the exercises originally proposed by von Neumann and Morgenstern.[13] Although the interval properties of the data obtained using the gamble have been assumed, they have not been empirically demonstrated.[20] A variety of other problems with the gamble also have become apparent. For example, it has often been stated that the standard gamble has face validity because it approximates choices made by medical patients.[47] However, treatment of most chronic diseases does not approximate the gamble. There is no known product that will cure a patient with arthritis nor one that is likely to kill him or her. In other words, the decision-making experience of the patient is not likely to include an option that has a realistic gamble. Further, the cognitive demands of the task are high.

TIME TRADE-OFF

The concept of probability is difficult for most respondents and requires the use of visual aids or props to assist in the interview. Thus, an alternative to the standard gamble, which is also consistent with the von Neumann and Morgenstern[13] axioms of choice, uses a trade-off in time.[48] Figure 3 demonstrates the trade-off for a chronic disease state. Here, the subject is offered

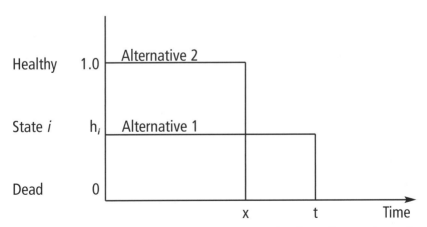

Figure 3. Time trade-off for a chronic health state. $h_i = x \div t$, where h_i = preference value or utility for state i; state i = chronic health state; t = life expectancy for an individual with chronic health state i; x = time at which respondant is indifferent between alternatives 1 and 2.

a choice of living in health state i (chronic health state considered better than death but less desirable than perfect health) for time t (life expectancy for an individual with chronic health state i) or perfect health for time x. Times x and t are followed by immediate death. Time x is varied until the respondent is indifferent between the two alternatives. Presumably, all subjects would choose a year of wellness versus a year with some health problem. However, by reducing the time of wellness and leaving the time in the suboptimal health state fixed (such as one year), an indifference point can be determined ($h_i = x \div t$; hi is the utility or preference value for chronic health state i). For example, a subject may rate being in a wheelchair for two years as equivalent to perfect wellness for one year ($1 \div 2 = 0.5$). The time trade-off is theoretically appealing because it is conceptually equivalent to a QALY.

PERSON TRADE-OFF

The person trade-off technique allows comparisons of the numbers of people helped in different states. For example, respondents might be asked to evaluate the equivalencies between the number of persons helped by different programs. They might be asked how many persons in state B must be helped to provide a benefit equivalent to helping one person in state A. From a public policy perspective, the person trade-off approach is intended to incorporate social value information similar to that required as the basis for resource allocation decisions. Eric Nord,[33] one of the main proponents of person trade-off, has included this approach as an integral part of an alternative to CUA called *cost-value analysis*.

Differences Between the Methods

Several papers in the literature have compared preferences for health states as captured by different methods. Based on publicly available source documents, Tengs and Wallace[49] compiled an extensive list of utilities/preference weights for hundreds of health states. Along with the weights for defined health states, they listed the preference assessment method used, type of respondents/judges, and upper and lower bounds of the scaling method. Their results demonstrate the considerable variation in values for the same health states based on differing (and, at times, similar) methodologic approaches.

Differences in health state values have been reviewed by Nord.[50] In general, standard gamble and time trade-off methods give higher values than rating scales in most, but not all, studies. In about half of the studies reported, time trade-off yields lower utilities than standard gamble. In one of the earlier studies, Patrick et al.[51] found that person trade-off methods produced the same results as rating scales. However, these findings were not confirmed in more recent studies.[44] Magnitude estimation has produced results that are highly inconsistent across studies.[50]

The variability of health state utilities in comparisons of different studies is hardly surprising. The methods differ substantially in the questions posed to respondents. In summary, there is substantial debate about which technique should be used to acquire utility information. Results obtained from different methods do not correspond, although they typically have a high degree of similarity in the ranks they assign to outcomes. However, the differences in preferences yielded by different methods can result in different allocations of resources if the preferences are not obtained on a linear or interval response scale. For example, suppose that the difference between the effect of a drug and a placebo is 0.05 units of well-being as assessed by rating scales and 0.02 as measured by magnitude estimation. The benefit would have to last 20 years to produce 1.0 QALY if rating scale values were used and 50 years if magnitude estimation values were used. Aggregation of benefits necessarily requires an underlying linear response scale in which equal differences at different points along the response scale are equally meaningful. For example, the differences between 0.2 and 0.3 (0.1 QALY if the duration is one year) must have the same meaning as the difference between 0.7 and 0.8. A treatment that improves a patient's condition from 0.2 to 0.3 must be considered of equal benefit to a treatment that improves it from 0.7 to 0.8. Confirmation of this scale property has been demonstrated for rating scales, but not for other methods.[46,52]

Another difference between methods is the inclusion of information about uncertainty in the judgment process. Time trade-off, standard gamble, or person trade-off theoretically include some judgment about duration of stay in the health state. Magnitude estimation and rating scales typically separate utility at a point in time from probability. Considerably more theoretical and empirical work will be necessary to resolve these differences of approach.

Nord[53] has argued for quality assurance standards for QALY calculations. These recommendations were based on a review that revealed inconsistency in the methods used to assess utilities. According to Nord, the utility assessment typically lacked a theoretical or empiric basis. Apparently, this refers to inattention to economic theories. However, others have noted that some utility assessment approaches are based on different theoretical models and empiric results. For example, advocates for the use of rating scales offer evidence that the methods found theoretically and empirically justified by economists fail to meet the basic requirements for an interval response scale.[54] Nord et al.[55] suggested that the person trade-off be used as the standard against which other methods are compared. However, they did not offer evidence that data obtained using the person trade-off meet standards of reliability, validity, and interval scale property. Lenert and Kaplan[56] do offer evidence that rating scales have interval properties. In contrast to Nord, they argue that each method has some theoretical justification. It should not be a surprise that different methods produce different results because the methods ask different questions. Although it is desirable to develop standardized utility elicitation protocols, it is apparent that the lack of consensus will continue into the foreseeable future.

Whose Utilities or Preferences Should Be Used?

Choices between alternatives in health care necessarily involve preference judgment. For example, the inclusion of some services in a basic benefits package and the exclusion of others is an exercise in value, choice, or preference. There are many levels at which preference is expressed in the healthcare decision process. For example, an older woman may decide to cope with the symptoms of upset stomach in order to gain relief from the discomfort of osteoarthritis. A physician may order pelvic ultrasound to ensure against missing the very low probability that a 40-year-old woman has ovarian cancer. Or, an administrator may decide to put resources into prevention for large numbers of people instead of devoting the same resources to organ transplants for a smaller number.

In CUA, preferences are used to express the relative importance of various health outcomes. There is a subjective or qualitative component to health outcome. Whether we prefer a headache or an upset stomach caused by its treatment is a value judgment. Not all symptoms are of equal importance. Most patients would prefer mild fatigue (an adverse effect of treatment) to a severe headache (the symptom eradicated by treatment). Yet, providing a model of how well treatments work implicitly includes these judgments. Models require a precise numeric expression of this preference. CUA explicitly includes a preference component to represent these trade-offs.

Some models obtain preferences from random samples of the general population.[42,57] It is recognized that administrators ultimately choose between alternative programs. Community preferences may represent the will of the general public rather than those of administrators. Yet there is considerable debate about technical aspects of preference assessment. Some of the debate has to do with whose preferences are considered.

In most areas of preference assessment, it is easy to identify differences between various groups or individuals. It might be argued that judgments about net health benefits for white men should not be applied to Hispanic men who may give different weight to some symptoms. Preferences for movies, clothing, or political candidates differ for social and cultural groups; it is assumed that these same differences extend to health states. Some analysts have suggested that preference weights from the general population should be applied with caution to particular patient groups.[58]

Most studies do not support the common belief that preferences differ. Some small, but significant differences between demographic groups have been observed.[59] Studies have found little evidence for preference difference between patients and the general population. For example, Balaban et al.[60] compared preference weights obtained from patients with arthritis with those obtained from the general population in San Diego. They found a high degree of correspondence for ratings of cases involving patients with arthritis. Similar results were found by Hughes et al.[61] among HIV-infected patients. Studies also have shown a high degree of similarity in preferences provided by men versus women, the medically insured versus the uninsured, those ever in wheelchairs versus those never in wheelchairs, British versus Americans, citizens of Oregon versus those of California, and residents of three different European communities.[62]

It would be incorrect to say that there are never any mean differences in preference based on sociodemographic factors since significant differences in preferences have been observed in several studies. However, these differences have typically been small.[62] Further analysis will be required to determine whether these differences affect the conclusions of various analyses.

A related problem is the assumption that all people in the same health state should get the same score. Most approaches to utility assessment use the mean preference for a particular case to represent all individuals who meet a common definition. For example, suppose that the average utility for being in a wheelchair, limited in major activities, and having missing limbs is 0.50. The models would assign the same number to all individuals who occupy that state. However, there is substantial variability in how individuals view their own health. If individual preferences are used, there might be significant variation in scores across people with identical objective descriptions.[63] Despite the appeal of individualized preferences, they rarely lead to different treatment decisions than would be obtained from the use of aggregate preferences.[64]

Multi-Attribute Health Status Classification Systems

Although it is important to understand the various approaches to the measurement of health state utilities/preference values, some pharmacoeconomic researchers conducting a CUA will not measure health state utilities directly. They may use one of the existing multi-attribute health status classification systems for which the utility functions have been empirically derived. Three such instruments in common use are the Quality of Well-Being Scale (QWB), the Health Utilities Index (HUI), and the EuroQol Group's EQ-5D.

The QWB, developed at the University of California—San Diego, is a general quality-of-life instrument that includes symptoms or problems plus three dimensions of functional health status: mobility, physical activity, and social activity. Standardized preference weights for the QWB have been measured (using the category rating-scale method) and validated on a general population in San Diego.[65] Other investigators have reweighted the symptoms/problems and function levels of the QWB in specific populations, such as patients with arthritis[60] and HIV-infected subjects,[61] and have found the generalizability of the original weights to be very high. The QWB is now available in a self-administered form known as the QWB-SA.[66]

The HUI, developed at McMaster University, is another general instrument that describes the health status of a person at a point in time in terms of ability to function on a set of attributes or dimensions of health status. The original version (Mark I or HUI1) of the HUI consists of four attributes and a formula to calculate utilities.[67] The second version, HUI2, consists of seven attributes and formulas for the calculation of utilities and preference values.[68] The measurement of the preference values/utilities for the health status classification system was made with visual analog scales and the standard gamble technique. The most recent version, HUI3, has eight attributes: vision, hearing, speech, ambulation, dexterity, cognition, pain and discomfort, and emotion.[69] A multiplicative multi-attribute utility function for the HUI3 is available based on visual analog scale and standard gamble measurements from a random sample of the general population in Hamilton, Ontario, Canada.[70]

The EQ-5D, developed by a multidisciplinary team of European researchers (the EuroQol Group), was designed to be self-administered and short enough to be used in conjunction with other measures.[71,72] The first of the two parts is a descriptive system that consists of five dimensions (mobility, self-care, usual activities, pain/discomfort, anxiety/depression) that classifies subjects into one of 243 health states. A preference value for the self-reported health state is then assigned from a set of valuations that have been empirically derived. Although initial valuations for the EQ-5D health states were obtained in several country-specific population studies,[73-75] the most commonly applied valuation system or "tariff" is one developed in the United Kingdom using the time trade-off method.[57] The second part of the EQ-5D is a 20-cm visual analog scale that has endpoints labeled "best imaginable health state" and "worst imaginable health state" anchored at 100 and 0, respectively. The respondent is asked to draw a line to the point on the scale that reflects his or her current health state. This reponse is not used in the calculation of the preference-based health status score.

A more thorough evaluation of these three instruments is provided elsewhere.[7,76] Other preference-weighted health state classification systems identified by the USPHS's Panel on Cost-Effectiveness in Health and Medicine[77] for use in CUA include the 15D,[78] the Quality of Life and Health Questionnaire,[79] the Disability/Distress Index,[80] and the Years of Healthy Life measure.[81] The Panel did not specify the type of utility elicitation approach required, nor did it recommend one multi-attribute health status classification system over another for the Reference Case; however, it did provide general guidelines regarding these and other significant methodologic issues (eg, perspective, comparators, costs to include, discounting, sensitivity analysis).

From Health State Preferences to QALYs and Cost per QALYs Gained

For pharmaceuticals, as with most other healthcare interventions, the ultimate therapeutic endpoint or outcome is the enhancement of quality of life and/or length of life. Therefore, in theory, the most appropriate outcome measure would be QALYs. Once a means of eliciting or assigning preferences for health states has been determined, the next step in the calculation of QALYs is to account for time in the health states.

For example, let's consider a hypothetical clinical trial in which a new pharmaceutical (ie, Treatment) was compared with the standard pharmacotherapy (ie, Control) for severe osteoarthritis. A primary endpoint of the trial was functioning and well-being, or health-status, as measured by the QWB. The QWB was administered at baseline, six months, and 12 months. Figure 4 provides a graphic representation of the hypothetical results.[7] The randomization procedure provided two groups that began the trial at the same mean level of health status. From baseline to 12 months, the area between the two diverging curves represents the incremental QALYs produced by the new pharmaceutical for the average person in the Treatment arm of the trial. To calculate the area between the two curves at the end of the trial, the QALYs gained in the Control arm are subtracted from the QALYs gained in the Treatment arm. The nondiscounted QALYs gained in the Control arm are calculated with the following equation:

$$QALYs_C = [0.5(0.40 + 0.50)6 + 0.5(0.50 + 0.50)6] / 12 = 0.475$$

The nondiscounted QALYs gained in the Treatment arm are calculated with the following equation:

$$QALYs_T = [0.5(0.40 + 0.60)6 + 0.5(0.60 + 0.65)6] / 12 = 0.563$$

Subtraction of $QALYs_C$ from $QALYs_T$ results in the following:

$$QALYs \text{ gained} = 0.563 - 0.475 = 0.088$$

If 100 subjects were in the treatment arm for the full 12-month study period, 8.8 QALYs would have been the incremental gain over standard therapy. Although a clinical trial is not a real-world setting, incremental costs associated with the Treatment intervention could be determined and a *cost / QALYs gained* ratio could be calculated. Some economists argue that health outcomes that occur in the future must be discounted; however, discounting has little effect over a short interval such as one year.

Numerous published studies have used QALYs and CUA to evaluate the economic efficiency of healthcare interventions, including pharmaceuticals. An extensive review of CUAs published in English from 1976 to 1997 by Neumann et al.[82] found that the number increased markedly during that time. However, their assessment of the quality of the reporting of CUAs is discouraging, with only slight improvement over time, which reinforces the need for adherence to the recommendations of the Panel on Cost-Effectiveness in Health and Medicine. Of the 228 articles reviewed, 31.1 percent focused on pharmaceutical interventions, 18 percent focused on surgical procedures, and 12.3 percent addressed various diagnostic procedures. These findings suggest that CUA has a significant role in the economic evaluation of pharmaceuticals.

A common method of summarizing and comparing the results of CUAs is in the form of a league table. Table 1 shows selected interventions from a league table compiled by Chapman et al.[83] The league table includes CUA ratios that conform to selected Panel recommendations for the Reference Case (ie, adoption of a societal perspective, community or patient preference weights, use of net costs, appropriate incremental comparisons, and discounting of costs and QALYs at the same rate). These data are derived from a much larger league table that has been published on the Web (www.hcra.harvard.edu/medical.html). As can be seen from the pharmaceutical interventions shown in Table 1, the cost per QALY gained can vary widely and is extremely dependent on the target population.

There are many concerns regarding the manner in which league tables are constructed and applied.[83,84] As observed by Mason et al.,[85] the source studies in league tables often use various means of calculating QALYs and different years of origin, discount rates, settings, and types of comparison programs. Nevertheless, they concluded that, although league tables have

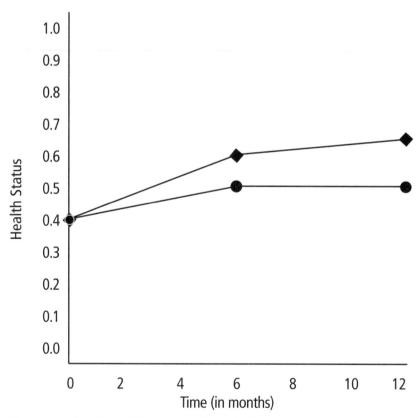

Figure 4. Quality-adjusted life-years gained through a hypothetical treatment intervention.[7] u = Treatment; l = Control.

serious limitations, the systematic comparisons that they provide are preferable to the alternative: reliance on the informal, unsystematic assessments made in the absence of data.

Summary

In a society in which healthcare resources are limited, it is essential that the resources available are used efficiently and eq-

Table 1. Cost per Quality-Adjusted Life-Years Gained: Selected Interventions[83]

Intervention vs Comparator (target population)	Cost/QALY[a] ($)
Warfarin vs aspirin (65-year-old pts. with nonvalvular atrial fibrillation and high risk for stroke)	cost-saving
Eradidate *Helicobacter pylori* empirically with omeprazole, clarithromycin, and amoxicillin vs no treatment (adults with dyspepsia presenting to primary care physicians)	1,400
Pneumococcal pneumonia vaccination vs no vaccination (people greater than 65 years old)	2,800
Captopril vs no captopril (70-year-old pts. surviving MI)	6,500
Fluoxetine vs imipramine (30-year-old women with one previous episode of major depression)	7,700
Warfarin vs aspirin (65-year-old pts. with nonvalvular atrial fibrillation and medium risk for stroke)	9,700
Captopril vs no captopril (60-year-old pts. surviving MI)	12,000
Tissue plasminogen activator vs streptokinase (pts. presenting within 6 hours after onset of symptoms of acute MI)	35,000
Captopril vs no captopril (50-year-old pts. surviving MI)	80,000
Warfarin vs aspirin (65-year-old pts. with nonvalvular atrial fibrillation and low risk for stroke)	450,000

MI = myocardial infarction; QALY = quality-adjusted life-year.
[a]Converted to 2002 United States dollars based on data at www.hsph.harvard.edu/cearegistry.

uitably. However, for this system to function effectively, data about costs and outcomes are essential. Resources should be used for programs that produce the greatest benefit for the greatest number of people. Lack of good information about input–output relationships in health care has led to enormous variations in costs and clinical practice patterns.[5] There has been little consensus on what constitutes good clinical practice. The integration of data on the quality of life with corresponding data on life expectancy yields a single index of health benefit, expressed in terms of QALYs gained. Our interest in life expectancy and quality of life arises from the fact that health care can influence either or both of these factors.

It is likely that the use of CUA will increase as the need to evaluate the benefits derived from very different healthcare interventions increases. This type of analysis will assist in ensuring that resources are allocated as efficiently as possible to serve health outcome goals. Resources will never be sufficient to provide all of the health care that might be given; there are finite resources and potentially infinite demands. CUA provides a systematic approach to comparing ways of using the resources most efficiently in the process of meeting those demands.

Pharmaceuticals are a critical component of contemporary medical care; they are the primary treatment modality for the majority of individuals with chronic conditions. Pharmaceuticals can produce QALYs by lengthening life, improving the quality of life, or both. However, in certain conditions (eg, some cancers), the pharmaceutical intervention (ie, chemotherapy) can be a double-edged sword: it can lengthen life while decreasing the quality of life during the treatment period.[86] Nevertheless, it is more common for pharmaceuticals to be prescribed to improve the quality of life in people who have conditions that are not life-threatening but are potentially debilitating (eg, arthritis, glaucoma). If conducted properly, CUA can be a powerful tool to more comprehensively evaluate the overall impact of pharmacotherapy. More and better CUA research is needed to document the relative value of pharmaceuticals compared with alternative medical interventions and to inform decisions as to the most efficient use of finite healthcare resources.

References

1. Neumann PJ, Weinstein MC. The diffusion of new technology: costs and benefits to health care. In: Gelijns AC, Halm EA, eds. The changing economics of medical technology. Washington, DC: National Academy Press, 1991:21-34.
2. Maynard A. Developing the health care market. Econ J 1991;101:1277-86.
3. Roper WL, Winkenwerder W, Hackbarth GM, Krakauer H. Effectiveness in health care: an initiative to evaluate and improve medical practice. N Engl J Med 1988;319:1197-202.
4. Starfield B. Primary care and health: a cross-national comparison. JAMA 1991;266:2268-71.
5. Weinstein MC, Stason WB. Foundations of cost-effectiveness analysis for health and medical practice. N Engl J Med 1977;296:716-21.
6. Sloan FA, ed. Valuing health care: costs, benefits, and effectiveness of pharmaceuticals and other medical technologies. Cambridge, UK: Cambridge University Press, 1996.
7. Drummond MF, O'Brien B, Stoddart GL, Torrance GW. Methods for the economic evaluation of health care programmes. 2nd ed. New York: Oxford University Press, 1997.
8. Patrick DL, Erickson P. Health status and health policy: allocating resources to health care. New York: Oxford University Press, 1993.
9. Drummond M. The role and importance of quality of life measurements in economic evaluations. Br J Med Econ 1992;4:9-16.
10. Gold MR, Siegel JE, Russell LB, Weinstein MC, eds. Cost-effectiveness in health and medicine. New York: Oxford University Press, 1996.
11. Stone PW, Chapman RH, Sandberg EA, Liljas B, Neumann PJ. Measuring costs in cost-utility analyses: variations in the literature. Int J Technol Assess Health Care 2000;16:111-24.
12. Hopkins A. Editor's introduction. In: Measures of the quality of life and the uses to which such measures may be put. London: Royal College of Physicians of London, 1992:iii-iv.
13. von Neumann J, Morgenstern O. Theory of games and economic behavior. Princeton, NJ: Princeton University Press, 1944.
14. Torrance GW, Feeny D. Utilities in quality-adjusted life years. Int J Technol Assess Health Care 1989;5:559-75.
15. Kaplan RM, Anderson JP. The general health policy model: an integrated approach. In: Spilker B, ed. Quality of life assessments in clinical trials. New York: Raven Press, 1990:131-49.
16. Kaplan RM, Coons SJ. Relative importance of dimensions in the assessment of health-related quality of life for patients with hypertension. Prog Cardiovasc Nurs 1992;7:29-36.
17. Coons SJ, Kaplan RM. Assessing health-related quality of life: application to drug therapy. Clin Ther 1992;14:850-8.
18. Weinstein MC, Stason WB. Hypertension: a policy perspective. Cambridge, MA: Harvard University Press, 1976.
19. Russell LB. Is prevention better than cure? Washington, DC: The Brookings Institution, 1986.

20. Froberg DG, Kane RL. Methodology for measuring health state preferences, II: scaling methods. J Clin Epidemiol 1989;42:459-71.

21. Froberg DG, Kane RL. Methodology for measuring health state preferences, III: population and context effects. J Clin Epidemiol 1989;42:585-92.

22. Froberg DG, Kane RL. Methodology for measuring health state preferences, IV: progress and a research agenda. J Clin Epidemiol 1989;42:675-85.

23. Froberg DG, Kane RL. Methodology for measuring health state preferences, I: measurement strategies. J Clin Epidemiol 1989;42:345-52.

24. Fanshel S, Bush JW. A health-status index and its applications to health-services outcomes. Operations Res 1970;18:1021-66.

25. Torrance GW. Social preferences for health states. An empirical evaluation of three measurement techniques. Socioecon Plan Sci 1976;10:129-36.

26. Carr-Hill RA. Allocating resources to health care: is the QALY (quality adjusted life year) a technical solution to a political problem? Int J Health Serv 1991;21:351-63.

27. Coast J. Developing the QALY concept: exploring the problems of data acquisition. Pharmacoeconomics 1993;4:240-6.

28. Harris J. Life: quality, value and justice. Health Policy 1988;10:259-66.

29. LaPuma J, Lawlor EF. Quality-adjusted life-years: ethical implications for physicians and policymakers. JAMA 1990;263:2917-21.

30. Loomes G, McKenzie L. The use of QALYs in health care decision making. Soc Sci Med 1989;28:299-308.

31. Mehrez A, Gafni A. Quality-adjusted life years, utility theory, and healthy-years equivalents. Med Decis Making 1989;9:142-9.

32. Mehrez A, Gafni A. The healthy-years equivalents: how to measure them using the standard gamble approach. Med Decis Making 1991;11:140-6.

33. Nord E. Cost-value analysis in health care: making sense out of QALYS. Cambridge, UK: Cambridge University Press, 1999.

34. Ubel PA, Nord E, Gold M, Menzel P, Prades JLP, Richardson J. Improving value measurement in cost-effectiveness analysis. Med Care 2000;38:892-901.

35. Raiffa H. Decision analysis: introductory lectures on choices under uncertainty. Reading, MA: Addison-Wesley, 1968.

36. Bell DE, Farquhar PH. Perspectives on utility theory. Operations Res 1986;34:179-83.

37. Howard RA. Decision analysis: practice and promise. Manag Sci 1988;34:679-95.

38. Parsons T. The structure of social action. Vol. 1. New York: Free Press, 1937:241-9.

39. Arrow KJ, Debreu G. Existence of equilibrium for a competitive economy. Econometrica 1954;22:265-90.

40. Arrow KJ. Social choice and individual values. New York: Wiley, 1951.

41. Keeney RL. A group preference axiomatization with cardinal utility. Manag Sci 1976;23:140-5.

42. Kaplan RM, Anderson JP, Ganiats TG. The Quality of Well-Being Scale: rationale for a single quality of life index. In: Walker SR, Rosser RM, eds.

Quality of life assessment: key issues in the 1990s. Lancaster, UK: Kluwer Academic Publishers, 1993:65-94.

43. Feeny D. A utility approach to the assessment of health-related quality of life. Med Care 2000;38(suppl II):II–151-4.

44. Nord E. The validity of a visual analogue scale in determining social utility weights for health states. Int J Health Plan Manag 1991;6:234-42.

45. Weinstein MC, Stason WB. Cost-effectiveness of coronary artery bypass surgery. Circulation 1982;66(suppl 3):56-66.

46. Anderson NH. Contributions to information integration theory. Vol. 1–3. Hillsdale, NJ: Erlbaum Publishers, 1991.

47. Mulley AJ. Assessing patient's utilities: can the ends justify the means? Med Care 1989;27(suppl):S269-81.

48. Torrance GW, Thomas WH, Sackett DL. A utility maximization model for evaluation of health care programmes. Health Serv Res 1972;7:118-33.

49. Tengs TO, Wallace A. One thousand health-related quality of life estimates. Med Care 2000;38:583-687.

50. Nord E. Methods for quality adjustment of life years. Soc Sci Med 1992;34: 559-69.

51. Patrick DL, Bush JW, Chen MM. Methods for measuring levels of well-being for a health status index. Health Serv Res 1973;8:228-45.

52. Hughes TE, Coons SJ, Kaplan RM, Draugalis JR. Evaluation of linearity of the Quality of Well-Being Scale using functional measurement theory (abstract). Qual Life Res 1994;3:47-8.

53. Nord E. Toward quality assurance in QALY calculations. Int J Technol Assess Health Care 1993;9:37-45.

54. Kaplan RM, Feeny D, Revicki DA. Methods for assessing relative importance in preference based outcome measures. Qual Life Res 1993;2:467-75.

55. Nord E, Richardson J, Macarounas-Kirchmann K. Social evaluation of health care versus personal evaluation of health states. Int J Technol Assess Health Care 1993;9:463-78.

56. Lenert L, Kaplan RM. Validity and interpretation of preference-based measures of health-related quality of life. Med Care 2000;38(suppl II):II–138-150.

57. Dolan P, Gudex C, Kind P, et al. A social tariff for EuroQol: results from a UK general population survey. University of York: Center for Health Economics, (discussion paper 138) 1995.

58. Ubel PA, Loewenstein G, Jepson C. Whose quality of life? A commentary exploring discrepancies between health state evaluations of patients an dthe general public. Qual Life Res 2003;12:599-607.

59. Kaplan RM, Bush JW, Berry CW. The reliability, stability, and generalizability of a health status index. In: Proceedings of the American Statistical Association. Washington, DC: ASA Social Statistics Section, 1978:704-9.

60. Balaban DJ, Fagi PC, Goldfarb NI, Nettler S. Weights for scoring the quality of well-being instrument among rheumatoid arthritics. Med Care 1986;24:973-80.

61. Hughes TE, Coons SJ, Kaplan RM, Draugalis JR. Reweighting the Quality of Well-being Scale in HIV-infected subjects (abstract). Qual Life Res 1994;3:79-80.

62. Kaplan RM. The Hippocratic predicament: affordability, access, and accountability in health care. San Diego: Academic Press, 1993.
63. O'Connor GT, Nease RF Jr. The descriptive epidemiology of health state values and utilities. Med Decis Making 1993;13:87-8.
64. Clancy C, Cebul R, Williams S. Guiding individual decisions. A randomized, controlled trial of decision analysis. Am J Med 1988;84:283-8.
65. Kaplan RM, Bush JW, Berry CC. Health status: types of validity and the index of well-being. Health Serv Res 1976;11:478-507.
66. Kaplan RM, Sieber WJ, Ganiats TG. The Quality of Well-being Scale: comparison of the interview-administered with a self-administered questionnaire. Psychol Health 1997;12:783-91
67. Torrance GW, Boyle MH, Horwood SP. Application of multi-attribute utility theory to measure social preference for health states. Operations Res 1982;30:1043-69.
68. Feeny D, Furlong W, Boyle M, Torrance GW. Multi-attribute health classification systems: Health Utilities Index. Pharmacoeconomics 1995;7:490-502.
69. Boyle MH, Furlong W, Feeny D, Torrance GW, Hatcher J. Reliability of the Health Utilities Index-Mark III used in the 1991 cycle 6 General Social Survey Health Questionnaire. Qual Life Res 1995;4:249-57.
70. Feeny D, Furlong W, Torrance GW, Goldsmith CH, Zhu Z, DePauw S, et al. Multiattribute and single-attribute utility functions for the Health Utilities Index Mark 3 system. Med Care 2002;40:113-28.
71. The EuroQol Group. EuroQol: a new facility for the measurement of health-related quality of life. Health Policy 1990;16:199-208.
72. Brooks R, Rabin R, de Charro F, eds. The measurement and valuation of healthy status using EQ-5D: a European perspective. Dordrecht, the Netherlands: Kluwer Academic Publishers, 2003.
73. Essink-Bot ML, Bonsel GJ, van der Maas PJ. Valuations of health states by the general public: feasibility of a standardized measurement procedure. Soc Sci Med 1990;31:1201-6.
74. Brooks RG, Jendteg S, Lindgren B, et al. EuroQoL: health related quality of life measurement. Results of the Swedish questionnaire exercise. Health Policy 1991;18:37-48.
75. Nord E. EuroQol: health-related quality of life measurement: valuations of health states by the general public in Norway. Health Policy 1991;18:25-36.
76. Coons SJ, Rao S, Keininger DL, Hays RD. A comparative review of generic quality of life instruments. Pharmacoeconomics 2000;17:13-35.
77. Gold MR, Patrick GW, Torrance GW, Fryback DG, Hadorn DC, Kamlet MS, et al. Identifying and valuing outcomes. In: Gold MR, Siegel JE, Russell LB, Weinstein MC, eds. Cost-effectiveness in health and medicine. New York: Oxford University Press, 1996:82-134.
78. Sintonen H, Pekurinen M. A fifteen dimensional measure of health-related quality of life (15D) and its applications. In: Walker SR, Rosser RM, eds. Quality of life assessment: key issues in the 1990s. Dordrecht, the Netherlands: Kluwer Academic Publishers, 1993:185-95.
79. Hadorn DC, Uebersax J. Large-scale outcome evaluation: how should quality of life be measured? I. Calibration of a brief questionnaire and a search for preference subgroups. J Clin Epidemiol 1995;48:607-18.

80. Rosser RM, Kind P. A scale of valuations of states of illness: Is there a social consensus? Int J Epidemiol 1978;7:347-58.

81. Erickson P, Wilson RW, Shannon I. Years of healthy life. Statistical note no. 7. Hyattsville, MD: National Center for Health Statistics, 1995.

82. Neumann PJ, Stone PW, Chapman RH, Sandberg EA, Bell CM. The quality of reporting in published cost-utility analyses, 1976–1977. Ann Intern Med 2000;132:964-72.

83. Chapman RH, Stone PW, Sandberg EA, Bell C, Neumann PJ. A comprehensive league table of cost-utility ratios and a sub-table of "panel-worthy" studies. Med Decis Making 2000;20:451-67.

84. Petrou S, Malek M, Davey PG. The reliability of cost-utility estimates in cost-per-QALY league tables. Pharmacoeconomics 1993;3:345-53.

85. Mason J, Drummond M, Torrance G. Some guidelines on the use of cost effectiveness league tables. BMJ 1993;306:570-2.

86. Smith RD, Hall J, Gurney H, Harnett PR. A cost-utility approach to the use of 5-fluorouracil and levamisole as adjuvant chemotherapy for Dukes' C colonic carcinoma. Med J Aust 1993;158:319-22.

Health-Related Quality of Life: An Overview

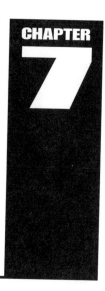

CHAPTER

7

Kathleen M Bungay,
J Gregory Boyer,
and John E Ware Jr

Traditionally, health has been considered from a medical point of view. From this perspective, discussions of health have been concerned with the activities associated with repairing injury, alleviating pain, and eliminating illness. As medical science has advanced and the conditions under which we live improve, this narrow view of health has become insufficient. Today's health professionals and their patients increasingly are faced with decisions that require a broader definition of health, a definition that considers the patient's entire life, not simply the biological manifestations of the chronic or acute condition under treatment.

Although this more complete view of health has received much attention during the past decade, it is not a new concept. As long ago as 1948, the constitution of the World Health Organization defined health as more than freedom from disease; instead, it expanded the boundaries of health to include complete physical, mental, and social well-being.[1] Most contemporary health practitioners and health services researchers have adopted this expanded view of health and now strive to consider the impact that a disease and its treatment have on patients' lives. The traditional medical approach is essential; however, patients,

, and policy-makers increasingly are demanding explana-
; to how the medical care provides/promotes health. These
_......ations must encompass more than laboratory results and
clinical opinions. Information about physical and social functioning and mental well-being is also required to answer the questions now being posed.

These nonclinically defined components of health are the focus of a number of studies. An entire area of research has
evolved to capture and evaluate data necessary to provide insights into patient outcomes. This area of study is known as
health-related quality of life (HRQOL) and is particularly relevant in today's healthcare environment.

In the new era that we are entering, information about functional status, well-being, and other important health outcomes
will be used both by policy analysts and managers of healthcare
organizations. Policy analysts will compare the costs and benefits of competing ways of organizing and financing health cares
to obtain the best value for each healthcare dollar spent. The information also will be used by clinician investigators evaluating
new treatments and technologies, as well as by healthcare practitioners trying to achieve the best possible patient outcomes.
The primary source of new information on general health outcomes is standardized patient surveys. These tools are becoming
accepted by clinicians, but have been serving researchers effectively during the past decade.

HRQOL is a specifically focused area of investigation within
the larger field of health services research and/or quality-of-life
research. Standardized questionnaires are used to capture
HRQOL data in a variety of research settings by self-adminis-
tration, telephone interview, personal interview, observation, or
postal survey. In the jargon of this field of research, these standardized questionnaires are often called instruments, tools, surveys, scales, or measures; these terms are used interchangeably
in the literature. *Psychometrics*, the science of testing questionnaires to measure attributes of individuals, is fundamental in
the study of HRQOL.

While quality of life refers to an evaluation of all aspects of
our lives, including such things as where we live, how we live,
how we play, and how we work, HRQOL encompasses only those

aspects of our lives that are dominated or significantly influenced by our personal health or activities performed to maintain or improve health.[2] Advances in medical science have encouraged this attention to HRQOL because medical care is no longer limited to providing only death-averting treatments. Today, maintaining or restoring quality of life is an important therapeutic goal for many medical conditions, among them arthritis and diabetes—conditions having no cure but for which medical treatment is targeted at controlling disease progression and symptoms. The use of HRQOL measures to capture appropriate data offers a way to monitor disease effects and treatment impacts in terms that are relevant to patients and that reflect the quality of their lives.

Historical View

The use of standardized surveys to assess functional status and well-being can be tracked back over 300 years. Methodologic interest, however, has been greatest during the last half of the twentieth century.[3] The psychometric techniques of scale construction, now more widely used in the healthcare field, have been available for most of the past century.[4-6] The study of methods to measure HRQOL began with physicians' attempts to measure patient functioning. The Karnofsky Functional Status Assessment[7] and the New York Heart Association Classification[8] were among the first instruments developed to capture data about a patient's level of physical activity. The first health status instruments sought to distinguish among patients' functional states and included symptoms, anatomic findings, occupational status, and activities of daily living. These early instruments were significant because they provided a standardized approach for physicians to document the consequences of patient care being provided. The early tools found application in inpatient studies designed to evaluate the functional status of patients with severe disabilities.

The first modern health status questionnaires appeared in the 1970s when social scientists and clinical experts came together with a common research agenda to answer questions about the consequences of the medical care provided. Most health measures prior to the 1970s were not based on methods of scale construction. The early tools were quite long, but the data they captured were valid, reproducible, and relevant. Their focus was multidimensional, providing assessments of physical, psychological, and social health.[9] The development, refinement, and use of the early instruments helped to establish the foundation for today's studies.[10] Many of these early measures are still popular and will be familiar to many readers: Quality of Well-Being Scale,[11] Sickness Impact Profile,[12] the Health Perceptions Questionnaire,[13] and the OARS[14] (Older American Resources and Services) methodology. Tools of more recent origin include the Duke–University of North Carolina Health Profile,[15] the Nottingham Health Profile,[16] and the Medical Outcomes Study 36-Item Short-Form Health Survey (MOS SF-36).[10]

Common to all of these assessment tools is a theoretical framework that views the measurement of biologic functioning as an essential but inadequate component for comprehensively evaluating health. Beyond the documentation of organ system functioning, central to the traditional medical view of health, lies the need to assess general well-being and behavioral functioning. This broader assessment of health is necessary because the basic biological abnormalities can extend into a person's behavioral functioning and sense of well-being, disrupting the person's HRQOL.[9] The analogy often given of the impact a disease can have on a person's life is that of a rock dropped into the center of a still pond, sending out ripples over the entire surface of the water. All of the variables detailed in Figure 1 must be addressed in an HRQOL assessment if a comprehensive understanding of the patient's condition is to be achieved.

The interest in HRQOL was greatly expanded in 1989 when the United States Congress passed the Omnibus Budget Reconciliation Act.[17] This legislation required the Secretary of Health and Human Services to establish a broad-based, patient-centered outcomes research program, the Agency for Healthcare Research and Quality. Still an active research agenda, the objective of this initiative is to monitor the effectiveness of specific medical treatments by including assessments of patients' functional status, general well-being, and satisfaction with the medical care provided. In addition to research, the agency promotes clinical practice guidelines, database development, and information dissemination efforts.

Additionally, researchers in both academia and private industry interested in evaluating alternative medical, surgical, and pharmacologic treatments have adopted HRQOL assessments as a valid approach for documenting the consequences of using medications. These specialized researchers look forward to including HRQOL findings in their economic assessments of competing therapeutic options.

Components of Health-Related Quality of Life Measures

HRQOL focuses on aspects of quality of life that are specifically related to personal health and activities to maintain or improve that level of health. Health is just one of the 12 domains of life identified by Campbell[18] to be considered when researching and evaluating overall quality of life. The other 11 domains are community, education, family life, friendships, housing, marriage, nation, neighborhood, self, standard of living, and work. Thus, the term *health-related quality of life* has been adopted by researchers to set their research apart from the global concept of quality of life as identified by Campbell and to more accurately reflect the scope of their research.[19]

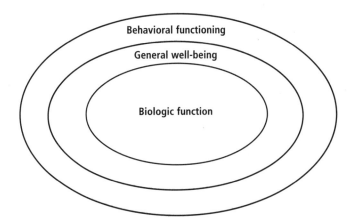

Figure 1. Health status concepts. The impact of a disease and its treatment often affects more than biologic funtioning. Biologic abnormalities and imbalances can impact other important areas of a patient's life, including general well-being and behavioral functioning. This impact is comparable to that of a rock hitting the surface of a still pond, sending ripples over the entire water surface.[13]

To provide an assessment of HRQOL, one of three approaches is usually taken. Researchers can either select tools that focus on general health status or they can choose tools that are more narrowly focused on specific aspects of the disease under study. For a comprehensive picture of a patient's HRQOL, it is often desirable to include both types of assessment tools—the general health and the disease-specific—in research projects having an HRQOL objective.

General Health Status Instruments

General health status instruments evaluate aspects of health relevant to all ages, races, sexes, and socioeconomic backgrounds. Questions in a general health status questionnaire are not defined by the disease or disorder under study. These questions have historically covered the full range of the state of disease or illness and have, therefore, emphasized the negative end of the health continuum. Increasingly, this limitation in older general health status instruments is being recognized, and outcomes researchers are now constructing general health status tools that extend measurements into the well-being end of the health spectrum.[20]

General health status tools are by definition multidimensional, generally evaluating at least four key health concepts: physical functioning, social and role functioning, mental health, and general health perceptions.

PHYSICAL FUNCTIONING

Physical functioning as it relates to HRQOL assessment generally refers to the limitations or disability experienced by the patient over a defined period. The questions focus on observable and important physical limitations easily noticed and evaluated by the patient or observer. Among such limitations are difficulties in walking, eating, or dressing. In the past, questions concentrated on the negative end of the physical functioning continuum and provided no insight into the "well" range of physical functioning (eg, playing sports, running).

To be comprehensive, measures of physical functioning should not be confined to limitations and disabilities; rather, these measures should include questions covering activities of daily living, energy level, satisfaction with physical condition, and ability to perform all level of activities—from the most basic to the most vigorous. Without questions covering the entire continuum of this domain, only persons with physical limitations or disabilities will be identified, evaluated, and segmented for research purposes. Any differences among respondents without significant physical limitations or disabilities will be lost by assessments that do not include the well end of the range.

In addition to physical limitations, specific concepts often included in general health status questions are physical abilities, days in bed, bodily pain, and physical well-being. Table 1 pro-

Table 1. General Health Concepts[21]

Concept	Definition
Physical functioning	
physical limitations	limitations in performance of self-care, mobility, and physical activities
physical abilities	ability to perform everyday activities
days in bed	confinement to bed because of health problems
bodily pain	ratings of the intensity, duration, and frequency of bodily pain and limitations in usual activities because of pain
Social and role functioning	
interpersonal contacts	frequency of visits with friends and relatives; frequency of telephone contacts with close friends or relatives during a specific period of time
social resources	quantity and quality of social network
role functioning	freedom from limitations due to health in the performance of usual role activities such as work, housework, and school activities
Mental health	
anxiety/depression	feelings of anxiety, nervousness, tenseness, depression, moodiness, and down-heartedness
psychological well-being	frequency and intensity of general positive affect
behavioral/emotional control	control of behavior, thoughts, and feelings during specific periods
cognitive functioning	orientation to time and place, memory, attention span, and alertness
General health perceptions	
current health	self-rating of health at present
health outlook	expectations regarding health in the future

vides basic definitions of these components of the physical domain of general health assessments.[21]

SOCIAL AND ROLE FUNCTIONING

Although social and role functioning are often thought of as a single entity and used interchangeably, they are distinct concepts in terms of HRQOL. Social functioning addresses the extent that a person participates in social interactions, as well as the satisfaction derived from these interactions and the social network established. Role functioning questions are concerned with a patient's duties and responsibilities that are limited by health.

Social functioning is defined as the ability to develop, maintain, and nurture mature social relationships. Social well-being is separated into two areas: the frequency of social contacts and the nature of those contacts within the social network or community. These areas must be considered together. Evaluating only the frequency of contacts in isolation from the nature of those contacts may offer no insight or the wrong insight into the person's state of social functioning. Therefore, including a person's assessment of the adequacy of his or her social network is essential when evaluating social functioning in the context of HRQOL. Belonging to a community, family, or neighborhood provides a strong sense of being wanted, loved, or valued[22] and has significant influence on assessments of mental as well as social health.[23]

Role functioning is concerned with the impact health has on a person's ability to meet the demands of his or her normal life role. Work for pay, homemaking duties, and schoolwork are covered by this concept. A role function assessment should identify everyday role situations or activities that can be directly affected or limited by disease, illness, or treatment. Although most role limitations are the result of physical health problems, role limitations have been observed both in the presence and absence of physical limitations.[24]

MENTAL HEALTH

Disease often affects behavioral as well as physical aspects of a person's life. Therefore, general health status assessments usually include questions covering aspects of psychological health. These questions typically focus on the frequency and intensity of symptoms of psychological distress. Anxiety and depression are common themes in mental health components of general health status instruments; however, scales focusing only on these two concepts do not adequately cover the full mental health continuum. Perceptions of psychological well-being, life satisfaction, and cognitive functioning also are needed if a comprehensive assessment of the mental health domain by an HRQOL instrument is to be achieved.[25] General health status questionnaires covering the mental health domain are not intended for use as diagnostic tools; however, some questions have been used as screens for certain disorders (eg, depression).[1]

GENERAL HEALTH PERCEPTIONS

General health perceptions address overall beliefs and evaluations about health. Questions covered in this area focus on health preferences, values, needs, and attitudes. Assessments of general health perceptions are necessary because they allow consideration of individual differences in reactions to pain, perceptions of difficulty, the level of effort required, or the degree of worry or concern about health.[1]

Unlike questions that focus on measures of limitations, pain, or dysfunction used to assess other health domains, questions covering general health perceptions address positive feelings or can be positively framed, allowing the full spectrum of HRQOL to be evaluated.

Disease-Specific Health Status Instruments

It is often necessary to focus on the particular impact that a certain disease has on patients. In such cases, general health status tools are inadequate for providing the information needed. To overcome this limitation, condition- or disease-specific measures often are used to supplement the general health status instrument. The more narrowly focused disease-specific measure requests detailed information on the patient's perspective on the impact of a disease and its treatment. Additionally, using disease-specific measures allows inclusion of domains of specific interest for the disease under study and the patients it affects.

Among areas previously investigated with disease-specific questionnaires are sexual and emotional functioning, nausea and vomiting, chronic pain, anxiety and depression, asthma, chronic obstructive pulmonary disease, cardiovascular disorders, hypertension, epilepsy, benign prostatic hypertrophy, end-stage renal disease, diabetes, cancers, AIDS, HIV infection, and migraine.[26-31]

Psychometrics

The literature is ever expanding with reports of general health and disease-specific HRQOL research. As with any field of research, the studies being reported meet various levels of scientific rigor. Readers of these reports must have a basic understanding of psychometrics to draw appropriate conclusions from HRQOL findings.

Psychometrics is the science of using standardized tests or scales to evaluate attributes of an individual. It is used in the field of health assessment to translate people's behavior, feelings, and personal evaluations into quantifiable data. These data must be both relevant and correct if they are to provide useful insights into HRQOL.

There are two psychometric properties that any measurement scale or instrument must possess: reliability and validity. Additionally, useful measuring scales must be sensitive to change and accepted by the investigators and respondents.

RELIABILITY

When measuring reliability, the scientist is concerned with the relationship between true variation and random error.[32] Evaluations assess the consistency and repeatability of measurements. Reliability is expressed as decimal values between 0.0 and 1.0, with values closest to 1.0 indicating little chance variance. A reliability estimate of 0.85 reveals that 85% of the observed variance in the data is true variance and 15% of the observed variance is the result of chance. If there was no chance variance or random error in the measurement, the reliability estimate would be 1.0.

Reliability estimates are useful because they allow the researcher to examine the consistency of results from different measures thought to evaluate the same thing.[33] These estimates can be obtained by capturing data using the same tool on repeated administrations or by using alternative forms of a measure.

Stability of the responses is desired when evaluating reliability using the same tool on different occasions with the same study population. This approach is commonly called the *test–retest procedure*. It is, however, usually inadequate as the only determinant of an instrument's reliability. This method assumes that, during the time interval between the two tests, there will be no recall of the original response, no change in the attribute being evaluated, and no change in the respondent. Because health and disease are dynamic processes, ensuring that no change in the respondent occurs between the original assessment and the repeated assessment is particularly difficult. The time interval between administration of the tests is critical and must always be known before one can have any confidence in a test–retest of reliability. Researchers relying on the test–retest method will most likely underestimate an instrument's reliability rather than overestimate it.[31]

The *alternative forms method* of estimating reliability avoids some of the problems inherent in the test–retest method. This approach requires that alternative, equivalent questionnaires be administered to the same individuals at the same time. The correlation between the scores provides an estimate of the reliability of the measure.

Rather than having equivalent forms of the same instrument (a difficult task!), a useful approach is the *split-half method*. As its name implies, this method compares the score derived from half of the items with the score obtained from the other half. Convenient approaches to accomplish this are to compute a scale score using the even-numbered items and a second score using the odd-numbered items. If the original measure has been developed appropriately to measure a single health concept, the correlation between the two halves should be strong (ie, close to 1.0).

An expansion of the split-half approach is the coefficient alpha estimate (often calculated using Cronbach's coefficient alpha). This estimate is essentially the average of all possible split-half correlations and is known as the *internal consistency reliability estimate*.[34]

It is important to note that reliability estimates are influenced by the number of items in the measure. Logically, the more questions asked about a particular subject, the more information will be gained from the inquiry. This trade-off between reliability and length of the measure is discussed in greater detail on page 163.

Acceptable reliability coefficients vary depending on what is being analyzed and to what end the findings will be used. Comparisons at the individual patient level require high reliability estimates (values >0.90). For group comparisons, reliability estimates between 0.50 and 0.70 are considered acceptable.[35]

VALIDITY

A number of key questions must be answered if researchers are to have confidence in the data captured using HRQOL instruments. All are related to the validity of the assessment. Do the questions in the instrument really measure the concept under study? Do respondents understand the questions being asked? Are the response categories appropriate for the questions?

Validity refers to the extent to which differences in test scores reflect the true differences in individuals under study. Although it is the goal to elicit observed differences that are indeed true differences among respondents, factors such as how the measure is administered, who administers it, where it is administered, and when it is administered can affect responses across study participants; these factors can add a degree of uncertainty to the findings of an HRQOL assessment. There are no standard guidelines for validating health measures.

However, standards established by the American Psychological Association,[36] the American Educational Research Association, and the National Council on Measurement in Education have found application in evaluating measures.[37]

The types of validation necessary and most applicable to HRQOL measures are content, construct, and criterion.[27]

Content Validity

Researchers measuring content validity are concerned with how well the health concept is captured by the items in the measure. A scale with good content validity is one that covers all aspects of the concept being addressed. To establish content validity, a comparison is made between the items included in a scale and some definitional standard for which there is general acceptance. This type of validation assumes the researcher has confidence in the definitional standard. Additionally, each item included in the scale must "appear" to measure the concept under study; this special type of content validity is commonly called *face validity*.

Construct Validity

The central question asked when determining construct validity is whether the health measure relates to other measures or variables in plausible ways. Evaluating scale scores in various patient groups known to differ in relevant ways (eg, age, sex) is a frequent approach for determining construct validity. Validity is supported when scale scores for each patient group reflect the known group differences. Hypothesized relationships between relevant clinical parameters and scale scores often are evaluated to establish construct validity.

Convergent and *discriminant validity* are special types of construct validity. For convergent validity, correlations should be high between similar or related measures of the same health concept. For discriminant validity, correlations should be low between scales evaluating very different health concepts. Observing these expected or hypothesized relationships is evidence of construct validity. For example, if an instrument has construct validity, items designed to measure physical activity, mobility, and physical functioning should have high correlations with each other and should each have low correlations with measures of mental health, such as anxiety or depression.

Criterion Validity

Criterion validity requires the comparison of a scale score with a gold standard. Unfortunately, there are no gold standards against which HRQOL measures can be evaluated. It is acceptable practice, however, to use longer, well-validated measures of HRQOL as criteria for evaluating the validity of shorter, newly developed measures. Because this approach uses a proxy as a criterion, it is more appropriately called criterion-related validity.[31]

For example, two external variables with known characteristics, such as resource use (dollars) and age (years), can be used to assess a relationship with physical and mental health concepts. An investigator would hypothesize and test that health status and resource use are negatively correlated; similarly, age and physical health should produce a negative correlation. Thus, resource use and age compared with patients' assessments of their physical and mental health are examples of useful ways to investigate the criterion-related validity.

A final word on validation is warranted. Without an understanding of the validity of an HRQOL scale, changes or differences in score are meaningless. Validation is, however, a continuous process. Each new use of an HRQOL scale provides new information about the interpretation and meaning of scores. Stewart[33] notes that "there is no one point at which a measure is considered valid." Certainly, a single study is inadequate to thoroughly provide validation of an HRQOL measure.

SENSITIVITY

Perhaps the least well studied and documented aspect of HRQOL measures at this time is that of sensitivity.[33] Researchers evaluating sensitivity are concerned with detecting the true changes that occur in a health concept over time. It is important when assessing sensitivity that measures of change over time cover the entire range of a particular health concept. That is, they should extend from severe limitations to well-being. This permits investigators a continuum of responses over which to detect changes. It has been suggested that sensitive measures should be stable in patients who do not change clinically and should shift in patients who do experience clinical changes.[38,39]

Sensitivity can be affected greatly by the simple choice of response options. Crude measures may use only the dichotomous yes/no response options. More advanced measures use graduated response categories, allowing respondents to record varying amounts of an attribute. An example of a frequently used graduated response option contrasted with a dichotomous yes/no response option is found in Table 2.

ACCEPTABILITY FOR USE

Both investigators and respondents will have valuable opinions about the acceptability of various HRQOL instruments. How easy the measure is to use, score, and interpret are valid concerns. The completion rate, the extent of missing data, and the number and nature of complaints about the tool are clues about the acceptability of the measure for use in a research or clinical setting. Acceptability also is expressed as respondent burden. Regardless of the administration format (self-administered, telephone interview, personal interview, observation, or postal survey), failure to consider respondent burden can doom any survey project.

Today's researchers strive to achieve a balance between an increase in reliability (achieved by asking more questions) and a decrease in respondent burden (achieved with fewer questions). Some short-form multi-item scales derived from much longer measures are now in use. These short forms achieve an acceptably high level of precision when compared with their longer parent versions and are much less burdensome to both respondents and investigators. The MOS SF-36[10,40] and the 17-item Duke Health Profile[41] are two examples of short-form scales. Advances in computer adaptive technology[42] will continue to allow health service research scientists to further decrease respondent burden. The adaptive technology presents sets of questions

---

Table 2. Example of Dichotomous and Graduated Response Options

Dichotomous
During the past 4 weeks, has nausea affected your daily function?
  Yes ○
  No ○

Graduated
How often during the past 4 weeks has nausea affected your daily functioning?
  all of the time   ○
  most of the time   ○
  a good bit of the time ○
  some of the time   ○
  a little of the time   ○
  none of the time   ○

specific to the individual patient and his or her responses to the initial questions. Patients only answer as many questions needed to achieve acceptable reliability of their answers to a certain concept. For example, the SF-36 Physical Functioning Scale contains 10 questions, many of which are not needed if a person answers that they are not limited in vigorous activities such as sports.

The Future of Health-Related Quality of Life Research

The agenda for the future of HRQOL research and its application is quite full. HRQOL measures appearing today are shorter and more user-friendly than earlier versions. These shorter tools are gaining acceptance in clinical practice as well as in industry and academic research. Future efforts require interpretation of patient scores and amalgamation of data from patient scores with traditional biological markers of disease. Future research will test the use of these combinations in therapeutic decision-making, as well as in monitoring therapy. Only through knowledge of the HRQOL of very healthy individuals, very disabled individuals, and those in between can findings from HRQOL research have meaning and find application. Establishing community norms and characteristic patterns within population segments also are important research objectives of many contemporary scientists.

The future research agenda focuses on the use of these instruments for three different, but interrelated purposes: to continue to measure or define health states, assist with monitoring patient care, and be used as information with which to manage an individual patient's care.

Each of these three purposes is illustrated with examples. Findings from the MOS have been instrumental in measuring and defining health. Information gained from the use of these tools in clinical drug trials has assisted in furthering that mission and has enabled the exploration of how to use HRQOL assessments as monitoring parameters. Finally, clinical application of HRQOL research is just beginning to be realized. The routine use of this information as a management tool in making decisions regarding therapy has yet to be fully implemented.

THE MEDICAL OUTCOMES STUDY

Much has been and continues to be learned about measuring and defining health from the Medical Outcomes Study (MOS).[43-45] In the MOS, a comprehensive approach to the assessment of health was first embraced. One of the major objectives of the MOS was to develop practical tools for monitoring patient outcomes and their determinants in routine medical practice. In particular, the study was designed to evaluate the impact of chronic disease on patient functioning and well-being and to determine whether key features of medical care are associated with more favorable patient outcomes.[46,47] This study is described more fully elsewhere.[48]

QUALITY OF LIFE RESEARCH IN CLINICAL TRIALS

Research on furthering the use of HRQOL instruments as a monitoring tool in clinical practice has been conducted in the context of clinical drug trials. However, clinical trial planning is driven largely by corporate needs to develop products and obtain regulatory approval to market them. With the recognition and demand for information about product attributes beyond traditional measures of safety and efficacy in the United States and abroad, the only practical opportunity to conduct patient-based research on a product's attributes has been to integrate HRQOL components with Phase II, III, or IV studies. The results of this combination have been synergistic. Both clinical practice and the science of psychometrics have benefited from the resulting information of these combined studies.

The current and future importance of the results from HRQOL studies depends, in large part, on how the information will be used, as well as whose perspective is being considered. In the regulatory setting, HRQOL endpoints are included in clinical trials both to enhance product approval and support promotional claims that will be made when the product is brought to market. To date, the Food and Drug Administration (FDA) has not published specific guidelines on when HRQOL endpoints are important for regulatory purposes.

Results of these clinical trials that include HRQOL data are increasingly present in both the general medical literature and in medical specialty journals from which clinicians derive new information for patient care decisions. Payers also are using the results of HRQOL studies. In the world of increasing cost consciousness, it is tempting to assume that the payer's concern is to minimize cost and the HRQOL benefits of a new product are not germane. Although clearly concerned with cost, payers are generally more interested in maximizing the value of healthcare purchases than in minimizing costs. The principal payers for health services in the United States are employers, who act as advocates for their employees on many fronts. Employers generally will not withhold health services for covered indications from employees unless the costs are shown to exceed the value of the services. Moreover, employers have unions, courts of justice, and government regulations to contend with if they are seen to be sacrificing employee health in an effort to economize in healthcare costs.

Acceptance of the relevance of the results of HRQOL studies to payer coverage and related decisions has paralleled acceptance within the community of practitioners. Many of the specific decisions about product or technology coverage and payment are made by medical directors or technology advisory committees who look to the same clinical journals for scientific, peer-reviewed evidence of HRQOL benefits. A final perspective is that of patients and organizations who represent patient interests. HRQOL results may become important support for disease areas where patient advocacy is strong, such as AIDS, cancer, and arthritis.

Strategic Considerations in Implementing HRQOL Assessments in Clinical Trials

The identification of potential uses for HRQOL data does not imply that an HRQOL assessment should be performed in every clinical trial. Deciding which trials should or should not include these assessments is an important strategic decision, especially in the case of complex, multinational clinical testing programs that involve many trials of the same product in varying formulations for different indications. Such decisions should be made with a clear idea of what purpose the HRQOL results will serve.

When recombinant epoetin alfa for treatment of anemia in end-stage renal disease was examined in Phase III clinical trials, for example, the FDA was concerned about how this therapy would affect the lives of those treated.[49] The principal clinical endpoint, change in hematocrit concentration, was seen as insufficient to gauge the human impact, and a major quality-of-life component was integrated into this pivotal clinical trial. In this instance, there was clearly a regulatory need for quality-of-life information. Because the vast majority of persons with this disease in the United States are covered by Medicare as part of the End-Stage Renal Disease Program, there was an important payer use for the data as well. Medicare program administrators were interested in the HRQOL benefits to the affected beneficiary population. This concern contributed to the decision to include HRQOL assessments in the Phase IV epoetin alfa studies.

Many HRQOL assessments focus on adverse effects rather than treatment effects. An example is the series of studies reported on the HRQOL of alternative antihypertensive therapies.[50,51] In this instance, the HRQOL consequences of adverse effects were highlighted in head-to-head comparisons of drugs with the same indications. The data reported could be useful for clinicians.

Another important strategic consideration for integrating HRQOL assessments in clinical trials is the compatibility between the clinical and HRQOL objectives. An example is a clinical study of a product indicated for treatment of skin ulcers. This is an area that generates considerable skepticism among payers. Thus, data showing improvement in HRQOL from a well-controlled study might have influenced payers to accept the product. The trial design specified that eligible patients would have wounds on opposing limbs, with one limb randomized to receive experimental treatment and the other conventional treatment. Although the design was created to reduce large variability introduced by outside factors in the clinical data analysis, the protocol was incompatible with designing a meaningful HRQOL assessment.

Although this is an extreme example, it illustrates that achieving compatibility between clinical and HRQOL study objectives is important when planning research. This is especially true when the purpose of collecting the information and reporting the results is to provide information to more than one party, such as regulatory agencies and payers or physicians.

Finally, real-world confirmation of findings from clinical trial results is becoming increasingly important among providers and payers charged with making cost-conscious decisions regarding the acquisition and financing of technology. To respond to this need, researchers will need to continue studies on HRQOL into Phase IV trials and independent effectiveness research to provide evidence of the durability of HRQOL benefits in clinical practice.

Using Health-Related Quality-of-Life Assessments in Routine Patient Care

Standardized measures capturing patient perspectives on their physical functioning, social and role functioning, mental health, and general health perceptions are likely to become more acceptable as an additional piece of evidence on which providers and their patients can make decisions about treatment and the treatment's efficacy. Mature theoretical models[52-55] and enhanced technology for use in measurement make the routine use of individual patient results in their own care more promising than ever before.

Two practical concerns of critics for the use of HRQOL assessments in individual patient care are respondent burden and reliability of scores obtained from shorter questionnaires. Current researchers struggle with the competing demands invoked by the everyday use requiring shorter forms and the reliability of a result obtained from fewer questions. Specifically, concerns are raised about the reliability and interpretation of the result since, with popular outcomes measures, the standard error around a single-person estimate is large and not satisfying enough to ensure stable conclusions.

Modern test theory offers the potential for individualized, comparable assessments for the careful examination and application of different health status measures.[53] One such theory is that of *item response theory* (IRT). Researchers report that IRT has a number of potential advantages over the currently employed *classical test theory* (CTT) in assessing self-reported health outcomes. Applications of the IRT models are ideally suited for implementing computer-adaptive testing. IRT methods are also reported to be helpful in developing better health outcomes measures and assessing change over time.[52]

Patients increasingly have more access to computer technology. It is thus becoming more practical to employ assessments using a computer. Patients answering questions about a health status concept using dynamic assessment technology are requested to complete only the number of questions needed (minimizes response burden) to establish a reliable estimate. The resulting scores for an individual are estimated to meet the clinical measures of precision.

Summary

The study of HRQOL requires a multidimensional approach. Assessments must include components that evaluate, at a minimum, the health concepts of physical functioning, social and role functioning, mental health, and perception of general health. Additionally, the full continuum of these concepts must be included, from the most limited to the most healthy. Approaches to capture HRQOL data include the self-administered questionnaire, personal interview, telephone interview, observation, and postal survey. The assessment instruments must possess acceptable reliability, validity, and sensitivity, and they must be accepted by the investigators as well as the participants. Psychometrics is an essential part of HRQOL research, especially in today's research environment that requires shorter, more focused measures.

Existing health outcomes measures drawn from CTT and emerging approaches based on IRT offer exciting opportunities for appreciably expanded applications in biomedical and health services research, clinical practice and decision-making, and policy development. The research agenda of measurement scientists includes challenges to (1) refine and expand measurement techniques that rely on IRT, (2) improve measurement tools to make them more culturally appropriate for diverse populations and more conceptually and psychometrically equivalent across such groups, (3) address long-standing isssues in preference- and utility-based approaches, particularly in the elicitation of preference responses and scoring instruments, and (4) enhance the ways in which data from outcomes measurement tools are calibrated against commonly understood clinical and lay metrics, interpreted, and made usable for different decision-makers.[56]

With these advances in measurement that promise to continue, knowledgeable clinicians will become the transportation for these measures to inclusion in patient care. It is suggested that interpretation is, in part, an issue of familiarity, and repeated applications[2] of the measures will lead to a better understanding. Ideally, better understanding of what patients tell their providers about their health status can be used for decision-making that requires patients to more actively and routinely participate in their own care.

References

1. Basic documents: World Health Organization. Geneva: World Health Organization, 1948.
2. Bungay KM, Ware JE. Measuring and monitoring health-related quality of life. Kalamazoo, MI: Upjohn, 1993.
3. Katz S, Ford AB, Moskowitz RW, Jacobson BA, Jaffe MW. Studies of illness in the aged. The index of ADL: a standardized measure of biological and psychosocial function. J Am Med Assoc 1963;185:914-9.
4. Guttman LA. A basis for rescaling qualitative data. Am Soc Rev 1944; 9:139-50.
5. Likert R. A technique for the measurement of attitudes. Arch Psychol 1932;140:5-55.
6. Thrustone LL, Chage EJ. The measurement of attitude. Chicago: University of Chicago Press, 1929.
7. Karnofsky DA, Burchenal JH. The clinical evaluation of chemotherapeutic agents in cancer. In: Macleod CM, ed. Evaluation of chemotherapeutic agents. New York: Columbia Press, 1949:191-205.
8. Criteria Committee, New York Heart Association. Nomenclature and criteria for diagnosis of diseases of the heart and great vessels. 8th ed. Boston: Little Brown and Company, 1979.
9. Ware JE Jr. Scales for measuring general health perceptions. Health Serv Res 1976;11:396-415.
10. Ware JE Jr, Sherbourne CD. The MOS 36-item short-form health survey (SF-36). Med Care 1992;30:473-82.
11. Fanshel S, Bush JW. A health-status index and its application to health-services outcomes. Operations Res 1970;18:1021-66.
12. Bergner M, Bobbitt RA, Kressel S, Pollard WE, Gilson BS, Morris JR. The sickness impact profile: conceptual formulation and methodology for the development of a health status measure. Int J Health Serv 1976;6:393-415.
13. Ware JE. Conceptualizing and measuring generic health outcomes. Cancer 1991;67(suppl 3):774-9.
14. Pfeiffer E, ed. Multidimensional functional assessment: the OARS methodology. Durham, NC: Duke University Press, Center for the Study of Aging and Human Development, 1975.

15. Parkerson GR Jr, Gehlback SH, Wagner EH, James SA, Clapp NE, Muhlbaier LH. The Duke–UNC health profile: an adult health status instrument for primary care. Med Care 1981;19:806-28.

16. Hunt SM, McEwen J, McKenna SP. Measuring health status: a new tool for clinicians and epidemiologists. J R Coll Gen Pract 1985;35:185-8.

17. Omnibus Budget Reconciliation Act, 1989. Public Law 101-239. Washington, DC: Government Printing Office, 1989.

18. Campbell A. The sense of well-being in America: recent patterns and trends. New York: McGraw-Hill, 1981.

19. Patrick DL, Erickson P. Assessing health-related quality of life for clinical decision making. In: Walker SR, Rosser RM, eds. Quality of life: assessments and application. Lancaster, England: MTR Press, 1988:9-49.

20. Ware JE Jr. Measuring functioning, well-being and other generic health concepts. In: Osoba D, ed. Effect of cancer on quality of life. Boca Raton, FL: CRC Press, 1991:7-23.

21. Ware JE Jr. Standard for validating health measures: definition and content. J Chron Dis 1987;40:473-80.

22. Greenley JR. The measurement of social support. In: Donald CA, Ware JE Jr, eds. Research in community and mental health. Greenwich, CT: JAI Press, 1984;4:325-70.

23. Wortman CB. Social support and the cancer patient: conceptual and methodologic issues. Cancer 1984;53:2339-62.

24. Sherbourne CD, Stewart AL, Wells KB. Role functioning measures. In: Stewart AL, Ware JE Jr, eds. Measuring functioning and well being: the Medical Outcomes Study approach. Durham, NC: Duke University Press; 1992:205-19.

25. Veit CT, Ware JE Jr. The structure of psychological distress and well-being in general populations. J Consult Clin Psychol 1983;51:730-42.

26. Patrick DL, Deyo RA. Generic and disease-specific measures in assessing health status and quality of life. Med Care 1989;27(suppl):S217-32.

27. Wu AW, Rubin HR, Mathews WC, Ware JE, Brysk LT, Hardy WD, et al. A health status questionnaire using 30 items from the Medical Outcomes Study: preliminary validation in persons with early HIV infection. Med Care 1991;29:786-98.

28. Juniper EF, Guyatt GH. Development and testing of a new measure of health status for clinical trials in rhinoconjunctivitis. Clin Exp Allergy 1991;21:77-83.

29. Juniper EF, Guyatt GH, Ferrie PJ, Griffith LE. Measuring quality of life in asthma. Am Rev Respir Dis 1993;147:832-8.

30. Schipper H, Clinch A, McMurray A, Levitt M. Measuring the quality of life of cancer patients. The functional living index—cancer: development and validation. J Clin Oncol 1984;2:472-83.

31. Meenan RF. The AIMS approach to health status measurement: conceptual background and measurement properties. J Rheumatol 1982;9:785-8.

32. Selitiz C, Wrightsman LS, Cook SW. Research methods in social relations. 3rd ed. New York: Holt Rinehart and Winston, 1976:169-97.

33. Stewart AL. Psychometric considerations in functional status instruments. In: Functional status measurement in primary care. New York: Springer-Verlag, 1990:3-26.

34. Cronbach LJ, Warrington WG. Time-limit tests: estimating their reliability and degree of speeding. Psychometrika 1951;16:167-88.

35. Helmstadter GC. Principles of psychological measurement. New York: Appleton-Century-Crofts, 1964.

36. Standards for educational and psychological testing. Washington, DC: American Psychological Association, 1985.

37. Ware JE Jr. Measures for a new era of health assessment. In: Stewart AL, Ware JE, eds. Measuring functioning and well-being: the Medical Outcomes Study approach. Durham, NC: Duke University Press, 1992:3-11.

38. Deyo RA, Patrick D. Barriers to the use of health status measures in clinical investigation, patient care, and policy research. Med Care 1989;27(suppl):5254-68.

39. Launois R. Quality of life: overview and perspectives. Eurotext 1992;28:3-24.

40. McHorney CA, Ware JE, Rogers W, Raczek A, Lu JFR. The validity and relative precision of MOS short- and long-form health status scales and Dartmouth COOP charts. Med Care 1992;30(suppl 5):MS253-65.

41. Parkerson GR, Broadhead WE, Tse CK. Comparison of the Duke health profile and the MOS short-form in healthy young adults. Med Care 1991;29:679-83.

42. Ware JE Jr, Bjorner JB, Kosinski M. Practical implications of item response theory and computerized adaptive testing: a brief summary of ongoing studies of widely used headache impact scales. Med Care 2000;38(9 suppl):II73-82.

43. Tarlov A, Ware JE, Greenfield S, Nelson EC, Perrin E, Zubkoff M. The Medical Outcomes Study: an application of methods for monitoring the results of medical care. JAMA 1989;7:925-30.

44. Stewart AL, Greenfield S, Hays RD, Wells K, Rogers WH, Berry SD, et al. Functional status and well-being of patients with chronic conditions: results from the Medical Outcomes Study. JAMA 1989;7:907-13.

45. Wells KB, Stewart A, Hays RD, Burnam MA, Rogers W, Daniels M, et al. The functioning and well-being of depressed patients: results from the Medical Outcomes Study. JAMA 1989;7:914-9.

46. McHorney CA, Ware JE, Lu JFR, Sherbourne CD. The MOS 36-Item Short Form Health Survey (SF-36): III. Tests of data quality, scaling assumptions, and reliability across diverse patient groups. Med Care 1994; 32:40-66.

47. Ware JE, Kosinski M, Keller SD. SF-12: how to score the SF-12 physical and mental health summary scales. Boston: The Health Institute, New England Medical Center, March 1995.

48. Stewart AL. The Medical Outcomes Study framework of health indicators. In: Stewart AL, Ware JE, eds. Measuring functioning and well-being: the Medical Outcomes Study approach. Durham, NC: Duke University Press, 1992:12-24.

49. Evans RW, Rader B, Manninem DC. The quality of life of hemodialysis recipients treated with recombinant human erythropoietin. JAMA 1990; 263:825-30.

50. Croog SH, Levine S, Testa MA, Brown B, Bulpitt CJ, Jenkins CD, et al. The effects of antihypertensive therapy on quality of life. N Engl J Med 1986;314:1657-64.

51. Testa MA, Anderson RB, Nackly JF, Hollenberg NK. Quality of life and antihypertensive therapy in men. N Engl J Med 1993;328:97-113.

52. Wilson IB, Cleary PD. Linking clinical variables with health-related quality of life. A conceptual model of patient outcomes. JAMA 1995;273:59-65.

53. Patrick DL, Chiang YP. Measurement of health outcomes in treatment effectiveness evaluations: conceptual and methodological challenges. Med Care 2000;38(9 suppl II):II-14–25.

54. Hays RD, Morales LS, Reise SP. Item response theory and health outcomes measurements in the 21st century. Med Care 2000;38(9 suppl):II-28–42.

55. McHorney CA, Cohen AS. Equating health status measures with item response theory: Illustrations with functional status items. Med Care 2000;38(9 suppl II):II-43–59.

56. Lohr KN. Health outcomes methodology symposium: summary and recommendations. Med Care 2000;38(9 suppl II):II-194–208.

Decision Analysis and Pharmacoeconomic Evaluations

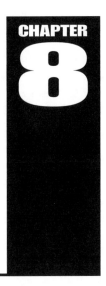

CHAPTER

8

Judith T Barr and
Gerald E Schumacher

ecisions. They are a fact of everyday life. Whether at
home or in clinical practice, decisions must always be
made. From a decision as mundane as whether to go to a
movie or a concert to a more complicated clinical consideration
of which antibiotic to select, decisions span a range of complexity. Using the techniques of reasoned guess, gut reaction, or intuition in our decision-making process, our usual course of action
is to implicitly consider the decision, its options, and possibly
the near-term consequences of the alternatives. If other considerations are recognized, they are somehow factored into the process in an ad hoc juggling act. This chapter demonstrates that
the decision process can be improved and that decision analysis
can be an important tool in pharmacoeconomic evaluations.

What Is Decision Analysis?

Our intuitive decision-making capabilities are limited, and we
rarely attempt an explicit examination of all factors affecting a
decision and its outcome. However, our decisions can be improved
through the use of the explicit structure and quantitative techniques of decision analysis—a systematic approach to decision-

making under conditions of uncertainty. Since few decisions are accompanied with absolute certainty of the consequences of their outcomes, decision analysis can be used to assist the decision-maker to (1) identify the available options when faced with a decision, (2) predict the consequences or outcomes of each option, (3) assess the likelihood or probability of the identified possible outcomes, (4) determine the value of each outcome, and (5) select the decision option, given the considerations that have been built into the decision, that is expected to produce the best outcome. Decision analysis not only forces an explicit, orderly, and careful consideration of a variety of important issues, but also provides insight into the process of decision-making.

Decision analysis is explicit, forcing one to structure the decision and identify the consequences of the possible decision outcomes. It is quantitative, forcing one to assign numbers to probability estimates and outcome valuations. Finally, it is prescriptive, with the analysis identifying the route that should be taken to maximize the expected value of the decision constructed.

The origins of decision analysis, as well as many of the techniques presented in this book, can be traced to the British during World War II when principles of game theory, systems analysis, and operations research were applied to decisions involving allocation of scarce resources. By the 1950s, these techniques were combined in the business world into the evolving field of decision analysis. The late 1950s saw the beginning of medical applications,[1] and the approach reached the medical literature in the early and mid-1970s.[2-4] Cost-benefit, cost-effectiveness, and cost-utility are extensions of decision analysis technology.[5]

Decision analysis is now an integral component of business school curricula as universities prepare future managers to make better allocative and strategic decisions. From Raiffa's[6] classic lectures to decision support computer packages, decision analysis is now central to modern business and economic decisions, more recently expanding into healthcare fields. A 1987 review article identified nearly 200 decision analysis citations from the clinical literature.[5] These analyses were performed to structure decisions related to one or more of 13 categories of clinical problems. In the medical community, decision analysis is being institutionalized. The Society for Medical Decision Making was established in 1977 and publishes its bimonthly journal,

Medical Decision Making, clinical decision consultation services have been established to provide assistance with complex patient-specific decisions,[7] and the American Association of Medical Colleges has recommended the inclusion of clinical decision analysis in the undergraduate medical curriculum.

Over the last 10 to 15 years, the application of decision analysis to clinical issues has continued to grow. Between 1990 and 2002, the National Library of Medicine classified nearly 1,500 articles in English using the index terms *decision analysis* or *decision analytic.* Over this period, an average of 61 percent of these articles also included *cost* as an index word; 31 percent, *drug*; and 22 percent *cost* and *drug.* Not only has the absolute number of articles increased (Figure 1), but the proportion of decision analytic articles including *cost* and *drug* (ie, pharmacoeconomics), singularly and in combination, has also increased. While this identification of pharmacoeconomic studies using decision analysis is not exhaustive, it clearly documents the growth of this field.

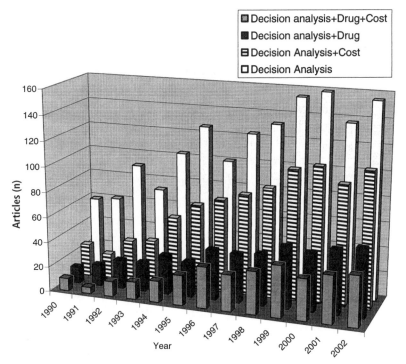

Figure 1. Trends in the use of decision analysis in the clinical and pharmacoeconomic literature.

Many factors contribute to this trend. Among them are the national concern about the increase in healthcare expenditures in general and pharmaceutical products in particular, development of decision analytic software, generation of new decision analytic researchers produced by new health economics and pharmacoeconomics educational programs, establishment of pharmacoeconomics and health outcomes divisions within the pharmaceutical industry, growth in the number of decision analytic publications within the journal *PharmacoEconomics*, and establishment of the International Society of Pharmacoeconomics and Outcomes Research and its journal *Value in Health*.

This chapter provides the opportunity to apply decision analysis to the process of combining the economic considerations of administrators with the associated health consequences of concern to clinicians. The steps and techniques of the decision analytic process are illustrated by their application to a teaching case concerning a decision facing a pharmacy and therapeutics (P&T) committee.

Decision analysis is a method with techniques to analyze situations. But perhaps more importantly, the use of decision analysis engenders the practitioner's attitude toward the problem or decision—to think more analytically; force the consideration of consequences of actions; explicitly recognize that uncertainty is present, estimate the degree of uncertainty, and assess the attitude toward risk; determine which are the relevant outcome measures; and value the preferences for alternative outcomes.

The Case

The following simplified teaching case serves as an introduction to the terminology and mechanics involved in the performance of a decision analysis.

Alphazorin and omegazorin are the only Food and Drug Administration–approved members of a new (fictional) class of antibiotics. Both are effective against gram-negative bacteria that are resistant to multiple antibiotics and block the transfer of extrachromosomal resistance factors between bacterial cells. In clinical trials, 95 percent of the cases of gram-negative septicemia were susceptible to alphazorin; 88 percent were susceptible to omegazorin. Although omegazorin has a higher incidence of drug-associated toxicity, the concentrations of both must be maintained within a narrow therapeutic range. Toxic adverse effects for both include diarrhea and vomiting (gastrointestinal [GI] toxicity), hepatic enzyme alterations (hepatotoxicity), and platelet inhibition (hematotoxicity).

The initial expenses of a 10-day course of intravenous alphazorin administered every eight hours are $1,650 for the direct costs associated with drug acquisition and storage and $540 for dispensing and administration ($18/dose); for intravenous omegazorin administered every six hours, the respective costs are $1,050 and $720 ($18/dose). Although alphazorin has the higher costs, it also has the higher percentage of successfully treated cases of gram-negative bacteremia and a lower incidence of drug-associated toxicity. Important characteristics for each antibiotic are summarized in Table 1.

The P&T committee has decided to approve the addition of only one of these antibiotics to its formulary, but which one? How can it combine all of the factors necessary to reach its decision: the cost of the antibiotics, the difference in susceptibility/

Table 1. Characteristics of Alphazorin and Omegazorin

CHARACTERISTIC	ALPHAZORIN	OMEGAZORIN
Cost of 10-day course of therapy ($)	1,650	1,050
Dosage regimen	every 8 hours	every 6 hours
Resistance rate (%)	5	12
Drug-related toxicities		
gastrointestinal symptoms	7	10
hepatotoxicity	1.5	3.5
hematotoxicity	0.4	1.5
Subtherapeutic response rate (%)	10	15
Characteristics of SDC at COL_t (%)		
predictive value positive	80	90
predictive value negative	90	85
Characteristics of SDC at COL_s (%)		
predictive value positive	90	87.5
predictive value negative	80	90

COL_s = subtherapeutic cutoff level; COL_t = toxic cutoff level; SDC = serum drug concentration.

resistance rates, the varying toxicity and subtherapeutic response rates, and the classification accuracy of the serum drug concentrations? The committee will organize the elements of the formulary selection, considering patient survival as well as the economic impact.

Six major steps are involved in the decision analytic process.

1. Identify the decision, including the selection of the decision options to be studied. Bound by the time frame of the decision, determine from which perspective the decision is to be made and the outcome measures to incorporate into the analysis.

2. Structure the decision and consequences of each decision option over time.

3. Assess the probability that each consequence will occur.

4. Determine the value of each outcome (eg, in dollars, quality-adjusted life-years saved, utilities).

5. Select the option with the highest expected outcome.

6. Determine the robustness of the decision by conducting a sensitivity analysis and varying the values of probabilities and outcomes over a range of likely values.

As with any teaching case, a number of simplifying assumptions occur here to allow focus on the basic decision analytic principles and processes in the case before applying the technique to more complicated "real world" situations. For example, in the section, "Who Will Be the Decision-Maker?," the committee had included survival as an outcome variable in the analysis. However, in this fictional case, survival is equal because the subpopulation of patients who fail on either alphazorin or omegazorin can be rescued with another antibiotic, betasporin. This third antibiotic is 100 percent effective, but is restricted to second-line use by the infectious disease service. Clearly, such a drug does not exist, but it does permit the design of this teaching case so that all patients will survive the septicemic episode. With survival as the effectiveness outcome, both options are equally effective during this episode of care. Therefore, by including betasporin, decision analysis can be used to structure a cost-minimization analysis since the noneconomic outcomes in each option are equal.

Each of the six steps is developed in the following sections. Simplying assumptions are clearly identified. Throughout the chapter, the definitions and conventions of clinical decision analysis presented by Weinstein and Fineberg[8] are used. DATA 4.0

(TreeAge Software Inc., Williamstown, MA) is applied to structure and analyze the case.

Identify and Bind the Decision

The ground rules of the decision are set at this stage. The following questions must be considered for any case using decision analysis: Who will be the decision-maker, and what perspective will be considered? What is the decision, and what options will be considered? Over what time span will the consequences be analyzed? Answers to these questions are necessary at this time to properly structure the decision and collect the appropriate data.

WHO WILL BE THE DECISION-MAKER?

This question is asked primarily to determine from what perspective the analysis is to be conducted. In the alphazorin/omegazorin case, is it from the point of view of the pharmacy department, the P&T committee, the hospital, an insurance company, a health maintenance organization, or society? If the decision's impact on the financial resources of a unit is considered, the type of unit will make a difference as to whether to measure costs or charges, which costs or charges to include, and over what time period they should be collected. For example, if the decision is being considered based on the financial impact to the pharmacy department, only the drug acquisition costs and pharmacy-associated direct costs of the drug's storage, dispensing, administration, and monitoring would be included. On the other hand, a health maintenance organization would consider all inpatient and outpatient charges and costs related to the entire episode of care for which it is likely to be held financially responsible. An insurance company would be most interested in the episode-of-care charges covered under the terms of the insurance policy. From a societal perspective, all direct and indirect medical and nonmedical costs would be included.

In this case, the analysis must be structured, on behalf of the P&T committee, from the hospital's perspective. Since the survival outcome is equal with the two options, the committee wants to select the option that minimizes costs to the hospital. Therefore, from the hospital's perspective, the decision analysis should include, in addition to the drug-related costs, the costs of all hospital goods and services during the hospitalization period. However, since the P&T committee already has decided to add one of the drugs to the hospital formulary, it is not necessary to calculate the non–drug-related costs of an uncomplicated, 10-day hospital stay for intravenous treatment of similar gram-negative infections because they are the same for both alphazorin and omegazorin. Rather, the additional direct costs associated with the drugs and the consequences of their respective therapies will be included: drug acquisition, storage, and dispensing; drug administration; and additional monitoring and laboratory costs, hospital stay, and pharmacokinetic and infectious disease consultations due to bacterial resistance, adverse toxic or subtherapeutic consequences of the antibiotic, or misclassification errors of the serum drug concentrations.

WHAT IS THE DECISION, ITS OPTIONS, AND THE DECISION CRITERIA?

In addition to new drugs being considered, pharmacoeconomic standards encourage the analyst to include the present standard of care as a comparator. However, in this teaching case, the P&T committee has decided to add one member of the new antibiotic class to its formulary. Therefore, the question to address is: Which of the two antibiotics will be added to the formulary? The decision tree will be constructed and the analysis performed to answer this question. The decision options are alphazorin and omegazorin.

What decision criterion is to be used to select between the two antibiotics? The criterion is linked to the type of analysis to be performed. If cost and lives saved are selected, it would be a cost-effectiveness study; if cost and utilities are measured, it would be a cost-utility assessment. All of the previously described pharmacoeconomic analyses can use the steps and structure of clinical decision analysis; only the unit of outcome measurement would differ.

For this illustrative example, the *decision analysis process* has been simplified by considering only economic costs. As stated earlier, this simplifying assumption is that, although the efficacy of the two drugs differs, the overall episode-of-care survival rates are equal. When an organism is resistant to either alphazorin or omegazorin, the course of therapy is switched to the restricted antibiotic betasporin, resulting in equal effectiveness (survival) in the overall episode of care. Therefore, because the committee's selected measure of outcome effectiveness is equal in both options, this analysis is a cost-minimization study and only economic costs will be considered as the outcome measure. If noneconomic outcomes were not equal, then outcomes expressed in units of effectiveness or utilities also would need to be measured.

To standardize the analysis, gram-negative septicemia should be selected as the base case since it is representative of the type of infections to be treated with these antibiotics. Thus, the decision criterion is clarified: given equal survival rates, the analysis will direct the decision-maker to the antibiotic that results in the lower expected cost for treatment of this septicemia.

Decision analysis uses the structure of a *decision tree* to organize the elements involved in the decision. A decision tree starts with the choice alternatives. In the "scientific notation" of decision analysis, a *choice node* (a square) indicates a point in time when the decision-maker can select one of several options or actions. The initial choice node, also called the *root node*, is placed at the far left and designates the beginning of the decision tree; the possible options (alphazorin and omegazorin) then originate as *branches* to the right of this initial choice node. This tree will provide an explicit structure for this cost-minimization study. The start of the decision tree is displayed in Figure 2.

Following the selected decision criterion, the branch option with the lower expected cost will be the antibiotic selected for addition to the formulary.

OVER WHAT TIME SPAN WILL THE ANALYSIS APPLY?

Generally, an analysis is performed over a finite period of time (eg, one week, one month, one year). However, when pa-

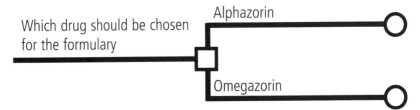

Figure 2. Initial choice (root) node of decision tree to choose between alphazorin and omegazorin for addition to hospital formulary.

tients with a condition are treated for varying periods of time, another approach is to use the length of the treatment as the period of time. This variable time approach, or episode of care, is the period span over which this analysis is conducted. The decision analysis begins with the initiation of either antibiotic to treat gram-negative septicemia (simplifying assumption: analysis limited to culture-confirmed cases) and ends with resolution of the infection.

Developing a Decision Tree

STRUCTURE THE DECISION AND ITS CONSEQUENCES OVER TIME

The structure of the tree is one of the most powerful features of decision analysis. The decision-maker is forced to explicitly structure the situation, thus changing the unexamined, intuitive process into one in which the thought process is made explicit. In laying out the tree prods, the decision-maker identifies the relationships that exist between the decision options and the consequences of selecting each alternative. The tree becomes a tool to assist in thinking through a decision, as well as to assist in communication among individuals and departments working on the same analysis. With a decision tree, coworkers can identify where they agree or disagree in the considered alternatives and consequences, suggest additional consequences that must be included in the tree, or recommend that a branch be trimmed.

Given the decision options originating from the initial choice node, the consequences of each action now must be determined. These consequences are chronologically structured over time in a decision tree by asking a series of "what if" questions. This section structures the decision tree and details the consequences of the actions.

The alphazorin branch of the decision tree is presented in Figure 3; the omegazorin portion appears in Figure 4. This structure may be used as a template to insert probabilities converted from results of a clinical trial, assign cost outcomes to each consequence, and calculate the preferred course of action.

What if patients with septicemia are given alphazorin? First, the outcome at this branch is no longer under the control of the decision-maker; some patients will respond and some will not. A *chance node*, indicated by a circle, is inserted in the appropriate branch and notes the point in time when the decision-maker loses control of the decision process. This indicates that future events are beyond the control of the decision-maker and the outcome is uncertain. In this case, the chance node is inserted in both the alphazorin and omegazorin branches, and the responding/nonresponding consequences or branches are identified (nodes A and M, respectively).

In the responding branch of the alphazorin tree, if the fever recedes and the laboratory results indicate response to the antibiotic, the balance of the 10-day course of therapy may continue uneventfully or the patient may develop toxicity (node B). Three principal types of toxic reactions occur (node C): GI effects such as

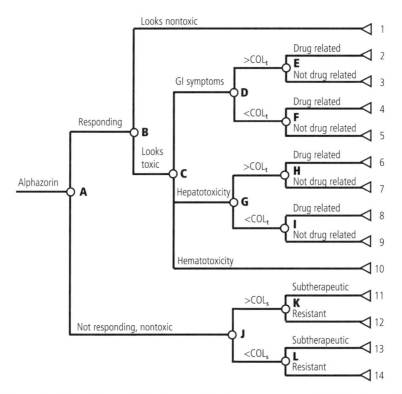

Figure 3. Alphazorin branch of decision tree showing consequences of selecting alphazorin, chance nodes identified, and decision paths numbered. COL$_s$ = subtherapeutic cutoff level; COL$_t$ = toxic cutoff level; GI = gastrointestinal.

nausea, vomiting, and diarrhea, which usually occur on day 2 of therapy; hepatotoxicity, with elevated liver function enzymes and reduced liver function (day 3), and hematotoxicity (day 5).

However, not all toxic symptoms in these patients are related to the antibiotic; rather, they can be associated with other medications or related to the nature of the patient's underlying illness. Serum drug concentrations provide additional information as to whether the toxicity is drug related. Therefore, a chance node with two branches follows each of the indicated toxicities—either the concentration is above or below the toxic cutoff level (COL$_t$). This occurs at nodes D and G in Figure 3 and nodes P and S in Figure 4.

It is rare when a test clearly separates one patient population from another; generally, there are areas of overlap.[9] As shown in Figure 5, three patient classifications are associated with serum drug concentrations: subtherapeutic, therapeutic, or toxic. How-

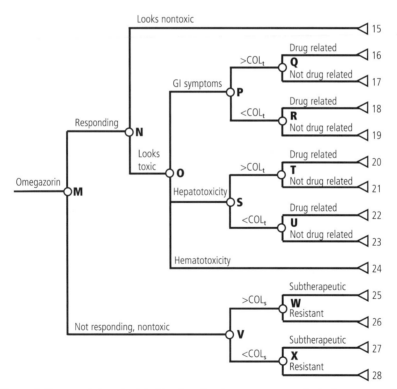

Figure 4. Omegazorin branch of decision tree showing consequences of selecting omegazorin, chance nodes identified, and decision paths numbered. COL$_s$ = subtherapeutic cutoff level; COL$_t$ = toxic cutoff level; GI = gastrointestinal.

ever, setting a COL_t and a subtherapeutic cutoff level (COL_s) does not clearly separate these three classifications, and classification errors will occur. Referring to the COL_t, most of the concentrations above it are associated with drug-related toxicities (true positive in Figure 5), but some patients with non–drug-related toxic symptoms also have high concentrations (false positive). Most concentrations below the COL_t are associated with a therapeutic response (true negative), but there are some patients who have concentrations below the COL_t who do have drug-related toxicities (false negative). The same overlap and resultant misclassification errors also occur between the subtherapeutic and therapeutic classifications.

Therefore, to display both the correct and incorrect classifications based on the COL_t, a chance node with drug- and non–drug-related toxicity branches follow, all greater than COL_t (nodes E, H, Q, and T in Figures 3 and 4, respectively) and less than COL_t (nodes F, I, T, and U in Figures 3 and 4, respectively). Additional consequences occur at many of these branches; for example, the misclassification of concentration below the COL_t as non-drug related when the symptoms really are associated with drug toxicity can lead to continuation of the antibiotic, development of more serious adverse effects, and longer hospital stays. To simplify the decision tree, such additional consequences are not further detailed as branches in this case, but are considered explicitly in the cost-implication section.

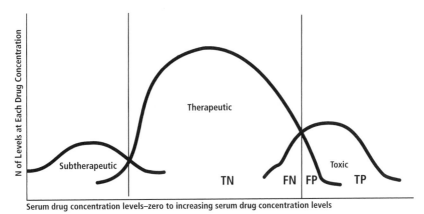

Figure 5. Frequency of patients whose response is subtherapeutic, therapeutic, and toxic. FN = false negative; FP = false positive; TN = true negative; TP = true positive.

In the "not responding" branch of the decision tree, serum drug concentrations are used to distinguish between two patient populations: those with bacterial infections that are susceptible to the antibiotic but who are receiving inadequate dosages, resulting in subtherapeutic concentrations, and those with bacterial infections that are resistant to the antibiotic. Again, the concentration is used to differentiate between the populations, but misclassification errors can also occur when the COL_s is applied.

In the subpopulation of nonresponding patients, most concentrations above the COL_s are from patients with resistant organisms; however, some are from patients who, while the concentration is above the COL_s, have subtherapeutic responses (nodes K and W). Rather than receiving the needed dosage adjustment, the antibiotic will be changed unnecessarily, thereby increasing the hospital stay and inducing additional charges. On the other hand, most patients with concentrations below the COL_s have susceptible infections and the dosage needs to be increased (nodes L and X). However, patients with low concentrations and resistant organisms are placed at risk because, rather than switching to a more appropriate antibiotic, the dosage is increased in response to the low drug concentration and the course of ineffective therapy is lengthened.

The alphazorin and omegazorin sections of the decision tree, with all options and drug selection consequences chronologically arranged from left to right, are now complete. All decisions under the control of the decision-maker are indicated by choice nodes; all outcomes left to chance and beyond the control of the decision-maker are indicated by chance nodes. For each drug selection, there are 14 possible courses of care or decision paths (indicated by a number on the right side of each path). A *decision path* is a sequence of actions and events beginning with the decision at the initial choice node and chronologically following the consequences of that decision in a unique line from left to right through subsequent chance and/or choice nodes.

Although the inclusion of serum drug concentrations and the interpretation of whether the results indicate drug or non–drug-related toxicities add to the complexity of this decision tree, they explicitly must be recognized as elements of the complete decision process. To assume that all toxic symptoms are drug related or that all concentrations above the COL_t are toxic introduces error into the pharmacoeconomic analysis. It is important to recognize that clinical decision analyses that incorporate diagnostic tests also must include the possibility that the test results do not cleanly separate patients with disease from those without disease. A good exercise is to examine a published pharmacoeconomic assessment and translate it into the decision tree format. Most likely the consequences of the decision are not completely specified, and if diagnostic tests are included in the management of the disease, the uncertainty associated with them is not factored into the decision process.

The consequences of selecting alphazorin or omegazorin are represented by the same structure. If the consequences are the same, why are the two antibiotics not considered equal? First, the likelihood or probability of occurrence of each of the consequences differs between the two drugs; second, the cost of the antibiotics, as well as the cost of each decision path, differs. These issues are examined in the following two sections.

ASSESS PROBABILITIES

At each chance node, there is a 100 percent probability that something will happen, but how does one determine how often each possibility is likely to occur? Published clinical trials, Phase III trial data from the manufacturers or other sources of data are sources for this information.

However, for this teaching case, the results of a large, randomized, blinded clinical trial (fictional) comparing alphazorin and omegazorin in a population of patients with gram-negative septicemia are presented. The probabilities associated with the various consequences for each antibiotic have been calculated from this trial: half of the patients received alphazorin and the other half omegazorin. The first 1,000 patients with gram-negative bacteria confirmed by culture receiving alphazorin comprise the alphazorin probability data set. The same method was used for the omegazorin probability estimates. The patient conditions and consequences in the clinical trial are representative of the patients at a hospital selecting one of these agents. The outcome results of the 2,000 patients are summarized in Table 2.

The sum of the probabilities of all consequences originating from a chance node must be 1.0; therefore, it is essential that all possible consequences be identified at each chance node. Because there is a 100 percent certainty that something will happen at each chance node, nodes with probabilities totaling less than 1.0 do not have all consequences identified and, thus, have been incompletely specified. The probabilities associated with each branch originating from a chance node are displayed adjacent to the respective branch in Figures 6 and 7.

Of the 1,000 patients receiving alphazorin, 850 (85 percent) responded with a reduction in temperature and change in hemato-

Table 2. Outcomes of Patients Receiving Alphazorin and Omegazorin

OUTCOME	NO. OF PATIENTS	PATH NO.
Alphazorin (n = 1,000)		
Responding	850	
no toxic symptoms	680	1
symptoms resembling toxicity	170	
gastrointestinal toxicity	131	
>COL_t	81	
drug related	65	2
not drug related	16	3
<COL_t	50	
drug related	5	4
not drug related	45	5
hepatotoxicity	35	
>COL_t	16	
drug related	13	6
not drug related	3	7
<COL_t	19	
drug related	2	8
not drug related	17	9
hematotoxicity	4	10
Not responding	150	
>COL_s	50	
subtherapeutic	10	11
resistant	40	12
<COL_s	100	
subtherapeutic	90	13
resistant	10	14

COL_s = subtherapuetic cutoff level; COL_t = toxic cutoff level.

(continued on page 191)

logic parameters and 150 (15 percent) did not respond. The probabilities of response/nonresponse are entered in the decision tree on the two branches originating from the alphazorin branch at the first chance node (node A). Of the 850 responding patients, 680 (80 percent) had no toxic symptoms and 170 (20 percent) had possible drug-related toxicities (node B). Of the 170 patients with toxic symptoms, 131 (77 percent) experienced GI toxicity, 35 (20.6 percent) had elevated liver function enzymes suggestive of drug-related hepatotoxicity, and 4 (2.4 percent) had a marked reduction in platelet function (node C).

OUTCOME	NO. OF PATIENTS	PATH NO.
Omegazorin (n = 1,000)		
Responding	730	
no toxic symptoms	495	15
symptoms resembling toxicity	235	
gastrointestinal toxicity	164	
$>COL_t$	102	
drug related	91	16
not drug related	11	17
$<COL_t$	62	
drug related	11	18
not drug related	51	19
hepatotoxicity	56	
$>COL_t$	36	
drug related	32	20
not drug related	4	21
$<COL_t$	20	
drug related	3	22
not drug related	17	23
hematotoxicity	15	24
Not responding	270	
$>COL_s$	110	
subtherapeutic	10	25
resistant	100	26
$<COL_s$	160	
subtherapeutic	140	27
resistant	20	28

Table 2. Outcomes of Patients Receiving Alphazorin and Omegazorin (continued)

COL_s = subtherapeutic cutoff level; COL_t = toxic cutoff level.

Serum alphazorin concentrations were determined in all patients with toxic symptoms. Eighty-one of 131 patients (62 percent) with GI symptoms had serum drug concentrations above the COL_t (node D). At node G, 16 of 35 patients (45.7 percent) with hepatotoxicity had concentrations above the COL_t, and 4 of 4 patients with hematotoxicity had concentrations above that level. However, as discussed earlier, the COL_t cannot be used to clearly identify patients with and without drug-related toxicities.

Measures of a test's predictive ability, predictive value–positive (PV^+) and predictive value–negative (PV^-), can be helpful. PV^+ answers the question: Given a positive test result, what is the probability that the patient has the disease? For tests involving therapeutic drug monitoring, the question translates to: Given a concentration above the COL_t, what is the probability that the concentration is from a patient who has drug-related

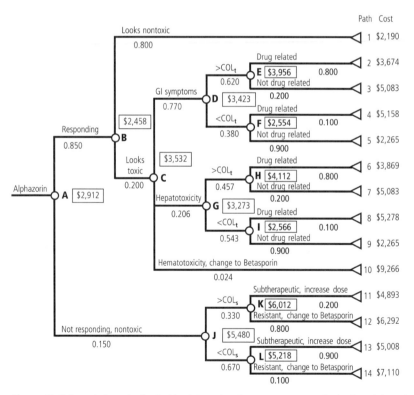

Figure 6. Alphazorin branch of rolled-back tree showing consequences of selecting alphazorin, chance nodes, cost of each path, and expected costs at node. COL_s = subtherapeutic cutoff level; COL_t = toxic cutoff level; GI = gastrointestinal.

toxicity? For serum alphazorin concentrations, the PV⁺ is 80 percent (nodes E and H). Conversely, the probability that a concentration above the COL_t is from a patient whose toxicity is not drug related is presented by the mathematical expression 1 — PV⁺, or 20 percent for alphazorin.

Similarly, the PV⁻ answers the question: Given a negative test result, what is the probability that the patient does not have the disease? For therapeutic drug monitoring, that question translates to: Given a concentration below the COL_t, what is the probability that the concentration is from a patient who does not have drug-related toxicity? For serum alphazorin concentrations, the PV⁻ is 90 percent. The probability that a concentration below the COL_t is from a patient with a drug-related toxicity is 1 — PV⁻, or 10 percent (nodes F and I).

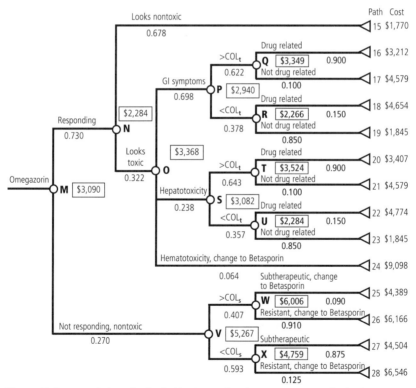

Figure 7. Omegazorin branch of rolled-back tree showing consequences of selecting omegazorin, chance nodes, cost of each path, and expected costs at node. COL_s = subtherapeutic cutoff level; COL_t = toxic cutoff level; GI = gastrointestinal.

In the nonresponding population, 100 of 150 patients (67 percent) had serum drug concentrations below the COL_s; the remaining 50 (33 percent) had results above the COL_s (node J). At this lower cut-off level, the PV⁺ is the proportion of concentrations below the COL_s that are from patients receiving a therapeutic dosage but who have a subtherapeutic response (90 percent for alphazorin). Ten percent of results below the COL_s are associated with resistant organisms (node L). PV⁻ is the proportion of concentrations above the COL_s that are from patients with resistant organisms, or 80 percent for alphazorin. The remaining 20 percent are from patients whose concentrations are above the COL_s and need a higher dosage to obtain a therapeutic response (node K).

Different probabilities are associated with the population receiving omegazorin (Figure 7). Fewer of the causative organisms were susceptible to this drug (88 percent vs 95 percent), and there was a higher incidence of drug-related toxicity (15 percent vs 8.9 percent). Of the 1,000 patients receiving this medication, 730 (73 percent) responded (node M); 495 of these (67.8 percent) had no toxic symptoms, while 235 (32.2 percent) did (node N). Of the patients with possible toxicity, 164 (69.8 percent) had GI symptoms, 56 (23.8 percent) had elevated liver function enzymes, and 15 (6.4 percent) had marked platelet dysfunction (node O).

At nodes Q and T, 90 percent of the results above omegazorin's COL_t are from patients with drug-related toxicities (PV⁺ = 0.90), and at nodes R and U, 85 percent of results below the COL_t are from patients without drug-related toxicities (PV⁻ = 0.85). In the nonresponding population, of the 59.3 percent with results below COL_s, 140 of 160 patients (87.5 percent) are receiving an insufficient dosage and 12.5 percent have resistant organisms (node X). Of the 110 patients (40.7 percent) with results above the COL_s, 100 (91 percent) are associated with resistant organisms and 9 percent with subtherapeutic responses (node W).

The information presented in Table 2 is useful for translating clinical data into probabilities for various chance nodes to determine and insert probabilities into Figures 3 and 4 and then compare the probabilities with those in Figures 6 and 7. The antibiotic's susceptibility rate cannot be entered at the "responding" nodes (A and M) because some patients with susceptible organisms did not initally respond due to subtherapeutic amounts of the antibiotic (J and V). When these drug concentrations are increased, the patients respond and contribute to the overall susceptibility rates of 95 percent for alphazorin and 88 percent for omegazorin.

The probabilities at each node must be calculated based on the appropriate subpopulation. The probabilities for each subsequent node in a decision tree are based on a subset of the population coming into that node; these are called *conditional* probabilities. For example, at node A, the probabilities are based on all 1,000 patients. However, at node B, the probabilities are based only on the 850 patients who advance to node B; the probabilities at node B are conditioned upon the patients who initially responded to alphazorin. When performing other decision analyses, one must determine upon what population a probability is conditioned: Is a value of 15 percent adverse effects based on 15 percent of the original population, 15 percent of the successfully treated patients, or 15 percent of some other subpopulation?

One final cautionary note should be raised about probabilities and other data from clinical trials that are incorporated into pharmacoeconomic studies in general and decision analyses in particular. The probabilities used in this example come from an ideal, fictional database, one rarely found in the clinical literature. However, this example, as well as data from most published clinical trials that are incorporated into pharmacoeconomic analyses, heavily rely upon results from *efficacy* trials (can it work?) that are conducted under strict experimental control. Efficacy trials are not representative of general clinical practice when *effectiveness* (does it work?), not efficacy, is established. In efficacy trials, patients with comorbidities frequently are excluded, tertiary care site and clinical specialists provide the care, and adherence is encouraged and tightly monitored. Results from efficacy trials may not be directly applicable to routine practice with general practitioners or patients with comorbidities, as well as when adherence may not be optimal.[10] As most clinical decisions are based on the cost and consequences of effective rather than efficacious care, it is essential that the collection of this type of patient outcome probability information becomes routine practice. An accurate cost-impact assessment is not possible unless it is linked to the probabilities of clinical consequences. Until pharmacoepidemiologic data are available, literature reports and meta-analyses of randomized clinical trials are the preferred source of probability estimates. Expert opinions, Delphi techniques, and methods of probability estimation are less reliable.[11,12]

VALUE OUTCOMES

To value the economic outcomes, the monetary value of drug, drug-related, and drug-induced costs per case of septicemia must be determined. The drug costs include the direct expenses of drug acquisition and storage: a 10-day course costs $1,650 for alphazorin and $1,050 for omegazorin. Drug-related costs consist of an $18 direct cost each time either drug is administrated. Alphazorin is administered every eight hours, resulting in a cost of $540 for 10 days of therapy; omegazorin is administered every six hours, costing $720 for the same length of therapy. When a change of therapy is indicated because of suspected bacterial resistance, a 10-day course of intravenous betasporin is initiated, resulting in $1,800 in drug and $360 in drug-related costs.

Drug-induced costs are expenses incurred from the follow-up created by less-than-optimal response to either alphazorin or omegazorin. These costs, calculated by the input component method and incorporating direct expenses, include $1,000 per extra day of hospital stay, additional laboratory tests ($75/serum drug concentration, $65/liver function enzyme tests, $60/platelet count), component therapy ($360/packed red blood cell transfusion and platelet concentrate), $115 per pharmacokinetic consult, and $400 per infectious disease and hematology consultations.

The costs of drug, drug-related, and drug-induced inputs required for each decision path in the alphazorin section of the decision tree are summarized in Table 3 and, for the omegazorin tree, in Table 4. The path costs are entered at the right of each path on the decision trees in Figures 5 and 6.

CHOOSE THE PREFERRED COURSE OF ACTION—CALCULATE THE EXPECTED COST FOR EACH DECISION OUTCOME

How does one combine the various decision options, probability estimates, and outcome valuations to choose the preferred course of action? How does one "solve" a decision tree?

First, it is necessary to break the decision tree into its component parts and analyze smaller sections. This is done in reverse order of the tree's development, starting from the right and working back to the initial decision or choice node on the left. The process is called *averaging out and folding back* since each path's outcome value is weighted by its probability of occurrence (averaging out) working from right to left, from outcomes to options (folding back).

At each chance node, outcome values (costs) are combined with and weighted by their respective probability of occurring. This yields an expected cost at each chance node. For illustration, a section of the alphazorin limb of the decision tree (paths 2–5) is reproduced in Figure 8. Starting on the top right with patients who have GI symptoms and drug concentrations above the COL_t, 80 percent will have alphazorin-related toxicity with an associated average cost of treatment of $3,674. However, 20 percent of the patients with high concentrations will not have drug-related toxicity; their dosage will be reduced unnecessarily, resulting in an average cost of $5,083 for path 3. To calculate the expected cost of patients with GI symptoms and with alphazorin concentrations above the COL_t (node E), the cost of each outcome is weighted by the probability of its occurrence and then added to the weighted costs of all other outcomes originating from the same chance node. The expected cost at each chance node appears in a bubble attached to the respective node in the tree.

$$(80 \text{ percent} \times \$3,674) + (20 \text{ percent} \times \$5,083) = \$3,956$$

For patients with GI symptoms and concentrations below the COL_t, 90 percent of the symptoms were non-drug related at a cost of $2,265. However, 10 percent of these concentrations will be from patients with drug-related toxicity. Their dosage will be continued, leading to additional toxicity and extended hospitalizations at an average cost of $5,158. The expected costs of patients with GI symptoms whose concentrations are below the COL_t (node F) are calculated as follows:

$$(10 \text{ percent} \times \$5,158) + (90 \text{ percent} \times \$2,265) = \$2,554$$

The next step back to the origin, or left, of the tree requires determination of the average expected cost of all patients with GI symptoms. At the next chance node, the expected costs of patients with serum drug concentrations above and below the COL_t are combined with their respective probability of occurring. There is a 62 percent probability that the concentration

Table 3. Outcome Costs ($) Associated with Consequences of Alphazorin-Treated Septicemia

PATH	CLINICAL CONDITION AND TREATMENT	DRUG	DRUG-RELATED	DRUG-INDUCED					TOTAL
				1[a]	2[b]	3[c]	4[d]	5[e]	
1	Uncomplicated response	1,650	540						2,190
2	GI symptoms, >COL$_t$, drug related, dosage adjusted	1,815	594	1,000	150		115		3,674
3	GI symptoms, >COL$_t$, non–drug related, dosage reduced unnecessarily, then readjusted	1,980	648	2,000	225		230		5,083
4	GI symptoms, <COL$_t$, drug related, delay in dosage adjustment	1,980	648	2,000	300		230		5,158
5	GI symptoms, <COL$_t$, non–drug related, therapy continued	1,650	540		75				2,265
6	Hepatotoxicity, >COL$_t$, drug related liver toxicity, dosage adjusted	1,815	594	1,000	150	195	115		3,869
7	Hepatotoxicity, >COL$_t$, non–drug related, dosage reduced unnecessarily, then readjusted	1,980	648	2,000	225		230		5,083
8	Hepatotoxicity, <COL$_t$, drug related, delay in dosage adjustment	1,650	540	2,000	150	270	230		5,278
9	Hepatotoxicity, <COL$_t$, non–drug related, therapy continued	1,650	540		75				2,265
10	Drug related hematotoxicity, drug switched (4 days of alphazorin, 10 days of betasporin)	2,460	576	4,000		1,200	230	800	9,266
11	Not responding, >COL$_s$, subtherapeutic response, organism sensitive, drug increased	1,980	648	2,000	150		115		4,893
12	Not responding, >COL$_s$, resistant, drug switched (3 days of alphazorin, 10 days of betasporin)	2,295	522	3,000	75			400	6,292
13	Not responding, <COL$_s$, subtherapeutic response, organism sensitive, dosage increased	1,980	648	2,000	150		230		5,008
14	Not responding, <COL$_s$, resistant, switch to betasporin (3 days of alphazorin, 10 days of betasporin)	2,625	630	3,000	225		230	400	7,110

COL$_s$ = subtherapeutic cutoff level; COL$_t$ = toxic cutoff level; GI = gastrointestinal.
[a] Extra hospital day, $1,000/day.
[b] Drug concentration, $75 each.
[c] Extra laboratory costs including component therapy.
[d] Pharmacokinetic consultation, $115 each.
[e] Hematology or infectious disease consultation, $400.

Table 4. Outcome Costs ($) Associated with Consequences of Omegazorin-Treated Septicemia

PATH	CLINICAL CONDITION AND TREATMENT	DRUG	DRUG-RELATED	DRUG-INDUCED					TOTAL
				1[a]	2[b]	3[c]	4[d]	5[e]	
15	Uncomplicated response	1,050	720						1,770
16	GI symptoms, >COL_t, drug related, dosage adjusted	1,155	792	1,000	150		115		3,212
17	GI symptoms, >COL_t, non–drug related, dosage reduced unnecessarily, then readjusted	1,260	864	2,000	225		230		4,579
18	GI symptoms, <COL_t, drug related, delay in dosage adjustment	1,260	864	2,000	300		230		4,654
19	GI symptoms, <COL_t, non–drug related, therapy continued	1,050	720		75				1,845
20	Hepatotoxicity, >COL_t, drug related liver toxicity, dosage adjusted	1,155	792	1,000	150	195	115		3,407
21	Hepatotoxicity, >COL_t, non–drug related, dosage reduced unnecessarily, then readjusted	1,260	864	2,000	225		230		4,579
22	Hepatotoxicity, <COL_t, drug related, delay in dosage adjustment	1,260	864	2,000	150	270	230		4,774
23	Hepatotoxicity, <COL_t, non–drug related, therapy continued	1,050	720		75				1,845
24	Drug-related hematotoxicity, drug switched (4 days of omegazorin, 10 days of betasporin)	2,220	648	4,000		1,200	230	800	9,098
25	Not responding, >COL_s, subtherapeutic response, organism sensitive, drug increased	1,260	864	2,000	150		115		4,389
26	Not responding, >COL_s, resistant, drug switched (3 days of omegazorin, 10 days of betasporin)	2,115	576	3,000	75			400	6,166
27	Not responding, <COL_s, subtherapeutic response, organism sensitive, dosage increased	1,260	864	2,000	150		230		4,504
28	Not responding, <COL_s, resistant, switch to betasporin (3 days of omegazorin, 10 days of betasporin)	2,115	576	3,000	225		230	400	6,546

COL_s = subtherapeutic cutoff level; COL_t = toxic cutoff level; GI = gastrointestinal.
[a] Extra hospital day, $1,000/day.
[b] Drug concentration, $75 each.
[c] Extra laboratory costs including component therapy.
[d] Pharmacokinetic consultation, $115 each.
[e] Hematology or infectious disease consultation, $400.

will be above the COL$_t$; that condition has an expected cost of $3,956. There also is a 38 percent probability that the concentration will be below the COL$_t$, with an expected cost of $2,554. Therefore, the expected cost of all patients with GI symptoms (node D) is

(62 percent × $3,956) + (38 percent × $2,554) = $3,423

The averaging out and folding back process continues until the expected costs are determined for the two branches originating from the initial choice node. These have been calculated and appear in Figures 6 and 7. The expected cost per patient of the alphazorin option is $2,912 and of the omegazorin option is $3,090. Thus, although the acquisition price of omegazorin is about $600 lower per patient than that of alphazorin, the institutional costs associated with omegazorin's higher resistance rate and increased drug-related toxicities augment omegazorin's total septicemia treatment costs to be more than those of alphazorin. If the P&T committee had based its decision on the lower acquisition cost, it would have selected omegazorin with the higher overall treatment cost. That decision would have reduced the cost impact on the pharmacy budget, but would have created higher overall costs for the hospital. By using decision analysis and adopting an institutional perspective that included the cost consequences, not just acquisition costs, of the two antibiotics, the committee can make a drug selection decision that will reduce the impact on institutional expenses. This analysis should be used to argue that, in this treatment decision, an increase in

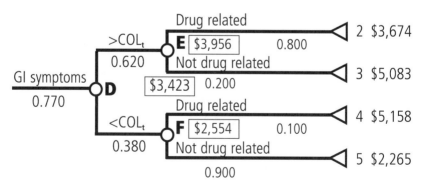

Figure 8. Section of alphazorin portion of decision tree. COL$_t$ = toxic cutoff level; GI = gastrointestinal.

the pharmacy's drug acquisition budget will result in a savings to the institution.

From the identification of the decision options, time frame, decision criteria, and objectives of the decision-maker through the structuring of the decision and identification of all consequences to probability assessment and outcome valuation, the selection now has had an explicit, structured, analytic, and quantitative assessment with a preferred action course identified: alphazorin should be added to the formulary.

Controversies in the Use of Decision Analytic Modeling in Pharmacoeconomic Studies

While decision analysis provided a useful approach and structure to the alphazorin/omegazorin case, controversies exist in the use of decision analytic modeling in pharmacoeconomic studies. The same controversies exist in the application of any retrospective pharmacoeconomic analysis—they are simply more visible in decision analysis because of the explicit and quantitative nature of the methodology and its decision tree.

These controversies have their roots in two very different approaches to pharmacoeconomic investigation: randomized clinical trials (RCTs) and modeling. Some have called it a clash of two cultures. The argument for the inclusion of cost studies within RCTs is that only the RCT can generate the type of true knowledge, free from bias and based on hypothesis testing, that is needed for advancement. On the other hand, the modeling proponents recognize "the necessity of various types of analytical models to enrich and broaden results from experimental research when it is available and to find substitutes for experimental data when it is not available."[13]

Even if all pharmacoeconomic analyses were derived from add-ons to RCTs, they still would have problems and not be directly applicable to clinical practices. O'Brien[10] identified seven threats to validity (several discussed earlier in the teaching case) when the economic evaluations of pharmaceuticals are added to RCTs, the primary purpose of which is to establish clinical efficacy. Several of these are inappropriate choice of comparison therapy and outcomes, inadequate time period and patient follow-up, excessive costs associated with the RCT protocol, and selected patient and provider populations. Although decision analysis is not perfect, O'Brien recommends the approach of "pulling together the many needed pieces of information from multiple sources and then stitching them together into a (hopefully) cohesive whole 'Frankenstein model.'"

Modeling in general, and decision analytic modeling in particular, can represent the real, non-RCT world with a decision tree and a synthesis of data from multiple disparate sources for approximations of effectiveness, consequences, and outcomes. Weinstein et al.[14] defines a healthcare evaluation model as "an analytic methodology that accounts for events over time and across populations that is based on data drawn from primary and/or secondary sources, and whose purpose is to estimate the effects of an intervention on valued health consequences and costs." When decisions need to be made before comprehensive data are available, a decision analytic model, incorporating the options and their consequences over time for the selected population, is the more efficient and effective method to assist the decision-making process. However, concern exists that investigators may introduce bias or even conflict of interest into decision analytic models. Many factors in the structure of and assumptions behind the model may influence the outcome. The selection of the decision options for consideration (Is the most current treatment option included?), the perspective of the analysis (Is it from the point of view of a third-party payer, an employer, or society?), the time period (Is it long enough to capture the adverse events?), whether patient adherence is included, and the outcome variables (biologic markers, cure, years saved, quality-adjusted life-years), as well as the underlying assumptions throughout the model, can be variables that influence the preferred option.

These concerns have led to worldwide interest in standardizing modeled analyses and the development of guidelines, consensus conferences, and modeling frameworks: the InterPORT Group,[15] the Panel on Cost-Effectiveness in Health and Medicine,[16] Consensus Conference on Guidelines on Economic Modelling in Health Technology Assessment,[17] and the International Society for Pharmacoeconomics and Outcomes Research (ISPOR) Task Force on Good Research Practices—Modeling Studies.[14] The validity of the decision analysis can be improved, and the potential for bias and conflict of interest can be reduced, by incorporating these guidelines into the design and conduct of pharmacoeconomic analyses, particularly decision analytic models.

For new decision analysts, the primary message from these guidelines is to be transparent in the design, structure, conduct, and reporting of the analysis. The assumptions behind the modeling approach and the values incorporated into the model should be fully described. Sufficient information should be included so that another person could replicate the study based on the information provided with the analysis. As always, the analysis should be explicit and transparent.

Applications of Clinical Decision Analysis in Pharmacoeconomic Studies

Decision analysis has been used to provide pharmacoeconomic information for a wide variety of clinical cases and health policy questions. To examine a representative sample of the published literature, we conducted a cross-sectional search of articles published in 2002. Using the terms "decision analysis," "decision analytic," "drug," and "cost," we identified 42 decision analytic pharmacoeconomic articles[18-59] indexed in the National Library of Medicine database. These studies cover a wide range of clinical issues—from treatment of constipation[21] and psoriasis[24] to whether to test, test then treat, or initially treat all patients for influenza,[18,48] kala-azar,[19] sore throat,[23] or possible *Helicobacter pylori* infection.[27,35,39] Other studies compare prevention strategies for rheumatic heart disease,[23] pelvic inflammatory disease,[28] influenza,[30,37] active tuberculosis,[33] venous thromboembolism,[36] gastric hemorrhage,[40] cirrhosis,[41] pulmonary embolism,[46] sudden cardiac death,[50] urinary tract infection,[52] or bacterial arthritis.[55]

While most are modeled studies and use data from many sources, some rely upon data derived from specific multicenter and international[21,29,34,36,42,50,54,57] or local[52] RCTs. Six used Markov models.[26,32,43,44,46,47] Some studies were conducted to support recommendations to justify local administrative changes (high-intensity hepatitis C clinic),[22] while others were performed to clarify national treatment policies (leishmania in Africa,[19] duodenal ulcer in India,[27] latent tuberculosis in the United States,[33] rheumatoid arthritis in Norway,[34] smoking cessation strategies in England,[49] malaria in South Africia,[58] and arthritis in Hong Kong[59]).

What are appropriate types of questions for decision analyses? If head-to-head randomized trials of decision comparators have not been conducted, a decision analytic model, based on other sources of data, can be used to structure such a comparison and include economic outcomes of interest. If RCTs have not included economic outcomes, then decision analysis can be used to structure the data from the RCT and include cost estimate information. Spath and O'Brien[50] compared results from modeled and trial-based analyses of the cost-effectiveness of implantable cardioverter defibrillator (ICD) therapy versus drug therapy for patients at high risk of sudden cardiac death. In this clinical condition, their study suggests that the five early, modeled, cost-effectiveness analyses based on observational data led to cost-effectiveness ratios for ICD that were much less than those obtained from data from four more recent prospective RCTs. Further comparisons of pharmacoeconomic studies based on modeled and RCT-based analyses are needed.

Brennan and Akehurst[60] summarized the major roles for decision analytic modeling in health economic evaluations. In a background paper for a 1999 Consensus Conference on Decision Analytic Modeling in Economic Evaluation of Health Technologies, they concluded that appropriate applications include:

1. extending results from a single RCT to relevant comparators: used to model the decision compared with "normal care" or "best alternative care" rather than the placebo comparator of the RCT;

2. extrapolating outcomes to the longer term: used when the decision requires a longer period of comparison than present in available RCTs;

3. translating from intermediate to final outcomes: used to model the extension of clinical physiologic or functional results to meaningful final outcomes such as survival, life-years extended, or quality-adjusted life-years;

4. generalizing from highly selective RCT populations to general populations: used to adjust RCT efficacy results derived from selected subpopulations, tightly controlled protocols, drug administration, and monitoring procedures to the effectiveness conditions of a general population.

The 42 articles cited above are a rich reference source for examination of the decision analytic literature. It would be useful to obtain a copy of one of these articles and perform a literature critique based on the following questions:

1. What are the decision options? Are all appropriate options considered, including usual care?
2. To what population are the results to be generalized? Is that population appropriate given the sources of data included in the analyses?
3. From what perspective is the analysis conducted? Who is the decision-maker, and is the perspective appropriate for the decision analytic question?
4. What is the time frame of the analysis? Is it of sufficient length to capture all important consequences? What side effects and adverse drug effects are included in the analysis? Is patient medication adherence structured into the analysis?
5. From what sources are the probabilities derived? Are the sources appropriate for the population being considered?
6. What costs are included in the analysis? Are they appropriate and complete given the perspective of the analysis?
7. What outcomes are included in the analysis? Are they appropriate for the pharmacoeconomic question?
8. Is the analysis transparent? What assumptions are built into the model? Could the analysis be reproduced given the appropriate information?
9. What is (are) the implication(s) of this study? What further questions need to be resolved?

Summary

Decision analysis can be used to structure the considerations and identify the elements of any type of economic study. However, decision analysis is more than a collection of mathematical calculations, probability estimates, and outcomes valuations. It engenders an attitude toward a decision—an attitude to think more analytically, to force the consideration of consequences of actions, to recognize explicitly that uncertainty is present, to estimate the degree of that uncertainty, to assess the attitude toward risk, to determine the relevant outcome measures, and to value the preferences for alternative outcomes.

A completed decision tree offers more than the answer to a question: it provides the underlying structure and assumptions behind the decision. If additional information becomes available that changes the consequences, probabilities, or outcomes of the question, the new information can be incorporated and the decision recalculated. Although structured, the decision analysis approach is flexible and offers many opportunities to improve the decision-making process.

References

1. Ledley RS, Lusted LB. Reasoning foundations of medical diagnosis. Science 1959;130:9-21.
2. Lusted LB. Decision making in patient management. N Engl J Med 1971; 284:416-24.
3. McNeil BJ, Keeler E, Adelstein SJ. Primer on certain elements of medical decision making. N Engl J Med 1975;293:211-5.
4. Kassirer JP. The principles of clinical decision making: an introduction to decision analysis. Yale J Biol Med 1976;49:149-64.
5. Kassirer JP, Moskowitz AJ, Lau J, Pauker SG. Decision analysis: a progress report. Ann Intern Med 1987;106:275-91.
6. Raiffa H. Decision analysis: introductory lectures under uncertainty. Reading, MA: Addison-Wesley Publishing, 1968.
7. Plante DA, Kassirer JP, Zarin DA, Pauker SG. Clinical decision consultation service. Am J Med 1986;80:1169-76.
8. Weinstein MC, Fineberg HV, eds. Clinical decision analysis. Philadelphia: WB Saunders, 1980.
9. Barr JT, Schumacher GE. Applying decision analysis in therapeutic drug monitoring: using the receiver-operating characteristic curves in comparative evolutions. Clin Pharm 1986;5:239-46.
10. O'Brien B. Economic evaluation of pharmaceuticals: Frankenstein's monster or vampire of trials? Med Care 1996;34:DS99-108.
11. Tversky A, Kahneman D. Judgment under uncertainty; heuristics and biases. Science 1974;185:1124-31.
12. Weinstein MC, Fineberg FV. Source of probability. In: Clinical decision analysis. Philadelphia: WB Saunders, 1980:37-74.
13. Luce BR. Policy implications of modeling the cost-effectiveness of health care technologies. Drug Info J 1995;29:1469-75.
14. Weinstein MC, Hornberger J, Jackson J, et al. Principles of good practice for decision analytic modeling in health care evaluations: report of the ISPOR Health Science Committee Task Force on Good Research Practice—Modeling Studies. Value in Health 2003;6:9-17.
15. Sonnenberg FA, Roberts MS, Tsevat J, et al. Toward a peer review process for medical decision analysis models. Med Care 1994;32:JS52-64.
16. Gold MR, Siegel JE, Russell LB, Weinstein MC, eds. Cost-effectiveness in health and medicine. New York: Oxford University Press, 1996.

17. Decision analytic modeling in economic evaluation of health technologies: a consensus statement. Consensus Conference on Guidelines on Economic Modelling in Health Technology Assessment. Pharmacoeconomics 2000;17: 443-4.

18. Blitz SG, Cram P, Chernew ME, Monte AS, Fendrick AM. Diagnostic testing or empirical neuraminidase inhibitor therapy for patients with influenza-like illness: what a difference a day makes. Am J Manag Care 2002;8:221-7.

19. Boelaert M, Le Ray D, van der Stuyft P. How better drugs could change kala-azar control. Lessons from a cost-effectiveness analysis. Trop Med Int Health 2002;7:955-9.

20. Choi HK, Seeger JD, Kuntz KM. A cost effectiveness analysis of treatment for methotrexate-naïve rheumatoid arthritis. J Rheumatol 2002;29:1156-65.

21. Christie AH, Culbert P, Guest JF. Economic impact of low dose polyethylene glycol 3350 plus electrolytes compared with lactulose in the management of idiopathic constipation in the UK. Pharmacoeconomics 2002; 20:49-60.

22. Dolder N, Wilhardt MS, Morreale A. Justifying a multidisciplinary high-intensity hepatitis C clinic by using decision analysis. Am J Health Syst Pharm 2002;59:867-71.

23. Ehrlich JE, Demopoulos BP, Daniel KR, Ricarte MC, Glied S. Cost-effectiveness of treatment options for prevention of rheumatic heart disease from group A streptococcal pharyngitis in a pediatric population. Prev Med 2002;35:250-7.

24. Ellis CN, Reiter KL, Bandekar RR, Fendrick AM. Cost-effectiveness comparison of therapy for psoriasis with a methotrexate-based regimen versus a rotation regimen of modified cyclosporine and methotrexate. J Am Acad Dermatol 2002;46:242-50.

25. Ewenstein BM, Avorn J, Putman KG, Bohn RL. Porcine factor VIII: pharmacoeconomics of inhibitor therapy. Haemophilia 2002;8(suppl 1):13-6.

26. Fendrick AM, Bandekar RR, Chernew ME, Scheiman JM. Role of initial NSAID choice and patient risk factors in the prevention of NSAID gastropathy: a decision analysis. Arthritis Rheum 2002;47:36-43.

27. Ghoshal UC, Das A. Management strategies for duodenal ulcer in India in the *Helicobacter pylori* era: an economic analysis. Nat Med J India 2002; 15:140-4.

28. Gift T, Walsh C, Haddix A, Irwin KL. A cost-effectiveness evaluation of testing and treatment of *Chlamydia trachomatis* infection among asymptomatic women infected with *Neisseria gonorrhoeae*. Sex Transm Dis 2002;29:542-51.

29. Glick HA, Orzol SM, Tooley JF, Remme WJ, Sasayama S, Pitt B. Economic evaluation of the randomized aldactone evaluation study (RALES): treatment of patients with severe heart failure. Cardiovasc Drugs Ther 2002;16:53-9.

30. Gupta RD, Guest JF. A model to estimate the cost benefit of an occupational vaccination programme for influenza with Influvac in the UK. Pharmacoeconomics 2002;20:475-84.

31. Halpern MT, Lipton RB, Cady RK, Kwong WJ, Marlo KO, Batenhorst AS.

Costs and outcomes of early versus delayed migraine treatment with sumatriptan. Headache 2002;42:984-99.

32. Hershman D, Sundararajan V, Jacobson JS, Heitjan DF, Neugut AI, Grann VR. Outcomes of tamoxifen chemoprevention for breast cancer in very high-risk women: a cost-effectiveness analysis. J Clin Oncol 2001;20: 9-16.

33. Khan K, Muening P, Behta M, Zivin JG. Global drug-resistance patterns and the management of latent tuberculosis infection in immigrants to the United States. N Engl J Med 2002;347:1850-9.

34. Kristiansen IS, Kvien TK. Cost-effectiveness of replacing NSAIDs with coxibs: diclofenac and celecoxib in rheumatoid arthritis. Expert Rev Pharmacoecon Outcomes Res 2002;2:229-41.

35. Ladabaum U, Chey WD, Scheiman JM, Fendrick AM. Reappraisal of non-invasive strategies for uninvestigated dyspepsia: a cost-minimization analysis. Aliment Pharmacol Ther 2002;16:1491-501.

36. Lamy A, Wang X, Kent R, Smith K, Gafni A. Economic evaluation of the MEDENOX trial: a Canadian perspective. Can Respir J 2002;9:169-77.

37. Lee PY, Matchar DB, Clements DA, Huber J, Hamilton JD, Peterson ED. Economic analysis of influenza vaccination and antiviral treatment for healthy working adults. Ann Intern Med 2002;137:225-31.

38. Maetzel A, Strand V, Tugwell P, Wells G, Bombardier C. Cost effectiveness of adding leflunomide to a 5-year strategy of conventional disease-modifying antirheumatic drugs in patients with rheumatoid arthritis. Arthritis Rheum 2002;47:655-61.

39. Ofman JJ, Dorn GH, Fennerty MB, Fass R. The clinical and economic impact of competing management strategies for gastro-oesophageal reflux disease. Aliment Pharmaol Ther 2002;16:261-73.

40. Ofman J, Wallace J, Badamgarav E, Chiou CF, Henning J. The cost-effectiveness of competing strategies for the prevention of recurrent peptic ulcer hemorrhage. Am J Gastroenterol 2002;97:1941-50.

41. Orlewska E. The cost-effectiveness of alternative therapeutic strategies for the management of chronic hepatitis B in Poland. Value Health 2002;5: 404-20.

42. Paladino JA, Gudgel LD, Forrest A, Niederman MS. Cost-effectiveness of IV-to-oral switch therapy: azithromycin vs cefuroxime with or without erythromycin for the treatment of community-acquired pneumonia. Chest 2002;122:1271-9.

43. Palmer CS, Brunner E, Ruiz-Flored LG, Paez-Agraz F, Revicki DA. A cost-effectiveness clinical decision model for the treatment of schizophrenia. Arch Med Res 2002;33:572-80.

44. Price MJ, Briggs AH. Development of an economic model to assess the cost effectiveness of asthma management strategies. Pharmacoeconomics 2002;20:183-94.

45. Saab S, Ly D, Han SB, Lin RK. Is it cost-effective to treat recurrent hepatitis C infection in orthotopic liver transplantation patients? Liver Transpl 2002;8:449-57.

46. Sarasin FP, Bounameaux H. Out of hospital antithrombotic prophylaxis after total hip replacement: low-molecular-weight heparin, warfarin, aspirin or nothing. Thromb Haemost 2002;87:586-92.

47. Silverberg K, Daya S, Auray JP, Duru G. Analysis of the cost effectiveness of recombinant versus urinary follicle-stimulating hormone in in vitro fertilization/intracytoplasmic sperm injection programs in the United States. Fertil Steril 2002;77:107-13.

48. Smith KJ, Roberts MS. Cost-effectiveness of newer treatment strategies for influenza. Am J Med 2002;113:300-7.

49. Song F, Raftery J, Aveyard P, Hyde C, Barton P, Woolacott N. Cost-effectiveness interventions for smoking cessation: a literature review and a decision analytic analysis. Med Decis Making 2002;22(suppl):S26-37.

50. Spath MA, O'Brien BJ. Cost effectiveness of implantable cardioverter defibrillator therapy versus drug therapy for patients at high risk of sudden cardiac death. Pharmacoeconomics 2002;20:727-38.

51. Stein K, Rosenberg W, Wong J. Cost effectiveness of combination therapy for hepatitis C: a decision analytical model. Gut 2002;50:253-8.

52. Stothers L. A randomized trial to evaluate effectiveness and cost-effectiveness of naturopathic cranberry products as prophylaxis against urinary tract infection in women. Can J Urol 2002;9:1558-62.

53. Stringer JSA, Sinkala M, Rouse DJ, Goldenberg RL, Vermund SH. Effect of nevirapine toxicity on choice of perinatal HIV prevention strategies. Am J Public Health 2002;92:365-6.

54. Thaulow E, Jorgensen B, Doyle J, Casciano R, Kopp Z, Arikian S, et al. A pharmacoeconomic evaluation of results from the Coronary Angioplasty Amlodipine Restenosis Study (CAPARES) in Norway and Canada. Int J Cardiol 2002;84:23-30.

55. Van Schaardenburg D, Kaandorp C, Krijnen P. Cost-effectiveness of antibiotic prophylaxis for bacterial arthritis. Expert Opin Pharmacother 2002;3:271-5.

56. Vidal-Trecan GM, Stahl JE, Durnad-Zaleski I. Managing toxic thyroid adenoma: a cost-effectiveness analysis. Eur J Endocrinol 2002;146:283-94.

57. Wahlqvist P, Junghard O, Higgins A, Green J. Cost effectiveness of esomeprazole compared with omeprazole in the acute treatment of patients with reflux oesophagitis in the UK. Pharmacoeconomics 2002;20:279-87.

58. Wilkins JJ, Folb PI, Valentine N, Barnes KI. An economic comparison of chloroquine and sulfadoxine–pyrimethamine as first-line treatment for malaria in South Africa: development of a model for estimating recurrent direct costs. Trans R Soc Trop Med Hyg 2002;96:85-90.

59. You JH, Lee KK, Chan TY, Lau WH. Arthritis treatment in Hong Kong—cost analysis of celecoxib versus conventional NSAIDs, with or without gastroprotective agents. Aliment Pharmacol Ther 2002;16:2089-96.

60. Brennan A, Akehurst R. Modeling in health economic evaluation. What is its place? What is its value? Pharmacoeconomics 2000;17:445-59.

Epidemiology and Pharmacoeconomic Research

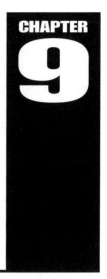

Paul E Stang
and Jacqueline S Gardner

There has been an explosion of interest in the methods used
to examine questions of cost and outcome of diseases. The
interest has come from many stakeholders in the healthcare system and process: managed care organizations and those
who control the delivery of care want to examine the natural
history of disease and its treatment in an effort to standardize
and optimize care (treatment guidelines and disease management programs), pharmaceutical and device companies want to
show how their products affect both the course and cost of illness to gain formulary and market position, consumers (and
clinicians) are striving to understand the target disease and the
risk–benefit of the various treatment options available to them,
and the evidence-based medicine movement is assessing all information to inform clinical decision-makers. Most of the mo-
mentum for this field has arisen from an interest in systematically examining the cost of disease versus the cost of therapy to
derive comparisons on which public policy and appropriations
decisions can be based.

Regulatory imperatives have now emerged in several countries that mandate economic analyses to justify approval for

marketing, as well as reimbursement and pricing of pharmaceuticals. Explicit in these mandates is the conduct of epidemiologic investigations to (1) reduce the volatility of the assumptions used in economic modeling, (2) generate estimates of market size, and (3) define source population parameters. Particularly interesting among these efforts are those that examine the entire spectrum of medicinal therapy, as the approval of these therapies is based on proof of safety and efficacy with relatively little attention to issues of access or cost. Given the wide availability of pharmaceutical products, the potential for their use in a wide range of disease indications (some of which may be outside of the intended patient population), and the new regulatory initiatives, it is important that the researcher understand the basic characteristics of the disease and of those affected by it before developing research plans to examine costs associated with and affected by drug therapy. Further, concise descriptions of the existing therapeutic alternatives, the way those therapies are used in the population, and their effects on the target diseases are critical in analyzing the cost of both current and new therapies.

Epidemiology is a relatively old science and discipline. It has enjoyed renewed enthusiasm because of its application for determining the baseline and current state of diseases within populations, describing characteristics of patients with particular diseases, and identifying exposures that have a positive or negative impact on the occurrence and outcome of the diseases. Much of the enthusiasm has been fueled by the availability of large clinical datasets based either on healthcare claims or on the evolving electronic medical record system. The role of epidemiology is complementary to that of economics; it encompasses rubrics ranging from health services research to pharmacoepidemiology, outcomes research, and clinical epidemiology (Figure 1). The resulting information is useful not only to the economist, but often has broader public health and policy implications.[1] The impact of interventions on cost also must be effectively linked to their impact on health.[2] As has been repeatedly demonstrated in macroeconomics, supplementing economic analyses with population-based epidemiology effectively addresses the benefits and risks of alternative approaches while placing these impacts into a public health perspective.[3] Table 1 illustrates the use of epidemiologic data for pharmacoeconomic applications.

This chapter examines the basic tools of epidemiology and how they contribute to our general understanding of the economics of disease. Specifically, this chapter shows how epidemiology can and should be used effectively in studies evaluating the economic impact of medicinal therapy. As part of the broad aegis of epidemiology, *pharmacoepidemiology*, or the study of the effects of drugs within populations, is discussed with respect to its role in pharmacoeconomic studies.

Basic Principles of Epidemiology

Epidemiology is a discipline whose goal is to describe the distribution of diseases and exposures in populations and to draw conclusions regarding associations between the exposures and the diseases. Epidemiologists use a range of methods—from systematic surveillance and simple descriptive reporting to rigorous multivariate analyses—to determine whether a particular characteristic or cluster of characteristics may be associated with or predictive of a given outcome. Epidemiologic studies can be observational (no active exposure manipulation by the investigator) or interventional (the exposure is manipulated, as in clinical trials). Often, data collected for another purpose, such as medical records or insurance claims, can be used. *Interventional studies*, in particular, clinical trials, use random allocation of

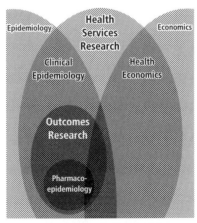

Figure 1. The relationship between economics and epidemiology. Reprinted with permission of H Guess.[1]

Table 1. The Epidemiology/Pharmacoeconomics Data Exchange

Epidemiologic Data	Examples	Major Pharmacoeconomic Applications
Disease frequency	incidence, prevalence demographics	new cases arising from intervention, magnitude of affected population, identification of high-risk groups and potential payer burden, quality-of-life parameters
Comorbidities, confounders, and effect modifiers	comorbid diseases, lifestyle factors (eg, smoking, alcohol)	spectrum of disease and additional sources of potential costs, additional risk factors or consequences of disease, identification of high-risk groups, quality-of-life parameters, economic risk, and medical decision modeling
Disease natural history	outcomes including survival, changes in disease over time, changes in use of services over time, distribution of risk factors	course of disease and costs over time, trends in ascertainment and technology used, referral patterns, length and outcomes of illness, QALYs, DALYs, risk assessment of outcomes, quality-of-life parameters, economic risk, and medical decision modeling
Utilization of services	healthcare-seeking behavior and predictors, disease-specific and total usage, type (site, specialist) of services	proportion of those who do not seek care but may still be impacted by disease, predictors of healthcare-seeking behavior, interventions and therapies used, referral patterns
Therapy	effectiveness and adverse effects of current therapies, observational study of new drug over time in a population	adverse effect risk/cost data; utilization under current therapies; adverse effects of comorbid conditions; naturalistic usage and disease data on new therapy as it enters population; risk of using inappropriate, addictive, or dangerous medications due to lack of effective therapies; quality-of-life parameters; estimate long-term outcomes; identify comparators for economic studies
Diagnostic issues	diagnostic criteria severity, accuracy of ascertainment, trends over time in coding	ability to look at increased costs due to missed diagnosis, issues of severity of disease and relationship to costs, severity as a marker for utilization, extent of under-ascertainment of disease

DALY = disability-adjusted life-years; QALY = quality-adjusted life-years.

(continued on page 215)

treatment to control for the effects of known and unknown co-variates. *Observational studies* must systematically collect these data to examine and control their effects in the analysis.

Clinical trials also are noteworthy for their short duration and unrealistically standardized monitoring, which often limits their generalizability and usefulness in examining issues related to utilization of services, changes in quality of life, or detection of effects from long-term use.[4] Clinical trial sample sizes also are based on the power necessary to detect efficacy differences and may not be large enough or cover populations broad enough to robustly address economic questions. These data can possibly be obtained through observational studies, as these studies often involve much larger, more diverse populations for longer periods of observation. This gives the economist a mechanism to compensate for the power lost in clinical trial data. However, observational studies are limited to products already being marketed.

One of the roles of epidemiology is to protect economic studies from biases.[5] Pharmacoeconomics must assume a cause–effect relationship between drug treatment and disease indication. It is important to understand all of the phenomena that are relat-

Table 1. The Epidemiology/Pharmacoeconomics Data Exchange (continued)

Epidemiologic Data	Examples	Major Pharmacoeconomic Applications
Risk (or benefit) assessment	rate of outcomes attributable to disease (attributable risk data), modeling of outcomes based on disease natural history	modeling of outcomes and their costs and consequences, economic risk and medical decision modeling, link manifestation of disease to outcome
Biomarkers, genetic markers	marker for disease subtype or to identify specific genotypic population	more precise and focused cost estimates of disease, outcome, and transitional probabilities
Clinical threshold	clinically meaningful difference	modeling, thresholds for pharmacoeconomic analysis

ed to the disease and the therapy prior to assessing baseline costs and eventual changes with therapy. For instance, patients with headache may be consuming a very small amount of resources directly related to the headache pain, but may be tremendous consumers of other medical services for associated diseases or symptoms resulting from their chronic disease or its therapy. In the case of headache, patients may be seeking treatment from internal medicine for gastrointestinal symptoms resulting from stress and chronic use of nonsteroidal antiinflammatory drugs, as well as from psychiatry for their comorbid depression and anxiety. It would be important to examine the changes in utilization and costs of these associated services with the introduction of a new headache therapy, as they may contribute substantial burden to the patient and the cost of the disease. Economic models become more robust by using realistic epidemiologic data on risk factors, treatment alternatives, and outcomes.

EPIDEMIOLOGY NOMENCLATURE

It is important to understand the nomenclature used in epidemiology. *Prevalence* is a measure of frequency that reflects the number of people at a given point in time who have a particular disease or exposure of interest. Prevalence can be based on a particular day, previous week, previous month, previous year, or lifetime prevalence, which reflects whether or not the subject has ever had the condition in question. Prevalence estimates are usually obtained using cross-sectional or one-time sampling techniques, including interviews administered either by telephone or in person, self-administered questionnaires as in a mail survey, or review of records or databases for the number of cases of a condition on record at any point in time. Prevalence in a broad sense represents the current disease burden from a population perspective.

Incidence reflects the number of new cases arising in a population in a given period of time. Incidence estimates are much more difficult to obtain because they necessitate observing a population over a period of time to identify new cases that arise or performing repeated prevalence estimates in the same population over a given period of time to differentiate between existing cases and cases of new onset. Incidence is a very powerful measure because it allows one to project population estimates into the future. Incidence reflects the emerging disease burden.

Incidence is not dependent on survival, as a case is identified and counted at the time it becomes a case. Prevalence is survival-dependent, as the patient must be able to be sampled at the given time point that prevalence is being measured. Prevalence estimates for a disease with varying lengths of survival will include only patients who have survived long enough to become a prevalent case. It is this "survival of the fittest" that may present a problem in using prevalence figures, as these cases do not represent all patients who have contracted the disease and certainly do not carry with them the total economic burden that the disease exacts on the population. The denominator in both prevalence and incidence estimates is the population at risk for experiencing the outcome of interest. If we are interested in outcomes among people taking a particular drug, we would want to assure ourselves that the denominator consists only of people exposed to the drug for a given period of time. Hence, our prevalence or incidence estimate will have meaning and be generalizable to a known target population.

Case fatality rate or dropout is important only insofar as it affects the ability to identify cases, since people who die or are lost to follow-up may not be captured in a prevalence-based study. *Incident cases*, in contrast, provide a realistic starting point from which to follow patients and the course of their disease and will not be affected by case fatality. This is especially important when looking at health service utilization over time, in establishing temporal trends, or when constructing quality-adjusted or disability-adjusted life-years (QALYs, DALYs), as disability and utilization of services may vary across the duration of the disease.

Inherent in the denominator of incidence is the concept of time, expressed as *person-time*, as each person may contribute a different amount to the length of observation. This allows us to include the contribution of all patients in the incidence estimate, regardless of how long they remain under observation. This concept is important in the quantification of utilization of services and calculation of cost associated with a disease, and it is the key strength of disease natural history studies.

STUDY DESIGNS

A discussion of epidemiologic study designs, complete with their advantages and disadvantages, is beyond the scope of this chapter. Those most commonly used are ecologic, cross-sectional (prevalence), cohort, and case–control study designs, although registries and simplified (or naturalistic) clinical trials have become more common in recent years. Interested readers are referred to classic textbooks on the subject.[6]

Observational study designs have long been the object of scorn by the clinical trial community and largely ignored by the evidence-based movement. However, recent work has shown that well-designed observational studies approximate the effects of treatment as well as randomized controlled trials.[7,8] Because observational data directly reflect healthcare delivery, they are ideal for evaluating healthcare effectiveness.[9] The data derived from studies using each design offer unique advantages in given situations. Less often addressed is the way in which the data are presented and interpreted. Nonetheless, discussions about analytic techniques also will be deferred.

For economic studies, the cohort or simplified/naturalistic trial design is favored for several reasons: cohorts are good observational approximations of real life and the natural course of disease that clearly define the temporal relationship between exposures and outcomes. They resemble clinical trials in their direction but tend to be much larger and, as such, are able to detect smaller differences between groups. Case–control studies have been used in economic analysis with modest success.[10] These studies are of limited utility as they are capable of exploring only a single outcome; however, they may be useful in examining the economic impact of adverse drug effects.

Disease Natural History

Disease natural history is the backbone of modern epidemiology. It implies the ability to give a "cradle-to-grave" characterization of a disease in a population and has many applications across the drug development process.[11] This includes description of changes in the disease over time, modifiers of disease outcomes, comorbidities, use of services, and the effect of treatment. Severity indices are constructed using these data that are also crucial in the determination of DALYs and QALYs. Such a longitudinal picture is very difficult to obtain; however, with the advent of computerized medical data, structured medical record systems, and the plethora of longitudinal cohort studies, it is often possible to follow affected people for several years. When using these secondary datasets, one must remember that they represent specific populations, often linked by a common health insurance payer, that may reflect socioeconomic status, geographic region, or employment status. These characteristics may limit the generalizability of findings to the broad population base. However, if one is interested in payer-specific data (eg, Medicaid, health maintenance organization), it is appropriate to limit the scope of the project to a dataset derived from that payer. Longitudinal studies also facilitate the capture of total utilization of healthcare services in addition to identifying services that are disease-specific. These studies are often instrumental in identifying marginal cost differences and they facilitate cost–benefit analysis.[12]

ASCERTAINMENT

It is important for the epidemiologist to provide some insight into how well patients are captured or identified in the medical care system. The extent to which a given disease is identified in a population and the likelihood of individuals being correctly identified once they enter the healthcare system bear directly on disease burden, direct and indirect costs, and perhaps the effectiveness of therapy. Sensitivity, specificity, and predictive value analyses of existing diagnostic systems are helpful in determining issues of disease frequency and recognition. They also provide a basis for confidence in future work in automated data and some guidance in the interpretability of patient-reported symptoms and diagnoses. These analyses also may draw attention to the need for public health screening or clinician/patient education programs or have an impact on the development of clinical guidelines.

A diagnostic algorithm may need to be constructed to identify cases and may dictate the necessity for more stringent diagnostic criteria based on symptom cluster analyses. This is especially important in primary care diseases in which missed diagnoses may not be evident until time passes, symptoms and signs are explored in more detail, or until referral to a specialist. Such analyses can also examine symptoms most likely to improve or reduce the likelihood of a correct diagnosis. Even more problematic are diseases and conditions that are asymptomatic and therefore unsuspected by people who are affected by them.[13]

Patient motivations for seeking medical attention, their satisfaction with their medical care, and their longevity in the medical care system also should be captured while examining ascertainment issues. Ascertainment data can be used in developing medical decision models, as patients who are missed (false negatives) may be subject to a different treatment and utilization pathway. Similarly, quality of life may be impacted by misdiagnosis, perhaps resulting in inappropriate therapy and poor outcome.

EXPOSURE AND DISEASE COMORBIDITY

A key byproduct of a well-developed epidemiologic study is the identification of relationships among diseases or comorbid events. Chronic diseases rarely occur in isolation and are often manifestations of more diffuse disease processes. It is important to elucidate the relationship between the disease or risk factor under study and any comorbid conditions (consequent, concomitant, antecedent). Comorbidities are important when deciding on relevant quality-of-life measurements, as many chronic diseases have substantive impact on nonphysical complaints. Comorbidities also impact medical decision and economic models as the constellation of risks, therapies, and outcomes are defined and their impact on the burden of the disease becomes apparent. Comorbidities, as a feature of disease natural history, are particularly important data when defining drug effects. Adverse events may be attributed to a treatment when the event is actually part of the natural course of the target disease or comorbid conditions occurring in the target population.

The cost implications of comorbid conditions can be determined by examining the patient's total healthcare utilization rather than disease-specific utilization (this is essentially the way marginal costs are derived). For example, many diseases carry associated risks of comorbid psychiatric disease that may completely drive the patient's utilization of health care, as has been shown to be the case in functional bowel disease.[14] These psychiatric comorbidities are often poorly ascertained in clinical practice and hence poorly reflected in diagnostic codes. Similarly, it may be the comorbidities that affect patient quality of life or productivity—critical components of any economic analysis.

DISEASE AND RISK FACTOR TRENDS

It is also important for an epidemiologist to characterize trends in risk factors and outcomes because, as therapies change, the frequency and course of risks and diseases in populations change. Secular trends in our ability to diagnose and treat will affect any baseline estimates of disease cost, especially if the diagnosis is one of exclusion. Migraine headache, for example, has a high direct cost during the initial visits to the physician, as many expensive tests are ordered to rule out more life-threatening causes of headache.[15] Environmental triggers of the disease and the prevailing risk factor trends also should be studied, as these data are crucial for predicting trends in prevalence.

Many costs also are being shifted within the system as new technologies become part of the natural course of disease: balloon angioplasty, outpatient/day surgery, endoscopy, and lithotripsy are a few examples of how technologies are affecting cost of disease and use of services over time. Disease frequency, especially if there are susceptible populations or preferential distributions of diseases in populations (eg, high-risk groups), can affect both aggregate estimates of costs of the disease as well as estimated costs to the individual patient. These trends can be measured as true prevalence or incidence of disease in the population or as distributions of outpatient or inpatient treatments in a population. However, as with any of these data, ability to effectively and reliably identify people with the disease or disorder is critically important.

DISEASE SEVERITY

Disease severity is a particularly important issue in defining populations and ascribing costs (both fiscal and humanistic) to disease states. Severity has become synonymous with intensity of symptoms or, in the case of arthritis and neoplasia, a staged classification of pathophysiologic signs or objective evidence from radiographic or laboratory results. Although symptom intensity is an important component of disease severity, it often fails to discriminate the features and disability of those with higher levels of dysfunction. A well-constructed severity/impact index may become an effective link among physiology, clinical diagnosis, economics, and patient outcome, as well as a guide for interventions. There are many desirable features of a useful classification of severity: (1) ordered categories that are mutually exclusive and exhaustive corresponding to qualitative differences in severity, (2) biologic relevance, (3) based on simple measurements that can be obtained in a variety of settings, (4) defined to yield homogeneous groups, and (5) precise, reliable, and valid construction reflecting cross-sectional association with severity measures and predictive of patient outcomes.[16]

Item response theory provides the methodologic framework for the development of these scoring systems; however, the challenge is in determining what constitutes the various levels of severity and how well it reflects outcomes. Von Korff et al.[16] include several applications of a well-constructed chronic severity index (Table 2) and apply some of these principles to the con-

Table 2. Applications of Severity Classification[16]

Study Type	Application
Epidemiologic field survey	more complete and reproducible differential of global severity among classes; ability to segment population by level of dysfunction
Clinical trial	improvement in qualitative description of patients at baseline and enhancement of qualitative changes at follow-up between groups
Observational/natural history	case-mix adjustment at baseline and assessment of outcomes
Meta-analysis	aid in the classification of studies and assessment of outcomes over time
Clinical practice	improve prognostic advice and provide substantiation for treatment decisions and patient education
Clinical information and tracking system	ability to track patient progress over time with limited information

struction of a chronic disease score from automated pharmacy data.[17] It is generally assumed that people with more severe forms of disease are different from those with less severe disease, although there is rarely consensus on how severity levels are to be defined. The differences may be in intensity of symptoms or level of dysfunction that the patient experiences as a result of the disease. Level of dysfunction is a difficult parameter to measure because it may involve issues of humanistic impact and psychological well-being (eg, quality of life), consumption of health care (both disease-specific and general), and impact on work and play. Severity differences are not consistently reflected in healthcare costs because, when the disease is fatal, those with more severe (and rapidly fatal) disease may have lower direct and indirect costs over a period of time.

The ability to chart disease progression over time, control for severity in analyses, identify homogeneous patient groups, and target patients who could benefit most from intervention heighten the importance of severity assessment. The interplay between the epidemiologist and the pharmacoeconomist is particularly crucial in this arena, as severity may be the issue upon which all subsequent work and analyses are based and assessment of disease cost can be segmented. Hence, the measures should be complementary to both and useful to the practicing clinician and clinical trialist alike. If costs are related to severity, then trials may be able to directly translate the effect of a therapy that reduces severity from one level to another or prevents a disease from advancing to a more severe stage. Burden of illness measures should reflect both disease severity and disease frequency. Using this paradigm, statistics can be employed that reflect the impact of an intervention in a population reflecting both severity reduction and prevention of adverse outcomes.[18] Such efforts are limited by the quality of the data and their ability to support definitions of disease severity.

Analagous to severity is the consistent definition of changes over the course of illness. Exacerbations of illness, recurrence versus new episode, and disease progression are concepts embedded in the assessment of disease severity and natural history over time. Prior to any reasonable assessment of the costs of illnesses at these junctures is the thorough and precise understanding of their occurrence, definition, and relevance. This understanding draws largely on the epidemiologic tool chest.

Quantification of Risk

The epidemiologic concept of quantification of risk is very important to economic analysis. The magnitude of risk, that is, of an association between exposure and disease, is often represented as a ratio. For instance, people with hypertension may have a relative risk of 3.1 for experiencing a stroke. This means that they are three times as likely to experience a stroke as are people without hypertension. (Interestingly, Naylor et al.[19] showed that clinicians respond more favorably to data presented in relative terms.) However, people without hypertension also experience stroke, and the incidence of stroke among this population is known as the *background rate*. What may be of most interest to economists is the proportion of strokes attributable to hypertension. This measure, called an *attributable risk proportion* (Figure 2), reflects the amount of disease outcome (stroke) in the population that could be prevented if the exposure (hypertension) was eliminated. Hence, determining both the background rate and the attributable risk proportion through epidemiologic studies becomes important. The economist can then begin the daunting task of translating this information into the economic benefits of intervening and preventing the costly outcome of stroke.

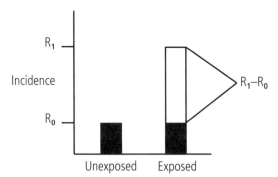

Figure 2. Calculation of risk attribution. Relative risk = $R_1 \div R_0$; Attributable risk = $R_1 - R_0$; Attributable risk proportion = $(R_1 - R_0) \div R_1$; R_0 = incidence of outcome in the unexposed; R_1 = incidence of outcome in those exposed.

The relative risk and attributable risk approach also can be applied to interpretation of adverse events that may be attributed to drug therapy, but are actually part of the clinical sequelae of the disease for which the drug was prescribed. This misattribution of adverse effects is known as *confounding by indication*. For example, among depressed people, there is a given risk of suicide or violent behavior. If these people are given a drug for depression, any observed incidence of this adverse behavior is often attributed to the drug when it may, in fact, be a predictable part of the disease process. The difficulty is in attributing a causal relationship on an individual basis, such as may be required in a medical safety review or in a court of law.

Anticipating these questions and determining the background rate of disease outcomes will provide valuable data for calculations of relative risk and attributable risk and the proper attribution of costs. This information may help either to defend or indict a drug exposure and will assist the economist in identifying disease features that add economic burden to the disease and perhaps to measure direct, indirect, or humanistic cost. Furthermore, these epidemiologic studies can be used to provide realistic data for predicting the outcomes of clinical and economic trials.

Unfortunately for many people, risk in the pharmaceutical development world has become synonymous with adverse events and, in particular, spontaneous adverse events identified after a drug is marketed. Because the nature and depth of any discussion of the topic would take volumes, it is important to note that such surveillance systems are hypothesis generating and intended to suggest areas for possible study. It is often difficult to separate true events from natural history and background rates, difficulties that are particularly evident when we consider the literature on the rates of adverse non-drug reactions.[20,21]

The Elusive Risk–Benefit Ratio

Recent political (high costs of health care, payers demanding value) and cultural (information empowerment of the consumer, highly visible tort litigation efforts, withdrawal of medications from the market) events have resulted in formal regulatory requirements to assess the risk–benefit balance of pharmaceutical products. Although risk–benefit ratio is a commonly used term, it is difficult to identify an accepted methodology that effectively addresses how this is best to be undertaken. The main issue is that benefits and risks are often expressed in different metrics, and combining the two concepts into a meaningful common metric is difficult. Economists have long used monetary values to accomplish these assessments. However, this approach is most relevant to payers and less so to patients, regulators, and providers. A salient review of current and proposed methods appears in a recent series.[22,23] There is great infrastructure in the pharmaceutical development life-cycle dedicated to identifying, codifing, and interpreting adverse events based mainly on anecdotal spontaneous adverse event reports. However, the study of benefit is undertaken in a more systematic manner through formal observational or clinical interventional studies. In the United States, the manufacturer's product package insert is the principal means of communicating risk and benefit about a pharmaceutical product. However, one needs only receive a single striking adverse event report to warrant an update to the package insert, while changes in benefit data constitute a formal claim and, as such, require formal hypothesis testing in two well-controlled trials. Hence, the balance is often not possible to communicate in the package insert.

These disparate approaches make it even more difficult to effectively combine data to assess the real benefit–risk balance of a product, although modeling does provide some of the necessary methodologic infrastructure.

OUTCOMES, MODELING, AND DECISION ANALYSIS

A key part of the evaluation of the impact of a new therapy is the determination of the full impact of the disease, the possible clinical decisions associated with it, and the expectation of various outcomes. If the disease under study is part of a constellation of related diseases, trials may be able to show that effective early detection and intervention can prevent other deleterious outcomes and offset their associated economic and humanistic toll (as would be the case in obesity studies that may show a reduction in psychiatric, metabolic, and cardiovascular outcomes with reduction in weight). Similarly, the unexpected positive effects of drug therapy[24] can be realized and quantified through epidemiologic studies, thereby providing a more balanced picture of a particular therapy and a new therapeutic avenue.

Because disease severity may greatly influence outcomes and clinical decision-making, appreciation of severity levels must be achieved and integrated into this process. Hence, the judicious application of epidemiologic data can be used in a number of decision-intensive settings, which helps to guide further research and arrive at informed decisions regarding disease and economic impact. These are the data used to make public policy decisions and, increasingly, new drug approvals. Modeling exercises rely on observational data to estimate the long-term effects, costs, and benefits of a new intervention in an unrestricted (ie, non-clinical trial) population. Sound population data are crucial, as the product of these models may guide future decisions on pricing, further clinical and economic research, and determinations of the impact of therapy.

Decision analysis models, including those used in utility analysis and medical decision-making, need reality-based data on risks, treatment alternatives, and outcomes. These can be obtained from good-quality epidemiology studies. Development of data that provide probabilities and risks of outcomes also can be powerful in the early planning phases of clinical trials. With these data, trials can be designed to capture some of these outcomes in comparison with existing therapies. These data also may be used to assess the feasibility of continuing development of a new compound or to determine necessary sample sizes.

A measure that can take research results and inform clinical decision-making is the *number-needed-to-treat* (NNT).[25,26] This measure quantifies the number of patients that one would need to treat with a given therapy until the benefit is realized in one patient. Similarly, the *number-needed-to-harm* (NNH) can be calculated for adverse effects related to a treatment. NNTs are specific to the patients being treated, the intervention and its duration, and the outcome measured.[27] The advantage of these measures is that they effectively bridge several related disciplines—epidemiology, economics, and clinical practice—while providing a clinically relevant metric for the physician. Defining thresholds for clinical relevance is at the heart of clinical epidemiology as it seeks to match changes in exposure and risk factors to quantifiable changes in outcome.

Several other areas of collaboration demand mention. The integration of epidemiology and pharmacoeconomics into quality-of-life research has been skillfully discussed elsewhere.[28] These authors cover issues of bias, methodologic techniques, analytic considerations, and the extension of inferences from quality-of-life research using epidemiology. Meta-analysis is another area to consider, as the insights derived may help to drive key decisions regarding thresholds, transitional probabilities, effectiveness, and safety issues (see Chapter 17). Finally, productivity research, or the impact of disease and its treatment on work effectiveness, is an area of keen interest with the rise of healthcare costs being borne by the employer–purchaser of health care. Studies have been undertaken in this area that are both prospective and use linked medical records.[29,30] Perhaps the most important aspect of this work is its immediate and proximal application to a defined population. However, it does introduce yet another perspective from an economist's point of view: that of the employer.

Resources for Epidemiologic Data

Epidemiology studies are designed to capture and characterize a population at a given point in time or over a designated period of time. For these data to be of maximum utility in assessing change due to a new therapy or technology, they should include the status prior to the availability of the new product or reimbursement scheme. In the case of new medicinal therapies, epidemiology studies should be undertaken when the compound is early in the development process. De novo prospective studies are the most expensive, logistically complicated, and time-intensive studies to undertake. Often, synthesis of the available literature may be sufficient to address many early data needs.

Opportunities to estimate the effects of therapy on long-term clinical outcomes may be available through clinical trials and ongoing large cohort studies (eg, longitudinal studies of aging). These studies may be used to capture information directly or it may be possible to add targeted questions. In clinical areas where complete ascertainment of disease may be an issue, these data sources are critical. This is especially true in mental health where population-based surveys have been undertaken that are focused on ascertainment, comorbidity, and use of services.[31]

Nonautomated alternatives exist, including the Rochester Epidemiology Project.[32,33] The researchers involved in this project have been performing population-based studies for years using a structured medical record system. Their ability to capture all healthcare encounters for the entire population of Olmsted County, Minnesota, has resulted in hundreds of studies to date. With the rising availability of electronic medical records, the depth of information may improve, but the length of observation and specific population base in many other systems may be limiting for the study of chronic disease.

Many fail to recognize the value of clinical trial data, especially data from the placebo group, in estimating disease or outcome frequency in the unexposed population (essentially the base rate). Although clinical trial data may be biased, they do offer some insight into subtleties that may not be apparent in the normal clinical recognition and treatment of disease. For instance, it may be helpful to look at the natural history of laboratory changes in the placebo group across time in a clinical trial, as the intervals of testing will be consistent and there will be capture and recording of all medications, medical history, and other physiologic measurements. However, adverse events do occur and become attributed to placebo, an effect that is particularly apparent in trials of mental health interventions.[34] Additionally, patient-centered data (eg, quality of life or impact measures) may be available from clinical trials.

AUTOMATED DATA SOURCES

With the explosion in the computerization of data, especially medical and health service utilization data, vast amounts of information have become temptingly available to anyone clever enough to extract it from computerized files. Most of these data were created for reasons other than epidemiologic research. Most commonly, they were created by fiscal officers in healthcare settings to track financial data within their accounting systems. Whereas 20 years ago it was necessary for researchers to laboriously sift through reams of medical records data manually, the essence of those data can now be captured on computerized tape.

This convenience comes at a price, however, as there are ever-present coding errors, difficulties in substantiating diagnoses, and problems linking patients between databases (ie, often diagnostic codes appear in one database, medication codes in another, and hospitalization data in yet another). Furthermore, drug exposures indicated in such databases constitute evidence only of prescriptions dispensed or orders filled; they do not necessarily correspond to either evidence of drug consumption or the circumstances (eg, timing, dosage, route of administration) that might have occurred. Finally, tantamount to the logistical problems associated with electronic database resources are the problems of confidentiality, as data source managers are becoming more and more reluctant to allow access to interested parties outside of their own systems, a question that has attracted some attention from ethicists.[35]

An extensive discussion of the advantages and shortcomings of the individual computerized databases is beyond the scope of this chapter. Some detailed discussion of various epidemiology data sources can be found elsewhere.[6] However, methods of conducting valid epidemiologic analysis using these datasets are being improved and are evolving because the advantage of computerized data is their capture of a unique payer perspective on the disease in question. These databases capture a relatively large population and facilitate the collection of utilization data. One could examine trends in the use of medical services and medications over time, the relationships between interventions and outcomes, indirect measures of adherence to therapy, and patterns of prescribed and administered care.

In general, these data provide strong and relatively comprehensive capture of the direct cost of disease. They also provide the opportunity to assemble matched controls from which marginal costs and utilization (*attributable costs*) can be derived. Furthermore, issues pertaining to adverse drug reactions, treatment failures, and therapeutic interchanges can be addressed and appropriately quantified depending on the type of data captured in such systems. Additionally, exclusively through observational methods and computerized data, the impact of a new therapy can be monitored as it penetrates a market. This provides additional data, under real-world circumstances, for documenting the impact of new therapy on direct costs, indirect costs, and humanistic parameters.

Caution is warranted, however, as the allure of the computerized system carries with it some risks.[36] Recall that most systems were created by fiscal officers interested in streamlining the billing process and facilitating budget review. Several caveats govern epidemiologic studies using computerized administrative datasets. First, enrollee or eligible patient turnover may be high, thus compromising the potential for tracking individuals over long periods of time. For example, Ray and Griffin[37] found that, in Medicaid data, only 79 percent of their original cohort had no lapses in eligibility over a one-year follow-up period; this proportion was further reduced to 38 percent over five years. The reason for dropping out may not be as obvious or adverse-event related as is found in clinical trials because the eligibility criteria for the subject being carried on the database may have changed (eg, lost eligibility for Medicaid, left job so is dropped from health maintenance organization rolls). Further, exposures in these databases are related to organization-approved formularies, cost-sharing systems, and other non–therapy-related factors. Consequently, the exposures of interest may be missing from the database altogether or may be present in a pattern that does not necessarily reflect the true exposure. A general guideline has been proposed by the International Society for Pharmacoeconomics and Outcomes Research for evaluating research undertaken with claims data.[38]

Secondly, data quality and comprehensiveness may affect the ability to accurately capture disease information. Because only diagnostic codes are recorded, it will be unclear how the diagnosis was made and how accurately it reflects the patient's true disease state.[12] Coded diagnoses lack detail on severity and chronicity and, in many databases, the number of diagnoses available for any given episode may be restricted. Hence, information on comorbidities may be unavailable. Source record validation is essential to ensure accuracy of coding and perhaps to capture some of the additional data, including data on relevant risk factors such as smoking or obesity.

Often, the rigors of diagnostic ascertainment in a given disease are not apparent without access to source documents. This becomes a particularly important problem when data span changes in disease definition, therapeutic practices, or technologic advances. It is important to keep in mind that, for most purposes, one would like to obtain the current status of knowledge or state-of-the-art of the disease and its therapies rather than capture a historic perspective that may no longer be relevant. Additionally, in conducting studies within computerized databases, one assumes that the temporal relationship between drug dispensing and subsequent events is causal; however, this is pure conjecture.

Paradigms can be created to estimate adherence by looking at refill patterns, but at the end of the day, it remains unclear whether or how effectively patients took the medication. This may be especially true of device-delivered medications, such as inhalers or injections, whose effectiveness depends not only on the patients attempting administration of the drug, but also on their effectiveness in operating the device.

Finally, difficulties may arise when trying to attribute resource use because of the limitations in coding for administrative purposes. Similar problems arise when attribution of diagnostic tests or drug therapy is attempted, as the motivation for these tests and medications may be unclear or one test or visit may cover more than one medical problem. Misclassification in this respect can be minimized by making a priori decisions about which resources would potentially be affected by the disease or the therapy under study.

The federal government also conducts regular research on the United States population and makes the raw data available to the public. Notable among these government efforts are the National Health Interview Survey, an annual representative sample of the United States (over 40,000 households) with data on chronic diseases, healthcare utilization, and demographic characteristics (including days spent in bed or days of restricted activity due to particular chronic diseases). Government prevalence estimates are derived from these data. The National Health and Nutrition Examination Surveys, the National Medical Expenditure Survey, and several site-specific surveys can be accessed through the federal government at a modest price. Analysis of these datasets is somewhat complex because they are large and the weighting schemes are somewhat complicated, necessitating sophisticated software packages for analysis.

Summary data for many of the government datasets is available online from the National Center for Health Statistics Web site (www.cdc.gov/nchs). Other data resources, including large cross-sectional surveys or longitudinal studies (ie, Nurse's Health Study, Framingham) can be used to explore additional questions of interest. Multiple data sources can be merged as zip code level pollen count data with daily diary data to estimate the change in productivity associated with changes in pollen count among people with allergies.[39] The International Society for Pharmacoepidemiology (www.pharmacoepi.org/resources/policies) has produced guidelines for Good Epidemiology Practices that codify some of the key issues addressed in this chapter.[40]

Summary

Healthcare decisions are based primarily on a consideration of risk and benefit and secondarily on cost consideration. Epidemiologic techniques of examining frequency and distribution of exposures and outcomes in a population provide a good foundation from which to project disease and therapeutic costs to the broader population. It is important to understand the total spectrum of the disease, comorbidities, severity issues, current treatment and service utilization patterns, and effectiveness and consequences of current therapies in order to gauge the potential impact of a new treatment. Policy-makers base decisions on epidemiologic outcomes data in large part because they provide a realistic assessment of the population at large.

Epidemiology also offers the opportunity to elucidate particular issues in disease ascertainment and therapeutic alternatives and how these may affect specific payer systems as well as the population at large. Specifically, issues relating to primary care of medical disorders may provide some clues to the initial cost and capture of diseases in populations. Epidemiologic data are crucial in quantifying the burden of illness, identifying risks and outcomes, providing the basis for economic and medical decision models, and aiding in the prediction of outcomes in clinical trial samples.

With the computerization of medical care data and the ability to observe large populations, sophisticated sampling and modeling techniques become important in ascertaining and attributing disease and utilization relationships within these populations. These enable high-quality observational data to form the basis of more risk and economic decisions. Finally, prior to declaring any effective change in cost, one must thoroughly understand the baseline state from which that change occurred. This is clearly the realm of the epidemiologist, and it presents a wonderful opportunity to merge the sciences of epidemiology and pharmacoeconomics to determine the impact of therapeutic innovation on the diseases that burden modern society.

References

1. Guess HA, Stephenson WP, Sacks S, Gardner JS. Beyond pharmacoepidemiology: the larger role of epidemiology in drug development. J Clin Epidemiol 1988;41:995-6.
2. Spitzer WO. Drugs as determinants of health and disease in the population. J Clin Epidemiol 1991;44:823-30.
3. Sen A. The economics of life and death. Sci Am 1993;268:40-7.
4. Simon G, Wagner E, Von Korff M. Cost-effectiveness comparisons using 'real world' randomized trials: the case of new antidepressant drugs. J Clin Epidemiol 1995;48:363-73.
5. Chrischilles EA. The contribution of epidemiology to pharmacoeconomic research. Drug Info J 1992;26:219-29.
6. Strom BL, ed. Pharmacoepidemiology. 3rd ed. West Sussex, England: John Wiley and Sons, Ltd, 2002.
7. Benson K, Hartz AJ. A comparison of observational studies and randomized, controlled trials. N Engl J Med 2000;342:1878-86.
8. Concato J, Shah N, Horowitz RI. Randomized, controlled trials, observational studies and the hierarchy of research designs. N Engl J Med 2000;342:1887-92.
9. Black N. Why we need observational studies to evaluate the effectiveness of health care. BMJ 1996;312:1215-8.
10. Eisenberg JM, Koffer H, Glick HA, Connell ML, Loss LE, Talbot GH, et al. What is the cost of nephrotoxicity associated with aminoglycosides? Ann Intern Med 1987;107:900-9.
11. Stang PE. Disease natural history. In: Mann R, Andrews E, eds. Pharmacovigilance, Wiley Press, 2002: 97-104.
12. Fishman P, Von Korff M, Lozano P, Hecht J. Chronic care costs in managed care. Health Affairs 1997;16:239-47.
13. Chesson HW, Blandford JM, Gift TL, Tao G, Irwin KL. The estimated direct medical cost of sexually transmitted diseases among American youth, 2000. Perspect Sex Reprod Health 2004;36:11-9.
14. Guthrie E, Creed F, Fernandes L, Ratcliffe J, Van Der Jagt J, Martin J, et al. Cluster analysis of symptoms and health seeking behaviour differentiates subgroups of patients with severe irritable bowel syndrome. Gut 2003;52:1616-22.
15. Stang PE, Osterhaus JT, Celentano DD. Migraine: patterns of health care utilization. Neurology 1994;44(suppl 4):S47-55.

16. Von Korff M, Ormel J, Keefe FJ, Dworkin SF. Grading the severity of chronic pain. Pain 1992;50:133-49.

17. Von Korff M, Wagner EH, Saunders K. A chronic disease score from automated pharmacy data. J Clin Epidemiol 1992;45:197-203.

18. Chang MN, Guess HA, Heyse JF. Reduction in burden of illness: a new efficacy measure for prevention trials. Stat Med 1994;13:1807-14.

19. Naylor CD, Chen E, Strauss B. Measured enthusiasm: does the method of reporting trial results alter perceptions of therapeutic effectiveness? Ann Intern Med 1992;117:916-21.

20. Reidenberg MM, Lowenthal DT. Adverse nondrug reactions. N Engl J Med 1968;279:678-9.

21. Meyer FP, Troger U, Rohl F-W. Adverse nondrug reactions: an update. Clin Phamacol Ther 1996;60:347-52.

22. Holden WL, Juhaeri J, Dai W. Benefit–risk analysis: examples using quantitative methods. Pharmacoepidemiol Drug Saf 2003;12:693-7.

23. Holden WL, Juhaeri J, Dai W. Benefit–risk analysis: a proposal using quantitative methods. Pharmacoepidemiol Drug Saf 2003;12:611-6.

24. Lasagna L. Are drug benefits also part of pharmacoepidemiology? J Clin Epidemiol 1990;43:849-50.

25. Cook RJ, Sackett DL. The number needed to treat: a clinically useful measure of treatment effect. BMJ 1995;310:452-4.

26. Sackett DL, Richardson WS, Rosenberg W, Haynes RD. Evidence-based medicine: how to practice & teach EBM. New York: Churchill Livingstone, 1997.

27. McQuay HJ, Moore RA. Using numerical results from systematic reviews in clinical practice. Ann Intern Med 1997;126:712-20.

28. Sugano DS, McElwee NE. An epidemiologic perspective. In: Spilker B, ed. Quality of life and pharmacoeconomics in clinical trials. 2nd ed. Philadelphia: Lippincott-Raven, 1996:555-61.

29. Kessler RC, Mickelson KD, Barber C, Wang P. Effects of chronic medical conditions on work impairment. In: Ross AS. Caring and doing for others: social responsibility in the domains of family, work, and community. Chicago: University of Chicago Press, 2001.

30. Kessler RC, Stang PE, eds. Health and work productivity: emerging issues in research and policy. Chicago: University of Chicago Press (in press).

31. Kessler RC, Nelson CB, McGonagle KA, Liu J, Swartz MS, Blazer DG. Comorbidity of DSM-III-R major depressive disorder in the general population: results from the US National Comorbidity Survey. Br J Psychiatry 1996;168(suppl 30):17-30.

32. Kurland LT, Molgaard CA. The patient record in epidemiology. Sci Am 1981;245:54-63.

33. Kurland LT, Molgard CA, Schoenberg BS. Mayo Clinic records linkage system: contributions to neuroepidemiology. Neuroepidemiology 1982;1:102-14.

34. Hoffman LH, Stang PE. Adverse events associated with placebo. Econ Neurosci 2000;2:49-53.

35. Westrin CG. Ethical, legal and political problems affecting epidemiology in European countries. IRB: a review of human subjects research (Hastings Center) 1993;15:6-8.

36. Stang PE. I hear the data singing: considerations when the siren calls. New Med 1998;2:233-8.

37. Ray WA, Griffin MR. Use of Medicaid data for pharmacoepidemiology. Am J Epidemiol 1989;129:837-49.

38. Brooks J, Clark M, Crown W, Davey P, Hutchins D, Martin B, et al. A checklist for retrospective database studies—report of the ISPOR Task Force on retrospective databases. Value Health 2003;6:90-7.

39. Kessler R, Almeida D, Berglund P, Stang P. Pollen and mold exposure impairs the work performance of employees with allergic rhinitis. Ann Allergy Asthma Immunol 2001;87:289-95.

40. Guidelines for good epidemiology practices for drug, device and vaccine research in the United States. International Society for Pharmacoepidemiology, July 21, 1998. www.pharmacoepi.org/resources/goodprac.cfm

The Impact of Pharmacogenomics on the Cost-Effectiveness Ratio

CHAPTER 10

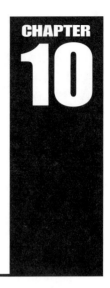

C Daniel Mullins,
Simu K Thomas,
and Jesse Cooke Jr

A great medicine is one that effectively treats or prevents disease and has no adverse effects.

Allen D Roses[1]

Pharmacogenomics is the application of the knowledge of individually inherited traits related to drug metabolism and disease susceptibility to prescribing and drug development; it promises new approaches to preventing and treating illness and drug design. One of the many advantages of pharmacogenomics is that it will enable healthcare providers to predetermine whether a patient is likely to respond well to a drug or will suffer from adverse reactions (ADRs). The benefit of pharmacogenomics on currently marketed drugs is that clinicians will be better equipped to select the best drug at the right dose for their patients.

The science of pharmacogenomics potentially increases the effectiveness of pharmacologic treatments in two ways: by enabling health practitioners to target therapy only to patients in whom an optimal response is likely and by selecting patients in whom there would be few, if any, adverse events. It is important to note, however, that currently pharmacogenomic tests are not commercially available, but rather are used only for research.

Regarding future drug development, the benefit of pharmacogenomics will be the potential identification of new drug targets (excluding antimicrobial agents, the number of human gene targets for drugs covering all therapeutic areas is around 500[1]; this figure is expected to increase from 3,000 to 10,000[2,3]). Thus, pharmacogenomics has the potential to increase the cost-effectiveness of drug therapies by either decreasing overall treatment costs, increasing effectiveness, or both. To determine whether pharmacogenomics will actually increase the cost-effectiveness of drug therapy, one must consider whether the costs and effectiveness remain the same, increase, or decrease.

There is a cost associated with performing pharmacogenomic tests. In some instances, these costs may be less than the cost savings associated with avoiding ineffective treatments. In such cases, all else being equal, pharmacogenomics would clearly reduce overall costs. In many cases, however, pharmacogenomic testing could increase the average cost of treatment. When pharmacogenomics increases both the effectiveness and the costs associated with drug therapy, the impact of pharmacogenomics on the cost-effectiveness ratio of the treatment is determined by the proportional change in these increases rather than the absolute change. This is essentially the same process used in the calculation of the incremental cost-effectiveness ratio as explained in previous chapters. This chapter outlines how pharmacogenomics may affect the costs, effectiveness, and the cost-effectiveness ratio of drug therapy interventions.

Pharmacogenetics and Pharmacogenomics—The Evolution

Before discussing how pharmacogenomics may affect the costs and effectiveness of pharmacotherapy, an overview of genetics terminology is in order. *Genotype* refers to the genetic constitution or makeup of an organism and is not directly observable. *Phenotype* refers to the observable properties of an organism as they have developed under the combined influences of the genotype of the individual and the effects of environmental factors (eg, hair color, eye color). The term *allele* refers to an alternative form of a gene, having a distinct genotype and, often, a distinct phenotype. Different alleles produce variations in inherited characteristics, such as eye color or blood type. A *polymorphism* is a common variation in the sequence of DNA among individuals. *Single nucleotide polymorphisms* (SNPs) are single-based differences in the DNA sequence that can be observed among individuals,[4] occurring in one percent or greater of the population, whereas mutations are rare, occuring in less than one percent of the population (usually, much less than one percent).

The terms *pharmacogenetics* and *pharmacogenomics* are often used interchangeably; however, they are not synonymous. The term *pharmacogenetics* was coined by Vogel[5] and refers to the science that is "the study of how genetic differences influence the variability in patients' responses to drugs,"[1] the use of which provides a better predictive model of patients' response profiles. Pharmacogenetic phenomena can be classified by combining pharmacologic and genetic criteria. From the genetic point of view, there are single gene effects (*monogenic*) and multiple gene effects (*polygenic*) that affect pharmacokinetics and pharmacodynamics, including biotransformation. A genetic polymorphism is the presence of several different forms of a trait, gene, or restriction site among individual members of a population. Variant forms of the same gene (alleles) involved with drug metabolism have been known for many years. Particularly significant are those of the cytochrome P450 family of enzymes (CYP2D6 and CYP2C19 are the main enzymes where polymorphism is of clinical significance in terms of drug metabolism).

Previously, toxicity and ADRs could only be linked to monogenic defects in enzymes involved with the metabolism of a specific drug. However, many problems with drug absorption, metabolism, toxicity, and elimination are, in fact, based on polygenic defects. Pharmacogenetics is the identification and investigation of the genetic factors underlying a particular defect. Pharmacogenetics is based, more or less, on observation.[6] A pharmacogenetic test relates to inherited characteristics (not disease-related) that are predictive of effective drug metabolism; thus, pharmacogenetics is the study of the hereditary basis of differences in responses to drugs. Genetic testing refers to testing regarding one's genetic predisposition to or susceptibility of a particular disease and is a measure of the probability of developing an inherited disease, based on the presence of genetic predisposition genes (eg, BRCA1/2 for breast cancer).

Pharmacogenomics is the application of the genomics principles and technology that evolved from the Human Genome Project to pharmacotherapy and drug development. Pharmacogenomics applies what is known about genetic variations in drug metabolism enzymes (pharmacogenetics) to the rest of the genome and is dependent upon the rapid and accurate sequencing tools that have evolved during the era of the Human Genome Project. Pharmacogenomics is the "use of DNA analysis to discover and assemble a comprehensive list of the variations within the human genome—specifically, the SNPs. SNPs are used to predict the use of new or existing therapeutic agents with maximal efficacy and minimal toxicity."[6]

The Problem with Good Medicine

Despite highly restrictive regulatory requirements for proving efficacy and safety, currently available medications are rarely effective in all patients; furthermore, ADRs are not uncommon, while optimum dose requirements for many drugs vary among individuals. Most effective medicines work in the majority of patients; some drugs work in only a small subset of patients. For example, 30 percent of schizophrenics do not respond to treatment with antipsychotics[7]; interferon B is only effective in one of three cases of multiple sclerosis.[8] Current chemotherapeutic regimens are not effective in most patients. For every drug, there are substantial numbers of patients who do not respond optimally.

Whether or not a drug is effective for its intended indication, it has the potential to cause harm. ADRs have been ranked between fourth and sixth as the leading cause of death in the United States with more than 100,000 avoidable deaths per year. ADRs represent a leading cause of hospitalization and a significant economic burden on the healthcare system. In a single year, more than two million patients are hospitalized for serious ADRs.[9] It is estimated that between $1.6 and 4.2 billion are spent each year in the United States for additional treatments to deal with ADRs in hospitalized patients[10]; the estimated cost of drug morbidity and mortality in an ambulatory setting is estimated to be $76.6 billion.[11]

Optimum dose requirements for many therapeutic agents vary considerably across individuals, thus affecting the effectiveness of therapy. For example, the daily required dose varies 40-fold for propranolol and 20-fold for warfarin.[12] Simvastatin has been found to be highly effective in reducing low-density lipoprotein cholesterol in a dose-dependent manner for the majority of individuals; however, about three to six percent of individuals have no response even at high doses.[13] Additionally, there is the issue of agents with a narrow therapeutic index, where toxicity is more likely and the cost of treating toxicities may be greater. Such instances include gentamicin ototoxicity and nephrotoxicity,[14] digoxin-induced dysrhythmias,[15,16] cyclosporine nephrotoxicity,[17] phenytoin-induced seizures,[18] and ganciclovir-induced neutropenia.[19] Medicines that effectively treat or prevent disease and have no adverse effects are rare. As tools for identifying and understanding diseases as well as the pharmacodynamics and pharmacokinetics of treatment become more sophisticated and precise, more specific treatments will be tailored to individual patients.

Genetic Differences in Drug Metabolism

Genetic morphism has been associated with three types of individual phenotypes, based on their extent of drug metabolism. Extensive metabolism (EM) of a drug is characteristic of the normal population; poor metabolism (PM) is associated with increased accumulation of administered drug, which leads to toxicity; and ultra-extensive metabolism (UEM) or increased drug metabolism is indicative of the need for increased dose requirements. Variability in the expression of genetic markers and enzymes can have a variety of therapeutic consequences in certain populations including:

1. no therapeutic effect due to ultra-rapid drug metabolism and clearance (UEM),
2. lack of prodrug activation,
3. toxic ADRs due to drug accumulation as a consequence of impaired metabolism (PM),
4. extended pharmacologic effect (PM),
5. exacerbated drug–drug interactions, or
6. metabolic activation to toxic products.[20,21]

Many principal enzymes in the human liver that are responsible for the metabolism of commonly prescribed medications are known to exhibit polymorphism in humans[22] (eg, CYP2D6) and affect the therapeutic management of up to 17 percent of individuals in some ethnic groups. The inter-individual variations of these enzymes have been demonstrated to be clinically significant for many drug classes. For instance, in the case of tricyclic antidepressants (eg, imipramine, desipramine, amitriptyline), both PM- and UEM-type individuals are at risk for ADRs. PM individuals given standard doses of these drugs will develop toxic plasma concentrations, potentially leading to unpleasant ADRs, including dry mouth, hypotension, sedation, and tremor, or in some cases, life-threatening cardiotoxicity. Administration of regular doses of these drugs to UEM patients would lead to therapeutic failure. UEM individuals can be successfully treated with higher concentrations of these drugs; however, in such instances, metabolites from alternate metabolic pathways may accumulate and contribute to toxicity. There are significant interethnic differences in the prevalence of PM individuals. For example, in American and European white populations, the prevalence of PM is five to ten percent, while the prevalence is 1.8 percent in African Americans, 1.2 percent in native Thais, 1.0 percent in Chinese, 2.1 percent in a native Malay population, and apparently absent in the Japanese population. The prevalence of UEM among the white population is seven percent.[24]

Pharmacogenomics as the Potential Solution

Pharmacogenomics aims to bridge the gap between gene discovery and drug development and is immediately applicable to clinical studies of existing drugs. The ability to select therapy that is patient specific is a byproduct of the enormous genetic mapping output of the Human Genome Project. The benefits of genomic testing are twofold in that patients can be tested for genetic predisposition to a particular illness as well as for their genetic predisposition to achieve an appropriate drug response with minimal ADRs. An alternative way of viewing the role of pharmacogenomics is that it holds the promise of "weeding out" patients who will not respond to therapy. As such, pharmacogenomics can help reduce costs to the healthcare system by avoiding costs for patients in whom a particular drug will not be effective.

Pharmacogenomics can be defined as molecular-based testing designed to predict physiologic response to specific drugs and monitor the response of the disease to therapy.[23] Using a genomic test to assess and prescribe a drug that is more efficacious to treat the individual is analogous to use of antibiotic sensitivity testing to prescribe the most effective antibiotic. Sensitivity testing for antibiotics is likely to be cost-effective because testing is relatively inexpensive, results can be obtained in a clinically relevant time frame, and the efficacy of the antibiotic is highly dependent on the sensitivity of the organism. Inappropriate use of an antibiotic could lead to severe consequences for the patient when infections are acute or drug resistance develops, thus leading to adverse health outcomes and costs. Pharmacogenomics identifies an area in which genetic screening for drug selection may provide significant benefits to the patient and could be of enormous economic importance. A physician could generate a pharmacogenetic profile of each patient and tailor drug use depending on the unique genetic makeup of each patient.

Potential Effect of Pharmacogenomics on Treatment—Examples

ACUTE LYMPHOBLASTIC LEUKEMIA

Childhood acute lymphoblastic leukemia (ALL) was a universally fatal disease until a few decades ago; however, with the advent of effective drugs, 75 to 80 percent of children with ALL survive at least five years from diagnosis. The backbone of maintenance therapy in most treatment protocols for ALL includes daily administration of oral mercaptopurine. In the years since the introduction of the drug, physicians have been plagued with problems because the drug is not effective in every child and causes serious and even fatal ADRs in some. Further investigation has revealed that about 10 percent of white and African American people carry a variant of the enzyme thiopurine methyltransferase (TPMT). This enzyme is responsible for the metabolism of mercaptopurine. The variant renders the crucial enzyme relatively ineffective; an additional one in 300 of these children lack the enzyme altogether.[24] When these patients are given the regular dose of the drug, they are unable to metabolize it and could experience ADRs that are often fatal due to immune system suppression.[25]

Physicians are now able to test routinely for activity of this enzyme in leukemic children. Children with especially high levels of TPMT who are UEMs are given doses up to 50 percent higher than normal to achieve a therapeutic effect. Those that possess the ineffective variant are given doses as low as one-fifteenth the normal dose, providing all of the anticancer efficacy of a normal dose without the extra ADRs that they would endure with higher doses.

ALZHEIMER'S DISEASE

The application of pharmacogenomics can be demonstrated using the development of drugs that prevent or slow the decline in mental function in patients with Alzheimer's disease. Initial experiments with tacrine were disappointing since, depending on dose and design, only 25 to 50 percent of patients with Alzheimer's disease responded to the drug and one in four patients suffered severe ADRs. Molecular studies indicated that response to tacrine depended upon the phenotype of the patients' apolipoprotein E (ApoE) gene. There are three phenotypes of ApoE: II, III, and IV. Patients with the ApoE IV phenotype respond poorly to tacrine and develop more ADRs than patients with the other two phenotypes.

This knowledge is invaluable when prescribing medication for patients with Alzheimer's disease and has proven important in trials of new drugs for the disease. Assuming a 40 percent response rate, one could use the genetic test in clinical practice to identify the four of 10 patients who would respond to tacrine optimally. Treating the remaining unresponsive six patients with an alternative therapy not only maximizes treatment across the entire group of patients, but also prevents ADRs that would be more likely to occur in those six patients who, without the pharmacogenetic test, would have been treated with tacrine.

SELECTIVE SEROTONIN-REUPTAKE INHIBITORS

Selective serotonin reuptake inhibitors (SSRIs) have emerged as leading oral antidepressant compounds. A critical molecular target of SSRIs is the serotonin transporter protein 5-HTT. Studies have demonstrated that a genetic polymorphism in the promoter of the 5-HTT gene influences the level of expression of that gene. Two allelic variants in the promoter have been described: a shorter form and a longer form. Smeraldi et al.[26] examined whether the polymorphism in the 5-HTT promoter influences the ability of patients to respond to fluvoxamine, a drug approved for use in obsessive–compulsive disorder, but also prescribed off-label for treatment of major depression. The researchers reported that patients with either one copy (heterozygotes) or two copies (homozygotes) of the long variant of the 5-HTT promoter showed a better antidepressant therapeutic response to this SSRI than did patients with a homozygous short variant of the 5-HTT promoter. Therefore, testing for this polymorphism in the 5-HTT promoter may prove important to identify patients most likely to benefit from SSRI therapy.

BREAST CANCER

Trastuzumab is indicated for the treatment of patients with metastatic breast cancer whose tumors overexpress the human epidermal growth factor receptor 2 (HER2) protein and who have received one or more chemotherapy regimens. Trastuzumab, in combination with paclitaxel, is indicated for treatment of patients with metastatic breast cancer who have not received chemotherapy and whose tumors overexpress the HER2 protein (observed in 25 to 30 percent of primary breast cancers).[27]

As previously mentioned, there are currently very few pharmacogenetic tests that are commercially available. However, a test that is comarketed with trastuzumab measures the level of the HER2 protein (a somatic mutation of the tumor)—not the genes that metabolize the drug—so it is not truly a pharmacogenomic test.

Impact of Pharmacogenomics on the Cost-Effectiveness of Treatment

The current emphasis on cost-effectiveness for new therapies encourages the production of medicines that maximize value for patients, providers, and insurers. The application of pharmacogenomics to the delivery of drugs has the potential to improve their value. Treating only predicted responders offers an efficient and economical solution to a growing concern over whether to offer or deny certain expensive medicines to all patients, knowing that a proportion of patients will not respond to the treatment.[28] The question that remains is, under what circumstances can the systematic discovery and analysis of genetic variety in drug response (pharmacogenomics) lead to more cost-effective drug development and treatment?

Several factors affect the costs and effectiveness of the application of pharmacogenomics to drug therapy management (Table 1). As mentioned previously in this chapter, the degree to which pharmacogenomics leads to more cost-effective treatment depends on the degree to which costs and effectiveness are changed. Again, the ratio of the change in costs to the change in effectiveness—not the absolute value of changes—will reflect how pharmacogenomics affects cost-effectiveness. To evaluate the aggregate effect of pharmacogenomics, one will want to consider when and how much costs and effectiveness will be increasing and/or decreasing.

There are several reasons why pharmacogenomics would increase costs; one of the most important is the cost of the drug itself. For example, pharmacogenomics may lead to increased drug costs since they will more than likely be produced as biologics, which are relatively expensive compared with traditionally manufactured synthetic drugs. Alternatively, there may be a decrease in drug costs if the costs of clinical development are reduced dramatically. The issue of patent extensions for new pharmacogenetically determined indications for existing drugs may keep drug costs elevated. Aggregate costs may increase if the number of people deemed treatable for any given disease is greatly expanded by both genetic testing and pharmacogenetic profiling. Thus, a payer may see dramatically increased drug costs for a particular disease category, such as cardiovascular disease.

In addition to drug costs, there are costs administration and interpretation of the pharmacogenetic test, follow-up, and those associated with false-positive and false-negative tests. The use of pharmacogenomics will tend to increase costs more substantially when there is a low prevalence of the genotype. In instances where pharmacogenomic testing increases costs, one may want to compare these costs with those of administering a drug of questionable safety. Nevertheless, these costs may outweigh the benefits of detecting a rare genotype.

In some instances, pharmacogenomic testing could actually lead to a decrease in costs. The cost of conducting the test may be more than offset by the reduced costs associated with treating a narrower, more responsive population. Costs may also decrease because of reduced ambulatory and inpatient costs to treat ADRs. Thus, cost savings from pharmacogenomic testing can be achieved by avoiding unnecessary use of expensive drugs

---

Table 1. Pharmacogenomic Factors that Affect Treatment Costs and Effectiveness

Cost increasing
  Increased drug cost because of increased biotechnology research and development
  Increase in size of the treatable population
  Decrease in size of the treatable population that results in orphan drug status
  Cost of genetic test, including those for technology development, test administration, analysis, interpretation, and dissemination of results
  Cost of genetic counseling, additional clinic visits, and further diagnostics
  Cost of treating the patients with false-positive test results
  Cost of treatment delay caused by false-negative genetic test results
  Low prevalence of the genotype

Effectiveness increasing
  Treatment focused on the population most responsive to treatment, with alternate therapies provided to those who are unlikely to respond
  High sensitivity and specificity of the genetic test in appropriately identifying the right population that would respond optimally to candidate drug
  High degree of association between genotype and phenotype

Cost decreasing
  Decrease in drug costs due to fewer drugs being abandoned in early development due to lack of safety or efficacy
  Smaller proportion of population to be treated
  Adverse events avoided in the population identified as not responsive to candidate drug
  Avoided costs of treatment failures
  Avoided costs of routine laboratory tests to monitor liver and/or renal function (eg, Zyflo, an asthma drug that caused hepatotoxicity, thereby requiring that patients be routinely monitored—the gene that is associated with this adverse event has been identified since the drug was marketed)
  Cost of genetic testing could be a one-time cost offering long-term savings, especially when the information can be used for choice of another drug therapy

Effectiveness decreasing
  Low degree of association between genotype and phenotype
  Less than optimal effectiveness of alternative therapies to which nonresponding patients are switched based on pharmacogenomic tests

that are unlikely to be effective in certain patients and by optimizing dosing in patients with atypical drug metabolism. Furthermore, there may be additional cost savings associated with genetic testing when the results can be used for other treatment decisions.

Pharmacogenomic testing may lead to increased treatment effectiveness. Contrary to popular thinking, the application of pharmacogenomics would not alter the population in whom a drug is effective. Rather, it would simply allow quicker identification of responders. Pharmacogenomic testing could replace a prolonged and expensive process of prescribing by trial and error.[29] Additionally, drugs may be developed to be effective in patients with various polymorphisms. Patients who are not the right candidates for a particular therapy would benefit not only by avoiding the harmful effects of that therapy, but also would benefit from earlier initiation of an alternative therapy. Pharmacogenomics can improve outcomes (effectiveness) by identifying responders and nonresponders, thereby leading to better directed therapies, shortened length of hospitalizations by more rapid resolution of acute illness, and reduced adverse effects and overall toxicity of drugs. In the instance of increased effectiveness, there are opportunity cost savings since resources will not be allocated to treat patients who are unlikely to respond. This process of targeted therapies would enable the provision of the right drug to the right patient, thus improving treatment effectiveness for the entire population.

Pharmacogenomic testing does not guarantee improved effectiveness. Genetic tests are both sensitive and specific; however, the presence of a particular genotype is not 100 percent predictive of drug response or ADRs. Concomitant drug use, food–drug interactions, adherence, and other nongenetic factors affect drug metabolism. Furthermore, effectiveness may be affected by the degree to which the genotype is predictive of phenotype. In some instances, phenotype may be influenced by factors other than genotype. In the case of Alzheimer's disease, phenotype–genotype discordance does exist when considering whether ApoE is a predictor of one's susceptibility to Alzheimer's disease. The association with Alzheimer's disease among ApoE IV homozygotes (odds ratio = 14.7) was higher than expected based on an observed odds ratio of 2.0 in heterozygotes.[30] Phenotype–genotype concordance was less frequent for ApoE II than for

ApoE IV. The ApoE II phenotype occurred at a frequency of 7.9 percent versus a genotype frequency of 4.9 percent, corresponding to a probability of 56 percent that an individual with ApoEII phenotype actually had the genotype. Finally, one must also consider the decreased effectiveness associated with therapeutic switches of nonresponders to less-than-optimal therapy in cases where there are not equally effective treatments for nonresponders.

In theory, the impact of pharmacogenomics could increase or decrease costs and effectiveness, as outlined above. In many instances, however, the likely impact is an increase in both the costs and effectiveness of treatment. In such cases, increases in the costs associated with genetic testing should be weighed against improved treatment effectiveness that would result from only treating patients in whom there would likely be a response to therapy. In the process of doing so, one should also consider the impact on nonresponders as well as responders.

Scenarios for the Cost-Effectiveness of Pharmacogenomics

In general, the use of pharmacogenomics will be cost saving as long as the method used for detecting genetic polymorphisms is less costly than the events being avoided or their sequelae. Pharmacogenomics will be cost-effective if the increased cost associated with genetic testing is less than the value of the improvement in health outcomes at the population level. The extent of cost-effectiveness when using pharmacogenomics in the therapeutic setting depends on several factors (Table 2).[31,32] The main point to consider is whether pharmacogenomic testing offers the ability to predict and prevent costly adverse events that are associated with a genetic polymorphism. It is worth noting that a polymorphism may or may not be a significant predictor of an ADR. Additionally, with some disease states, such as HIV, depression, and hypertension, ADRs are highly correlated to nonadherence and/or withdrawal from a medication[33-35] (eg, sexual dysfunction associated with antihypertensives[36,37]). Depending upon the disease, nonadherence or withdrawal may exacerbate a condition, thereby having economic consequences. When ADRs can be predicted and avoided, the long-term sequelae and costs associated with nonadherence can also be avoided. In some

Table 2. Scenarios for the Cost-effectiveness of Pharmacogenomics

When Pharmacogenomics Is More Cost-Effective	Assumptions	Example (Hypothetical)
Costly adverse events are associated with genetic polymorphisms and are predictable and preventable	existence of test for specific drug-related polymorphism polymorphism correlated with adverse event	hepatotoxicity resulting in hospitalization or death
Common, less severe adverse events that are highly correlated with non-adherence can be predicted and prevented	adverse reactions are genetically predisposed and result in drug therapy non-adherence nonadherence increases costly morbidity in the long term	angiotensin-converting enzyme inhibitors and cough antihypertensives and impotence extrapyramidal symptoms, common with many antipsychotics
A high dollar value is associated with therapy or there is a high opportunity cost of not receiving a more appropriate therapy	no viable therapeutic alternatives or effective therapies exist	Trastuzumab and breast cancer therapy patients who overexpress the HER2 protein tacrine and Alzheimer's disease
Drugs have a narrow therapeutic index with high patient variability	no viable therapeutic alternatives or effective therapies exist	histopathologically, patients receiving chemotherapy have a 40% response rate[27,28]
Events being avoided are more costly than the method used to detect them	events can be avoided using screens	current cost of genetic screening for disease costly and frequent laboratory tests to avoid hepatotoxicity
When Pharmacogenomics Is Less Cost-Effective	**Assumptions**	**Example (Hypothetical)**
Rare adverse events are predictable and/or preventable using existing technology	cost of screening for these events outweighs the cost of the events	agranulocytosis
Adverse events are neither costly to treat nor associated with nonadherence	occurrence of these lesser events does not create a cascade of events that leads to more costly outcomes	mild skin discoloration
Costs of genomic screening are more than those of the events being avoided	adverse effects are easily treated or dealt with by patients	dry mouth, flushing

cases, a therapy may have a very narrow therapeutic index based on genotype. In the case of trastuzumab, the drug is only effective in patients with breast cancer who are genetically predisposed to overexpression of the HER2 protein. In terms of cost, there is an opportunity cost involved when allocating treatment resources to a population that will not respond. Additionally, in the case of breast cancer, for example, there are costs associated with delaying treatment in patients who may inappropriately receive trastuzumab, particularly the costs of treating a more advanced stage of cancer.

The use of pharmacogenomics, however, may not be cost-effective when used to predict or prevent extremely rare adverse events. Nor will it be cost-effective to detect a polymorphism that has little or no correlation with drug metabolism and thus has little or no relation to whether the drug is toxic or ineffective.

Impact of Pharmacogenomics on Drug Development (Clinical Trials)

In addition to using pharmacogenomics in clinical practice to identify patients with anticipated drug response, the science could be used early in the drug development process to identify patients in clinical trials who are most likely to respond to the drug. Given that 80 percent of the compounds fail in clinical trials and industry spends $500 to $700 million for each new drug approval, considerable benefits may be reaped through the application of pharmacogenomics in the development of new drugs.[38] Drugs that previously would have been abandoned in early development because of failure to prove their safety and/or effectiveness may, in fact, proceed to approval as a result of identifying a priori the population to which the drug should be limited.

Suppose a promising new molecule is developed for the treatment of Alzheimer's dementia. During its early development, based on what is known about the genetic predisposition of certain people to Alzheimer's disease and what is known about how the drug is metabolized (ie, enzymes), it can be determined which patients will respond and in whom the drug will be toxic based on their pharmacogenetic tests. Subsequently, by being able to identify these patients, a reduced sample size will be needed because of the reduction in what would have otherwise been random variability. In Phases II and III clinical trials, only responders would be recruited, resulting in smaller trials that would be faster and more economical.

By focusing clinical trials on patients who are most likely to respond, drug development resources could then be allocated to those patients with continued unmet medical needs. In particular, molecules that show less than a 30 percent response rate in a large population, but have a clear efficacy in an identifiable population of patients, would become viable as they could be readily identified for development and clinical practice. Furthermore, the ability to target heterogeneous groups of patients for parallel drug development early, rather than waiting years for nonresponsive populations to emerge after extensive clinical use of the medicine, will be of significant economic benefit.

While pharmacogenomics could be used to select individuals who are most likely to respond to drug therapy, it could also be used to determine exclusion criteria for clinical trials. This may occur directly by excluding those who are unlikely to respond to treatment or indirectly by excluding patients who are at lower risk for disease progression. Although variation in disease susceptibility is commonly attributed to environmental exposures, genetic differences can also influence susceptibility. For instance, genes have been identified that protect against HIV infection, the development of AIDS, tuberculosis, malaria, and influenza. Winkler et al.[39] observed that survival after HIV infection varied by genotype, with approximately 30 percent of the least protected individuals surviving for 18 years versus 100 percent in the most genetically protected individuals. Such protective genes are beneficial to the individual carrier; however, they can adversely affect clinical trials by reducing the trial's power and increasing its duration since individuals with protective genes may never experience the endpoint or may progress toward the endpoint at a slower rate. Thus, inclusion of protected subjects in the trial could result in an overestimation of the true response rate. The rapid growth in knowledge about protective genotypes is increasing the feasibility of using genetic screening to remove genetically protected individuals from clinical trials.

The cost of genetic screening is an important consideration examining the impact of pharmacogenomics on clinical trials. Presently, genotyping costs between $100 and $600 per test.[40,41]

However, the United States Department of Commerce has awarded over $50 million in grants to aid in the development of quick genetic tests with target costs of $10 to $20 per test. These lower prices will probably apply to genetic tests that will be frequently used, such as those for determining whether one has the susceptibility gene for a common disease or tests that allow one to use genetic information to help determine the proper dosage of a common drug. As tests are developed, they could also be used for screening potential clinical trial participants.

Calculating the total potential savings and added costs due to genotyping shows that genotype screening will generally lower the costs of a trial. For example, Fijal et al.[42] demonstrated that, for a typical four-year clinical trial without genotypic screening, assuming 80 percent power and a five percent significance level, one would require 3,418 subjects. If five percent of the subjects have a screenable protective genotype, then 3,403 subjects would need to be screened and only 3,232 would need to be followed through the trial. If genotyping costs between $100 and $600 per test and per patient costs for a trial range from $6,000 to $12,000, then genotyping could add $340,300 to $2,041,800 to the trial, but could save $1,116,000 to $2,232,000 in total patient costs for the precluded 186 subjects. While genotyping will not necessarily lower costs in all situations, lower costs will lead to greater incentives to include genotype screening in clinical trials.

In a Phase II trial of a drug acting on the central nervous system, 450 patients were screened to ensure that only patients with the extensive metabolizer phenotype were included.[43] The overall cost savings associated with using this genotype screening criterion was estimated to be $143,000 (range 49,800 to 304,900). The use of genotype screening in this trial helped to avoid ADRs in patients with the poor metabolizer phenotype and substantially reduced the cost of conducting the trial by eliminating the need for additional healthcare resources that would have been used to treat these adverse events.

Impact on Future of Health Care

The potential implications of pharmacogenomics for the future of health care could be that each disease would be subdivided according to genetics rather than symptoms. Drug therapy will be targeted to act at or near the cause of a disease. Pharmacogenomics does not improve the efficacy of a given drug, but it helps in selecting patients who are likely to respond well. Thus, the ability to genetically define patient populations would help improve outcomes, and genetic prognostics will revolutionize treatment and improve cost-effectiveness.

Genetics-based tests that improve detection of diseases could preclude many of the unnecessary and overused procedures that are currently performed to confirm screening tests. The cost of pharmacogenomic testing should be compared with the benefits of detection, appropriate treatment, and issues important to society as a whole, including disease epidemiology and population management. High costs for unnecessary treatments can be demonstrated using the clinical testing for the genetic predisposition for cancer. In the United States alone, the annual cost of follow-up of positive prostate-specific antigen tests that do not result in a cancer diagnosis (false-positive rate of 75 percent) is estimated to be $750 million.[44] Similarly, the annual cost for follow-up for the 85 percent false-positive mammograms for breast cancer is estimated to be $850 million. For the 50 percent false-positive fecal occult blood test for colorectal cancer, unnecessary treatment is estimated at $800 million. The 75 percent false-positive atypical squamous cells of undetermined significance on Pap tests for cervical dysplasia cost $4 billion.

Thus, for cancer patients who would otherwise be destined to have unnecessary biopsies due to false-positive screening tests, the overall savings of using an appropriate molecular-based testing could approach $6.4 billion.[44] There is also considerable psychological morbidity associated with a false-positive test including counseling fees, drugs, and time lost from work by worried patients awaiting results of unnecessary biopsy procedures.

Current Challenges in Pharmacogenomics

The field of pharmacogenomics is evolving at a high pace; therefore, the existing knowledge in the area is limited and becomes outdated very rapidly. Identifying an effective therapeutic agent from genomic data is difficult and is further complicated by the fact that expression levels for many proteins change during disease progression. Currently, genomics companies offer genotyping services of SNPs using the Masscode system to genotype known SNPs (to date, approximately 40,000 have been identified) specific to their clients' requests and human genomic DNA samples provided by the clients. Some fear that the downside to designing clinical trials based on narrow patient populations is that the market potential of some drugs will be reduced because they will be targeted to smaller markets.[45] Also, the use of testing to determine which patients should participate in clinical trials may raise trial expenses. By contrast, it can be argued that prestratified clinical trials will be smaller and faster, thus yielding cost savings at the trial stage as well as in treating fewer drug toxicities and in prescribing fewer useless medications after marketing. In addition, removal of the small percentage of individuals who are likely to experience drug failure or complications could lead to a several-fold increase in a drug's market potential. This may occur because clinicians will have increased confidence in prescribing drugs to patients who are not currently treated; additionally, patients may be more motivated to adhere to a drug regimen that is less likely to cause adverse effects.

Like so many advances in genetics, pharmacogenomics raises important ethical questions with issues of genetic privacy and discrimination. People are nervous about their genetic profiles falling into the wrong hands. Patients could have varied reactions when a genetic test is required for prescription of an effective drug. Since some of the relevant gene patterns are ethnically linked, it raises issues of racial stereotyping and access to care. Another fear is that profit-conscious pharmaceutical companies may use pharmacogenomics to aim their drug development efforts toward genetic subgroups of people who can best afford to pay, further marginalizing the already underserved minorities.

Summary

The effects of pharmacogenomics on the cost-effectiveness ratio are speculative at best, as there are too many unknown factors at this time. This chapter presents examples to give the reader some idea of how pharmacogenomics could influence cost-effectiveness ratios. Medicines that work in all patients and have no ADRs are rare or nonexistent. Pharmacogenomics will enable health practitioners to individualize drug therapy by developing target-specific strategies to administer the right drug at the right dose to their patients. This approach will presumably improve effectiveness in the treated population and avoid suboptimal treatment of the patients who will not benefit from a particular drug, as well as avoid the use of a drug that is potentially toxic to a certain population.

Pharmacogenomics can assist ensuring that each patient receives the most appropriate therapy. Future developments in pharmacogenomics will have an impact on both the costs and effectiveness of drug therapy and therefore will alter the cost-effectiveness ratios of new drugs. Although the use of pharmacogenomics may offer cost-effective options for drug therapy decisions and development, a case-by-case economic analysis is warranted before making pharmacoeconomic decisions.

References

1. Roses AD. Pharmacogenetics and future drug development and delivery. Lancet 2000;355:1358-61.
2. Drews J. Genomic sciences and the medicine of tomorrow. Nature Biotech 1996;14:1518-9.
3. Drews J. Drug discovery: a historical perspective. Science 2000;287:1960-4.
4. Brookes AJ. The essence of SNPs. Gene 1999;234:177-86.
5. Vogel F. Modern problems of human genetics. Ergibb Inn Kinderland 1959;12:52-125.
6. Pfost DR, Boyce-Jacino MT, Grant DM. A SNP-shot: pharmacogenetics and the future of drug therapy. Trends Biotechnol 2000;18:334-8.
7. Emsley RA. Partial response to antipsychotic treatment: the patient with enduring symptoms. J Clin Psychiatry 1999;60(suppl 23):10-3.
8. Evidence of interferon beta-1a dose response in relapsing–remitting MS: the OWIMS Study. The Once Weekly Interferon for MS Study Group. Neurology 1999;53:679-86.
9. Lazarou J, Pomeranz BH, Corey PN. Incidence of adverse drug reactions in hospitalized patients: a meta analysis of prospective studies. JAMA 1998;279:1200-5.
10. Classen DC, Pestotnik SL, Evans RS, Lloyd JF, Burke JP. Adverse drug events in hospitalized patients. Excess length of stay, extra costs, and attributable mortality. JAMA 1997;277:301-6.
11. Johnson JA, Bootman JL. Drug-related morbidity and mortality: a cost-of-illness model. Arch Intern Med 1995;155:1949-56.
12. Lu AY. Drug-metabolism research challenges in the new millennium: individual variability in drug therapy and drug safety. Drug Metab Dispos 1998;26:1217-22.

13. Davidson MH, Stein EA, Dujovne CA, Hunninghake DB, Weiss SR, Knopp RH, et al. The efficacy and six-week tolerability of simvastatin 80 and160 mg/day. Am J Cardiol 1997;79:38-42.
14. Carvalho A, Fonseca C, Falcao F, Pereira TA, Freitas O, Parrinha A, et al. Individualized monitoring of the therapy with gentamycin using pharmacokinetic methods. Which method to choose? Acta Medica Portuguesa 1996;9:187-95.
15. Parker BM, Cusack BJ, Vestal RE. Pharmacokinetic optimisation of drug therapy in elderly patients. Drugs Aging 1995;7:10-8.
16. Evans WE, McLeod HL. Pharmacogenomics—drug disposition, drug targets, and side effects. N Engl J Med 2003;348:538-49.
17. Woo J. Therapeutic monitoring of cyclosporine. Ann Clin Lab Sci 1994; 24:60-8.
18. Parker BM, Cusack BJ, Vestal RE. Pharmacokinetic optimisation of drug therapy in elderly patients. Drugs Aging 1995;7:10-8.
19. Markham A, Faulds D. Ganciclovir. An update of its therapeutic use in cytomegalovirus infection. Drugs 1994;48:455-84.
20. Wolf CR, Smith G, Smith RL. Science, medicine, and the future: pharmacogenetics. BMJ 2000;320:987-90.
21. Tucker GT. Clinical implications of genetic polymorphisms of drug metabolism. J Pharm Pharmacol 1994;46(suppl 1):417-24.
22. Linder MW, Prough RA, Valdes R. Pharmacogenetics: a laboratory tool for optimizing therapeutic efficiency. Clin Chem 1997;43:254-66.
23. Ross JS. Financial determinants of outcomes in molecular testing. Arch Pathol Lab Med 1999;123:1071-5.
24. Relling MV, Hancock ML, Rivera GK, Sandlund JT, Ribeiro RC, Krynetski EY, et al. Mercaptopurine therapy intolerance and heterozygosity at the thiopurine S-methyltransferase gene locus. J Natl Cancer Inst 1999; 91:2001-8.
25. Andersen JB, Szumlanski C, Weinshilboum RM, Schmiegelow K. Pharmacokinetics, dose adjustments, and 6-mercaptopurine/methotrexate drug interactions in two patients with thiopurine methyltransferase deficiency. Acta Paediatr 1998;87:108-11.
26. Smeraldi E, Zanardi R, Benedetti F, Di B. Polymorphism within the promoter of the serotonin transporter gene and antidepressant efficacy of fluvoxamine. Mol Psychiatry 1998;3:508-11.
27. Press MF, Pike MC, Chazin VR, Hung G, Udove JA, Markowicz M, et al. Her2/neu expression in node-negative breast cancer: direct tissue quantitation by computerized image analysis and association of overexpression with increased risk of recurrent disease. Cancer Res 1993;53:4960-70.
28. Mather DB, Sullivan SD, Augustein D, Fullerton P, Atherton D. Incorporating clinical outcomes and economic consequences into drug formulary decision: a practical approach. Am J Managed Care 1999;5:277-85.
29. Roses AD. Pharmacogenetics and the practice of medicine. Nature 2000; 405:857-65.
30. Kardaun JW, White L, Resnick HE, Petrovitch H, Marcovina SM, Saunders AM, et al. Genotypes and phenotypes for apolipoprotein E and Alzheimer disease in the Honolulu–Asia aging study. Clin Chem 2000;46:1548-54.
31. Kumagai K, Shimizu K, Masuo K, Yamagata K, Tanaka T. Anticancer ef-

fects of preoperative chemotherapy on colorectal carcinoma. Dig Surg 1998;15:337-41.

32. Bissett D, Paul J, Wishart G, Jodrell D, Machan MA, Harnett A, et al. Epirubicin chemotherapy and advanced breast cancer after adjuvant CMF chemotherapy. Clin Oncol (R Coll Radiol) 1995;7:12-5.

33. Cohen JS. Avoiding adverse reactions. Effective lower-dose drug therapies for older patients. Geriatrics 2000;55:54-6, 59-60, 63-4.

34. Max B, Sherer R. Management of the adverse effects of antiretroviral therapy and medication adherence. Clin Infect Dis 2000;30(suppl 2):S96-116.

35. Michels KB. Problems assessing nonserious adverse drug reactions: antidepressant drug therapy and sexual dysfunction. Pharmacotherapy 1999;19:424-9.

36. Weiss RJ. Effects of antihypertensive agents on sexual function. Am Fam Physician 1991;44:2075-82.

37. Barksdale JD, Gardner SF. The impact of first-line antihypertensive drugs on erectile dysfunction. Pharmacotherapy 1999;19:573-81.

38. Housman D, Ledley FD. Why pharmacogenomics? Why now? Natl Biotechnol 1998;16:492-3.

39. Winkler C, Modi W, Smith MW, Nelson GW, Wu X, Carrington M, et al. Genetic restriction of AIDS pathogenesis by an SDF-1 chemokine gene variant. ALIVE Study, Hemophilia Growth and Development Study (HGDS), Multicenter AIDS Cohort Study (MACS), Multicenter Hemophilia Cohort Study (MHCS), San Francisco City Cohort (SFCC). Science 1998;279:389-93.

40. Dykes CW. Genes, disease and medicine. Br J Clin Pharmacol 1996;42:683-95.

41. 12th World AIDS conference: mutation count predicts response in drug-resistant HIV patients. Reuters Health Information Online 1998, July 1. www. reutershealth.com/frame2/arch.html (accessed 2002 Jul 9).

42. Fijal BA, Hall JM, Witte JS. Clinical trials in the genomic era: effects of protective genotypes on sample size and duration of trial. Control Clin Trials 2000;21:7-20.

43. Wallace M. Genotype screening—the impact on clinical trial costs. Annual meeting of International Society of Technology Assessment in Health Care 1999;15:412.

44. Ross JS. Financial determinants of outcomes in molecular testing. Arch Pathol Lab Med 1999;123:1071-5.

45. Evans WE, Relling MV. Pharmacogenomics: translating functional genomics into rational therapeutics. Science 1999;286:487-91.

Incorporating Pharmacoeconomic Research into Clinical Trials

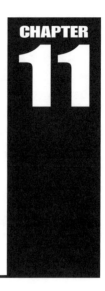

CHAPTER 11

Jane T Osterhaus
and Raymond J Townsend

As the United States and other healthcare systems continue to evolve, so do the requirements and expectations of decision-makers regarding "proof" of the value of pharmaceuticals. While some of the expectations have been transformed into specific requirements in other countries (eg, Australia, Canada, the United Kingdom), there are unwritten rules or expectations created not by edict, but by the marketplace. Regardless of the source of the incentive, it seems that greater efforts are being made in terms of trying to demonstrate more fully the value of pharmaceutical interventions.

It is important to remember that these evolving expectations are in addition to, not replacements for, the well-established requirements of safety and efficacy. Given that the basics of safety and efficacy have not changed markedly, the only place to start to understand the value of the drug is within the clinical trial process.

Pharmaceutical companies are increasingly being called on to document the value of their products, not only clinically, but also in terms of economic and humanistic value. This value can be measured via appropriate data collection and analysis techniques. Information collected early in clinical trials regarding the impact of a new product on the healthcare system can help determine its price and provide initial information to prospective purchasers regarding the value this new product will have versus current therapy. Once a product is on the market, its value must be continually assessed relative to its role in providing comprehensive pharmaceutical care.

Pharmacoeconomic Versus Traditional Research

Pharmacoeconomic research methods can be used to place value on therapies by identifying and measuring variables expected to be affected by healthcare interventions. Such research asks: What happened to the patient after an intervention? What impact did it have on the use of other healthcare resources? What were the outcomes? Was the patient relieved of symptoms? Was a condition cured, an illness prevented, or functional status restored? Until recently, such outcomes of medical care received little research attention. There is a paucity of data regarding the outcomes of medical care, surgical procedures, and behavioral interventions. Even diets generally are not thoroughly evaluated before they are incorporated into medical practice. In fact, drugs are considered to be the best paradigm for clinical outcomes in the United States because of the rigorous testing required for their approval.[1]

In order for a drug to be approved for marketing in the United States, safety and efficacy must be demonstrated, usually by presenting evidence from two adequate and well-controlled clinical studies. This experimental model is well established; safety and efficacy are critical factors to address, but that model, in outcomes terms, is incomplete. To obtain a complete assessment of the outcomes of healthcare procedures and treatments requires scientific evaluation in three dimensions: clinical, economic, and humanistic. Although economic and humanistic measures are not currently required for approval of a drug by the Food and Drug Administration (FDA), because of their mandate to regulate the promotion of pharmaceutical products, the FDA has demonstrated significant interest in the area. The FDA Modernization Act (FDAMA) was passed in November 1997; Section 114 became effective in February 1998. Section 114 created a new standard for healthcare economic information requiring "competent and reliable scientific evidence" (as opposed to data from adequate and well-controlled clinical trials) encompassing standards "widely accepted by experts in the relevant fields." The FDA has not yet published any formal guidance regarding Section 114. Health-related quality of life (HRQOL) is separated from healthcare economics, and the agency is working on developing guidance in both areas. This may have significant implications regarding how HRQOL and/or healthcare economic information generated from trials (or elsewhere) can be used in the United States. If the goal of incorporating pharmacoeconomic variables into clinical trials is to use the information via traditional means of promotion, the reader is encouraged to visit the FDA's Web site (www.fda.gov) to determine the current status of FDAMA and other guidances that may impact how pharmacoeconomic information can be used.

Additionally, committees making decisions on whether to include a drug in a health maintenance organization, hospital, or other formulary are gaining an appreciation for the importance of evaluating its use in the clinical, economic, and humanistic dimensions. Increasingly, these formulary committees and other purchasing groups are expecting pharmacoeconomic issues to be addressed in a standard fashion prior to approval or inclusion on the formulary.

How are the three dimensions of outcomes from pharmacotherapy measured? The clinical dimensions of safety and efficacy are evaluated during the drug development process in clinical trials. The economic and humanistic dimensions of outcomes are measured using research methodologies and data collection techniques within and alongside the traditional drug development process. Although the process of drug development has been described elsewhere,[2] a brief overview of the process will provide a better understanding of how and where pharmacoeconomic research fits into the process.

Clinical Research: The Drug Development Process

After basic animal research has been conducted and the preclinical studies have shown that a compound warrants further testing, a pharmaceutical candidate is then tested in humans.

This process is divided into three study phases. In Phase I studies, the drug is tested in small numbers of healthy volunteers to evaluate safety. If the drug appears safe, Phase II studies begin in patients who have the disease for which the drug is expected to be indicated. Phase II studies are designed to define initial efficacy parameters and optimal dosing of the drug using a small number of patients in various controlled clinical trials. After the demonstration of safety and initial efficacy, Phase III studies begin in large numbers of patients in controlled trials. Phase III studies are conducted to gather additional evidence for specific indications and usually are considered to be the pivotal safety and efficacy studies that support a New Drug Application (NDA).

The results of these three phases of studies, along with preclinical results, are compiled into an NDA or International Registration Dossier (IRD) and submitted to the FDA and other regulatory agencies worldwide with requests for approval to market the drug. While regulatory agencies are reviewing the data contained in the NDA/IRD, most companies initiate Phase IIIB studies to provide additional information regarding use of the drug. These studies usually involve a large number of patients, with safety and efficacy as major endpoints. They also address practical questions regarding the drug's use in more realistic situations.

Although this traditional method of evaluating drugs via safety and efficacy studies is well established, from an outcomes measurement perspective, it is incomplete. Because of the controlled nature of clinical trials, the safety and efficacy data obtained are likely to only approximate the effectiveness of the drug under real-world, or less-controlled, conditions. When conducting and interpreting clinical trials, it must be kept in mind that efficacy information indicates whether a drug can work under controlled conditions; it is the effectiveness of a product that is a measure of how the drug works in the real world, under average conditions created by, for example, nonadherence, use of concomitant therapy, or lack of access to care. Results obtained early in controlled trials may be compared and contrasted with results from Phase IV studies, which may have fewer controls, to determine the consistency of outcomes results. Pharmacoeconomic researchers and evaluators must keep in mind that data collected within any controlled study may not be representative of the drug effects experienced by all patients who take the drug. Study design and the pharmacoeconomic methods used will help to determine the degree to which data gathered will approximate what might be observed in the healthcare setting.

The shifts that are now occurring in the basic foundation of the medical care system necessitate incorporating pharmacoeconomic research within the context of clinical trial research. This chapter identifies issues and discusses considerations surrounding the incorporation of pharmacoeconomics into clinical trials. Establishing a benchmark, design issues, instrument selection and administration, data management, analysis and interpretation, and reporting of results are discussed.

Establishing a Benchmark

It is difficult to know whether a treatment has been successful if the natural course (condition without treatment) of the disease is unknown. The absence of baseline information markedly reduces the value of any information generated by the incorporation of pharmacoeconomics into an isolated clinical study since there is no benchmark with which to compare the results. Thus, it is crucial that a baseline be established before beginning the clinical research. Early incorporation of epidemiologic research and methods into the drug development and pharmacoeconomic research plans will aid in the interpretation of later study results. Epidemiologic research methods can be used to identify the natural course of the disease and current treatments, as well as provide information that will be useful in determining the burden of the disease to patients, healthcare systems, and society.

Before developing the research plan, a thorough review of the literature should be conducted. The literature search can be generated via MEDLINE using typical clinical search terms. Literature sources such as *Social Science Abstracts, International Pharmaceutical Abstracts*, government documents, and other databases also should be considered. However, not all information desired will be found in the literature; knowledge gaps can be identified from the literature review, providing a platform for the researcher to expand.

Identifying what is known about the condition and its current treatments helps focus the research effort. Questions of interest typically include: Who does the condition most affect? In what ways? Who bears the burden of the illness? For example, asthma may affect a child clinically and in terms of lost school days. However, in an economic sense, it may also affect a working parent or the parent's employer. Likewise, Alzheimer's disease has tremendous economic and humanistic consequences on the caregivers. Additionally, some diseases have no effective treatment, and the healthcare system can provide only minimal care for the patient. However, these conditions may incur costs outside of the healthcare system. Depending on the perspective taken, those costs may be as important as the costs incurred within the system. For example, the cost of AIDS is great in terms of the morbidity costs incurred outside of the healthcare system.

It is initially important to assess the humanistic factors affected by the disease to capture the total burden of the illness and establish baseline information. Likewise, patient satisfaction with specific aspects of current treatments or interventions should be considered and measured. These baseline humanistic (satisfaction, HRQOL) assessments may indicate the degree to which there is room for improvement from the patient's perspective. If baseline scores indicate minimal dissatisfaction or impairment, it is unlikely that an intervention will result in significant improvement in satisfaction or HRQOL, assuming valid, reliable, and precise instruments are used. For example, migraine headaches have been demonstrated to impact the quality of life of people who experience them compared with those who do not, even between headaches.[3] The HRQOL impact of nausea and vomiting associated with highly emetogenic chemotherapy has been documented.[4] Similar work has also shown that patients with osteoarthritis have a worse HRQOL (and therefore room for improvement) than those without that disease.[5] Baseline HRQOL assessment may involve cross-sectional data collection or longitudinal collection. Cross-sectional data collection provides a fingerprint of HRQOL at one point, with patients reporting their health status during the past week or month. Following a group of patients over time to collect longitudinal data can provide information about changes in health status during the measurement period.

It also is valuable to establish baseline levels of resource use. The basis for economic evaluation is an appropriate and complete assessment of the resources being used as opposed to dollars being spent. This is particularly true when collecting data from multiple locations and within environments where costs are subject to change. Resources used also represent, in part, the processes of care involved in patient diagnoses and treatment. Until recently, there have been only minimal attempts to link such processes of care to patient outcomes. If resources are limited, it is important for decision- and policy-makers to ensure that providers are using resources efficiently and effectively. If it is not known what or how much is being used to achieve an endpoint, it is impossible to know whether efficiencies are being attained. As resource use comes under greater scrutiny, it becomes more important to know what resources are involved in treating a condition to make proper use of the existing resources and ensure that new treatments are properly framed.

Although prospective studies may be required to capture the baseline data, there are other sources to consider. Some of these sources include patient diaries, government surveys, and medical charts. These sources can be used to conduct longitudinal studies to capture resource use over time. Various databases exist that can provide some information regarding resources used to treat conditions. These databases exist because many healthcare providers, including health maintenance organizations, have been paid based on the resources they use, so there is an incentive to provide such data. However, administrative databases do have shortcomings since they were not designed to provide complete outcomes information; they were designed to pay claims. If the condition is clearly and easily defined by a disease or treatment computer code, claims databases may provide information regarding the processes of care. However, medical claims data should never be assumed to be accurate. Appropriate validation techniques should be used to demonstrate the accuracy of the claims.

The importance of establishing appropriate and rigorous benchmarks for pharmacoeconomic assessment cannot be overstated. The management of outcomes is dependent on the ability to measure them, and measurement must have a frame of reference.

Study Design

RATIONALE

After benchmarks have been established, the next critical step is to incorporate pharmacoeconomic parameters into clinical trials. The goal of this step is to provide data that will demonstrate the value of the product or intervention from various perspectives. Pharmacoeconomic research attempts to answer the "so what" question to the observed clinical change; that is, it documents the economic and humanistic consequences of pharmacotherapy. Ideally, pharmacoeconomic and clinical study plans should be developed in tandem. The degree of pharmacoeconomic involvement will most likely be a function of the phase of research in which the study is being conducted, the clinical study design, the condition of interest, and the information gathered at baseline regarding the condition and its impact. Key questions to address include:

1. What is the primary purpose of the study?
2. Are economic and HRQOL measures of primary or secondary importance?
3. Why does this study need to be conducted? (eg, support registration, clinical experience)

The process defined to address these questions should be clear and transparent so that potential issues surrounding study design or bias are easily addressed.

OBJECTIVES

The pharmacoeconomic research question(s) should be defined in consideration of the clinical research question(s) raised. The questions should be clearly stated so that the study can be designed to answer the questions. Pharmacoeconomic research may be incorporated into a clinical trial as a secondary or primary objective. For example, if the study is a pivotal Phase III trial in which the primary goal is to measure safety and efficacy for an NDA/IRD submission, pharmacoeconomics may be considered as an "add on," and it is unlikely that the study will be (or should be) extensively modified to make it more appropriate for a pharmacoeconomics study.[6] On the other hand, a Phase IIIB or Phase IV study, with the primary intent of measuring

HRQOL or resource use in a general population with the condition under consideration, should be designed with the objective of answering a pharmacoeconomic question. Having a study designed primarily to collect pharmacoeconomic parameters does not mean that safety and efficacy are ignored; clinical data must be collected to associate resource use and HRQOL changes with the clinical response.

DESIGN ISSUES

The pharmacoeconomic endpoints should be clearly identified in the protocol. The protocol should be closely adhered to, and standard precautions should be taken to minimize potential biases or systematic error that may lead to erroneous conclusions. If the major purpose for conducting the study is to assess pharmacoeconomic changes with treatment, then completion of baseline pharmacoeconomic evaluations also should be part of the protocol's inclusion criteria.

When designing pharmacoeconomic studies, it is critical to adhere to sound scientific principles. Randomized controlled trials are generally considered to provide the strongest level of evidence of efficacy. Hence, clinical trials, especially those intended to be part of an NDA or supplemental NDA (sNDA) are typically randomized, double-blind, and placebo-controlled. However, other study designs (observational, pretest/posttest, modeling) may be better suited for evaluating a pharmacoeconomic question, where blinding may mask the actual use of resources or the impact of a means of drug administration on HRQOL. Observational studies are sometimes used by health services researchers if the goal is to evaluate resource use in a realistic setting for various populations using one intervention or another. The results must be interpreted cautiously and should not be viewed in isolation.

If resource use assessments are incorporated into the study, the perspective (eg, patient, society, employer) must be identified as well. Several perspectives may be of interest. As the healthcare system undergoes further shifts, some perspectives will no doubt be of greater interest than others. Clearly, society and patient perspectives are of interest because, as a society, certain types of healthcare resources, such as vaccinations, are highly valued, in part because of their external benefits. Third-party payer perspectives are of interest because of the decision-making power that they have in the current healthcare system.

It is difficult to collect resource use and other economic data that are representative of realistic situations in a clinical study designed primarily to assess safety and efficacy. This is particularly true for chronic conditions, such as hypertension, or studies designed to prevent disease that use intermediate outcomes as endpoints (cholesterol-lowering studies designed to reduce the incidence of coronary artery disease or studies on preventing the sequelae of osteoporosis). On the other hand, some clinical trials of acute conditions may very closely mimic reality (eg, treatment of sepsis). The researcher must be aware of the extent of the limits imposed by the clinical trial design and document them in subsequent publications or presentations.

Likewise, the extent to which humanistic data collected in controlled clinical trials are indicative of expectations in the true population of patients is a function of the type of patients enrolled in the trial and whether the study design reflects a realistic use of the drug. For example, an antihypertensive clinical trial may include only individuals with mild to moderate hypertension and exclude those with other preexisting conditions. Conversely, a study of migraine with strict enrollment criteria may enroll only patients with the most severe symptoms. The patients participating in a clinical trial may serve as a proxy or may provide an indication of what to expect in future use outside of trial conditions. If mildly affected patients show some improvement, one might expect to see larger improvements in patients affected more severely. If the intervention is linked with the improvement, results will indicate what aspects (economic or humanistic) have changed; this can be predictive of the expected results of future studies. The results from pharmacoeconomic evaluations in early clinical trials will allow for more focused research in later studies.

SAMPLE SIZE

In planning the design of a study, it is essential to determine the appropriate sample size. Sample size may be a function of efficacy parameters, specific HRQOL parameters, or economic parameters. If pharmacoeconomics is the primary objective of the study, the sample size should be estimated based on changes expected in those parameters. Currently, there is little information about sample size based on pharmacoeconomic parameters. Norms for the SF-36 Health Survey scales in the general United States population have been published by age and gender.[7] However, until more information becomes available, pilot studies with pharmacoeconomic parameters, or previous trials, also may provide useful data. As an alternative, clinical parameters may be used to generate sample sizes; however, such an approach does not guarantee an appropriate estimate. For example, the number of subjects needed to show a clinical difference in asthma treatment might be 40 based on forced expiratory volume in one second; however, a cost-effectiveness study might require 140 subjects if the power calculation is based on the expected difference in number of emergency department visits. Post hoc power calculations will provide support for future studies. Additionally, in cases where pharmacoeconomic measures were not used to estimate sample size, sensitivity analysis should be used to place the results obtained from a study in proper perspective.

INSTRUMENT SELECTION

Selection and design of the data collection instrument is another important aspect of this research plan. Recognizing the symptomatology of the condition and how the population is affected will enable the researcher to select or create an instrument to measure how an intervention might lessen the economic and humanistic burden of the condition in question. Instrument choice is critical. If HRQOL measures are to be included, the condition in question will be the determinant of whether a disease-specific instrument is required. If no appropriate instrument exists, an existing instrument may have to be modified or a new instrument designed. If it is not clear whether a disease-specific HRQOL instrument is needed, it is better to err on the conservative side and use one. A feasible approach is to use a standardized, validated core instrument to collect HRQOL measures, with customized additions to address the specific considerations warranted by the condition under study.

The issues of validity, reliability, and instrument sensitivity should be considered before an instrument is selected for use in baseline measurement and in a clinical trial. It is certainly possible to use a new instrument in a clinical trial without previous knowledge of its validity or reliability; however, the risk the researcher takes is that, after the fact, the instrument may be shown to lack those desired properties. Before using an instrument in a controlled trial, if possible, one should consider conducting a pilot test to verify that it is valid, reliable, and sensitive. If time does not permit it, one needs to consider the risks involved in ending up with data that are not usable.[8] Resource utilization questionnaires also should be carefully developed and tested prior to use within a clinical trial. Data to be collected directly from patients by use of these instruments require special considerations. Some points to consider before any instrument is selected are literacy and translation of clinical terms into language that the patients will understand. The number of items one intends to include will be a function of the disease of interest.

Proper administration of the data collection instruments also is important. The protocol should specify how data will be collected, who will collect them, the specific time(s) during the study that data will be collected, and who will provide the information. Investigators need to be informed of their responsibilities in providing and/or collecting data. Anticipating these questions and addressing them before data collection starts is important to the success of the data collection and, therefore, the study results.

Selection of investigators is another important consideration that affects the success of the study. The number of sites involved in a study may vary. Increasing the number of sites increases the potential complications from a management perspective. However, multiple sites are often needed so that sufficient numbers of patients can be enrolled within a reasonable time frame.

If the patient is the main source of pharmacoeconomic information, the burden placed on the patient needs to be considered. Most patients will not object to providing information; however, if the patients are going to be asked to provide information, they must be notified via informed consent. Patients should be told how much is expected of them, what they are to do, who will answer their questions, and other facts about the study and its effect on them. These issues must be clearly stated in the patient consent form.

Data Management

DATA COLLECTION

In most traditional clinical trials, data are collected in the practitioner's office, hospital, or clinic. Since the physician is usually the investigator and may be making decisions about clinical efficacy, this method is appropriate. Pharmacoeconomic data are frequently, but not always, collected from the patient. Knowledge of the disease helps indicate who can provide the most reliable information about its burden. The patient and the physician are often respondents of choice. However, if the trial involves children, elderly people with cognitive dysfunction, or patients with other mental impairment, the patient may not be the most ideal source of information. Rather, caregivers or parents may be more appropriate respondents.

There are also trade-offs between asking for information at the healthcare provider's site (eg, office, pharmacy) versus collecting it at home. Collecting data at the provider's office means that pharmacoeconomic data are collected at the same time that clinical data are collected. If questionnaires are completed at home, the ability to link the response with a clinical response may be a bit more difficult. On the other hand, patients or caregivers may feel rushed at the provider's site, especially if they are asked to provide additional information during the visit. The likelihood of obtaining complete responses is higher if the data collection forms are completed before the patient leaves the site, and the completeness can be checked by the investigator or another staff member. Also, if questions arise, someone is close by to answer them.

Another potential concern of asking questions at the provider's site is that the patient or caregiver may respond in the manner they think will please the provider as opposed to how they really feel. The issue of social response bias should not be ignored, but it should be kept in perspective. It is, in part, a function of what questions are being posed. If patient satisfaction with the provider is the issue, a social response is of concern. But if the questions focus on the patient's ability to work or attend school, response bias may not be as significant. Response bias is not limited to a physician's office; it also could occur in a home where a spouse may coach a patient as to the "right" responses.

Social response bias may be reduced by changing the data collection medium. A personal interview in a waiting room is not likely to generate any information that the patient considers confidential. Patient self-report via a paper-and-pencil format or computer may provide a better sense of security. There is no generally agreed-upon means to collect such data, as each method has its pros and cons, but whatever method is used, it is important to be consistent across all patients and throughout the study. For example, the SF-36 Health Survey, a commonly used, validated instrument, consistently generates higher scores when data are collected over the telephone as opposed to a paper-and-pencil completion.[9] If change over time is of interest, consistent use of one approach is most appropriate.

FREQUENCY OF DATA COLLECTION

How often should pharmacoeconomic data be collected? If change is to be measured, a baseline and final assessment are required, at a minimum. Additional data collection points will be a function of the trial design and the condition being evaluated. When making the frequency decision, one should consider the pattern of intervention, and whether measures can be concentrated on where the maximum response to treatment is expected. Distinguishing between early and late effects of an intervention may be useful. The frequency with which data are to be collected should be stated in the protocol. Conservative estimates are recommended as data can always be aggregated, but cannot be disaggregated any finer than the original data collection points. Patient burden should also be considered when making these decisions. For an acute treatment, a baseline and final assessment may be appropriate; for a long-term trial, more frequent measures may be necessary to reduce the time period for which patients are asked to recall drug effects.

DATA ENTRY

Proper procedures must be in place to ensure that data being analyzed are of acceptable quality. As with most studies, expected problems in the analysis of such data will surround missing data, multiple responses to single-item questions, illegible items, and stray marks. As the data proceed through data entry, quality assurance, and quality control, procedures such as how missing data are to be handled should be identified and then adhered to scrupulously. A code book should be developed addressing each variable to be entered and decisions made beforehand on how to deal with likely problems. When new problems arise with data entry (and they will), decide the response, be consistent, and note it in the code book.

In the case of HRQOL analysis where several items may comprise a scale, it will be important to state at what point missing items will negate the use of an observation. In the case of economic data, missing items may reduce the usable sample size. Lack of critical demographic information may mean that work status cannot be identified. Missing data can be minimized by using appropriate questionnaires that are easy to complete with minimal burden on the patient or caregiver.

Analysis and Interpretation

An analysis plan also should be developed and either stated in the protocol or maintained as a separate document. The data analysis methods included in the statistical section of the protocol will be dictated by the types of data collected. Variables should be identified that are hypothesized to change over time. As is the case for the clinical component of many studies, a single variable may not suffice as "the answer" for a pharmacoeconomic study. Therefore, primary and secondary measures should be identified. The more measures identified to be of primary importance, the larger the sample size needed and the greater the likelihood of having one measure reach statistical significance due to chance. In the case of resource use, variables of interest may be length of hospital stay or intensity of resource use.

Economic variables need to be evaluated as was determined before the study started. In the case of HRQOL measures, an index, a profile, or a battery of measures may be primary variables. If HRQOL is evaluated via a standard instrument, the instrument should be scored according to the developer's instructions. Multiple analyses of data not specified or planned for in the original study protocol will have less impact (seen as data dredging) than prespecified analyses, unless it is a pilot study intended to generate hypotheses as opposed to testing hypotheses.

The patients to be included in the analysis need to be identified. In some cases, the *intent-to-treat* sample is the appropriate choice. This typically includes all patients enrolled in the study, whether or not they actually followed the protocol, who received at least one dose of study medication. The intent-to-treat analysis is considered to most closely reflect actual use of a drug. Not everyone is adherent, and not every patient provides data for all collection points. Another option is to analyze only patients who completed the study *per protocol*. This subgroup may be of interest if HRQOL of an intervention is being evaluated (eg, there is interest in evaluating only patients who took the drug properly). Analysis of both intent-to-treat and per-protocol groups and a comment on the similarities and differences also is an option, but it is more time consuming.

There are a variety of methods by which pharmacoeconomic data may be analyzed. Clearly, which analytic method to use will be a function of what level of data is collected (eg, nominal, ordinal, interval), its distributional properties, and the number of time points at which data are collected (cross-sectional or longitudinal). Direct comparisons, trends, percent successes, survival analyses, repeated measures, and multivariate analyses all have been used. Whichever method is chosen, it should be stated and justified in the protocol. In general, it is best to keep the analysis as simple as possible. Results should be reported in unweighted averages, in standard form. If HRQOL is measured using a profile, each dimension should be reported separately. Treatment groups should be separated and analyzed by treatment.

Potential confounders of data also need to be considered. Before one can attribute an effect to a specific intervention, it is important to minimize the likelihood of that effect being due to other variables. Randomization into groups, control groups, adequate sample sizes, and appropriate control of baseline parameters help to minimize confounding.

Uncertainty can be addressed in two ways. Statistical methods can be used to address uncertainty that may be due to sampling techniques.

Sensitivity analysis can be used to address uncertainty due to lack of knowledge. Sensitivity analyses ask "What if?" and test the robustness of the data. When assumptions are made about certain parameters, sensitivity analysis quantifies how comfortable one can be with those assumptions. For example, there is no general agreement on the precise discount rate that should be used to discount future healthcare benefits or costs. Since the precise rate is unknown, it is reasonable to test study results with a low, high, and middle value. If study results vary widely, one can have less confidence in any single set of results. Sensitivity analysis can demonstrate the dependence of a conclusion on a certain assumption or that an assumption does not affect results significantly. It also can be used to establish a minimum or maximum value that a variable must possess for study results to be positive.

If the study is multinational, cross-cultural differences must be considered. Before clinical data such as blood pressure and laboratory values can be pooled for analysis, the data must be evaluated for homogeneity. In the same vein, neither HRQOL nor economic data should be pooled without cultural and homogeneity issues being taken into consideration. There may be substantial differences in HRQOL responses across cultures.[10-12] Thus, instruments need to be translated to ensure linguistic and conceptual equivalence. From an economic perspective, different countries may have different pricing policies, and the decision as to what monetary value to use is not always clear. It may be simpler to express economic evaluations in terms of resources used rather than in monetary increments, although some researchers have attempted to estimate country-specific cost-effectiveness from multinational trials.[13-15] Despite attempts to control for various parameters, differences may still exist and, in those cases, data should not be aggregated.

Reporting the Results

When reporting pharmacoeconomic data that were collected in clinical trials, it is useful to keep the presentation simple. If the initial questions asked were clearly stated, such an approach is realistic. One should avoid discussions of individual patients; rather, summary measures should be used to discuss the differences between treatments over time. One should be aware of potential censoring of HRQOL or economic results by death and/or early dropouts. For example, if patients in an osteoarthritis trial who do not experience pain relief are dropped from the study because the treatment is considered a failure, these patients may be using significantly more resources than subjects who are doing well and are still in the study. If the patients in whom treatment fails are lost to follow-up, it will be very difficult to trace the real impact of treatment due to limited knowledge of what happens to people in whom the treatment does not work. Likewise, the value of treatment may be underestimated if the patients in the placebo group are dropping out. The components of variance should be discussed and sensitivity analyses should be conducted so the reader can have an idea of the robustness of the data.

Conclusions

The decision to incorporate pharmacoeconomic parameters into a clinical trial depends on the healthcare environment and what information is being requested to make rational decisions about healthcare choices. Some regulatory agencies require and others are considering requiring economic information as a component of the drug approval and/or reimbursement process. Just as resource availability may limit a pharmaceutical company's ability to develop all of the potential drugs it has in its pipeline, resources also may limit the extent to which pharmacoeconomics will be incorporated into specific drug development programs. Realistically, some pharmaceutical products and healthcare interventions will be in greater need of pharmacoeconomic support than others. For example, drugs that are expected to be used for chronic conditions, to palliate symptoms, or slow the spread of an illness, but not cure it, are more likely to generate queries regarding their pharmacoeconomic benefit than a drug that cures an acute condition. Marketplace competition and demands also play roles in the decision. If a company plans to enter a market in which a number of similar drugs already exists, it may be sufficient to compete only on the basis of price as long as equal efficacy and safety can be demonstrated. HRQOL studies may be of interest only if there is a reason to suggest a difference in the adverse effects or functional status as a result of the intervention.

Pharmacoeconomics is a valuable tool used for making rational choices about pharmaceutical care interventions. Data can be collected in controlled trials before a drug has been approved, and such data can be very useful as long as certain caveats are acknowledged. Whatever pharmacoeconomic assessment is chosen, it is imperative that all aspects of the study be transparent and able to stand the tests of reproducibility and appropriate criticism.

References

1. Wennberg JE. Improving the medical decision making process. Health Affairs 1988;7:99-106.
2. Spilker B. Designing the overall project. In: Guide to planning and managing multiple clinical studies. New York: Raven Press, 1987:36-62.
3. Osterhaus JT, Townsend RJ, Gandek B, Ware JE Jr. Measuring the functional status and well-being of patients with migraine headache. Headache 1994;34:337-43.
4. Lindley CM, Hirsch JD, O'Neill CV, Transau MC, Gilbert CS, Osterhaus JT. Quality of life consequences of chemotherapy-induced emesis. Qual Life Res 1992;1:331-40.
5. Briggs A, Scott E, Steele K. Impact of osteoarthritis and analgesic treatment on quality of life of an elderly population. Ann Pharmacother 1999;33:1154-9. DOI 10.1345/aph.18411
6. Cady RK, Dexter J, Sargent JD, Markley H, Osterhaus JT, Webster CJ. Efficacy of subcutaneous cumatriptan in repeated episodes of migraine. Neurology 1993;43:1363-8.
7. Ware JE Jr, Snow KK, Kosinski M, Gandek B. SF-36 health survey manual and interpretation guide. Boston: The Health Institute New England Medical Center, 1993.
8. Young TL, Kirchdoerfer LJ, Osterhaus JT. A development and validation process for a disease specific quality of life instrument. Drug Info Assoc J 1996;30:185-93.
9. McHorney CA, Kosinski M, Ware JE. Comparisons of the costs and quality of norms for the SF-36 health survey collected by mail versus telephone interview. Med Care 1994;32:551-67.
10. Hurny C, Bernhard J, Gelberg RD, Coates A, Castiglione M, Isley M, et al. Quality of life measures for patients receiving adjuvant therapy for breast cancer: an international trial. Eur J Cancer 1992;28:118-24.
11. de Haes JC, Olschewski M. Quality of life assessment in a cross-cultural context: use of the Rotterdam Symptom Checklist in a multinational randomised trial comparing CMF and Zoladex (Goserelin) treatment in early breast cancer. Ann Oncol 1998;9:745-50.
12. Bullinger M, Alonso J, Apolone G, Leplege A, Sullivan M, Wood-Dauphi-

nee S, et al. Translating health status questionnaires and evaluating their quality: the IQOLA Project approach. International Quality of Life Assessment. J Clin Epidemiol 1998;51:913-23.

13. Schulman K, Burke J, Drummond M, Davies L, Carlsson P, Gruger J, et al. Resource costing for multinational neurologic clinical trials: methods and results. Health Econ 1998;7:629-38.

14. Willke RJ, Glick HA, Polsky D, Schulman K. Estimating country-specific cost-effectiveness from multinational clinical trials. Health Econ 1998; 7:481-93.

15. Jonsson B, Weinstein MC. Economic evaluation alongside multinational clinical trials. Study considerations for GUSTO IIb. Int J Technol Assess Health Care 1997;13:49-58.

Pharmacoeconomic Research in Medical Centers

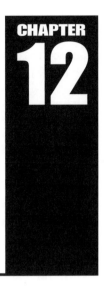

Nelda E Johnson,
Jan D Hirsch,
David B Nash,
and John J Schrogie

Conducting pharmacoeconomic analyses in a medical center setting is beneficial because the results can contribute to the ever-growing body of published research. More importantly, they can guide drug policy decisions for the formulary system and provide information for pharmacy budgeting.[1,2] By generating and using pharmacoeconomic data, medical center decision-makers are better informed about the total cost impact and outcomes of drug therapy and need not rely solely on information about drug acquisition costs. As demand grows for evidence-based, objective formulary decisions that consider the effects of new drugs on quality of life, satisfaction, and total health system costs, healthcare providers need to use the tools of pharmacoeconomics and outcomes research to make efficient, effective policy decisions. Data from pharmacoeconomic analyses can demonstrate the economic and humanistic value of pharmaceutical products, services, and programs and may prove essential as expensive new technologies diffuse rapidly into clinical practice.

This chapter describes some of the specific processes involved in designing and conducting pharmacoeconomic analyses in medical centers and illustrates some projects that can be completed in this setting. Additional discussion provides insight into the challenges that may be encountered when conducting pharmacoeconomic analyses in medical centers and highlights the future for this type of research.

Project Selection

In most medical centers, pharmacoeconomic and outcomes research projects usually need to be prioritized since the number of potential projects often outweighs the available time and resources available to conduct them. The greatest priority should be given to products with high acquisition costs or those with high utilization rates. New products that offer greater clinical benefit but cost significantly more than comparative therapy should be evaluated to determine whether the positive clinical outcomes offset the higher cost of the product. Final project selection should be based on discussions with physicians likely to prescribe new products, pharmacists responsible for medication use policies, and administrators in charge of the organization's quality initiatives.

If the results of the project will be used for anything other than routine healthcare operations, or if it could be considered to be a formal research project, steps should be taken to ensure the protection of patients' rights to privacy and confidentiality and to protect them from any risks associated with the research process. All research projects that use data from medical records or other individually identifiable health information from patient encounters should be submitted to and receive approval from the institution's internal review board or relevant research committee responsible for ensuring patient privacy and compliance with applicable local, state, and federal regulations and policies.[3]

Research Team Members

Conducting pharmacoeconomic analyses is best accomplished with an interdisciplinary team whose members have a broad range of expertise. Ideally, such a group would consist of physicians, pharmacists, nurses, pharmacoeconomic researchers, data analysts, information systems personnel, and a representative from the administrative staff. Using a team-based approach helps provide support for the project across different disciplines and helps ensure the development of a sufficiently sound or robust study that measures and evaluates important clinical and cost outcomes from different perspectives. It also helps to create support for collecting financial data, performing statistical analyses, and involving specialists in areas such as information systems or risk analysis.

Since the impetus for initiating pharmacoeconomic studies often originates from the pharmacy and therapeutics (P&T) or drug use policy committee in medical centers, collaborative efforts between physicians and pharmacists may already exist. Some organizations have created full-time positions for pharmacoeconomic analyses, and others have found that the addition of a data analyst technician greatly improves the efficiency of collecting and managing data.[4] Large integrated healthcare organizations and hospitals belonging to a network or consortium often have access to additional resources that support cost and outcomes studies.[5] One example is the United States Department of Veteran's Affairs (VA) Health Services Research and Development Service that supports several centers of excellence to help multidisciplinary teams of health services researchers assemble the resources and tools necessary for long-term research programs. Other resource centers provide technical assistance and consultation services to VA researchers for organizational and management issues, as well as for use of VA databases for outcomes research and economic analysis. A career development grant program has been implemented to facilitate the training and mentoring of new health services researchers at the VA.[6]

Study Design

Many different types of analyses fall under the umbrella of pharmacoeconomic research including cost-minimization, cost-benefit, cost-utility, and cost-effectiveness analyses. Any one of these methods might be appropriate for determining the value of an intervention in a medical center; however, the specific design will depend on the particular perspective and research question posed for the analysis. The perspective used for studies conducted in a medical center may need to consider several unique perspectives since decision-makers often come from diverse backgrounds and have varied interests. As such, both economic and humanistic outcomes may need to be measured to fully consider all relevant perspectives and adequately determine the value of the product, service, or program being evaluated. Investigators must be knowledgeable about current pharmacoeconomic methodologies and select the most appropriate technique for each analysis—especially for quality-of-life analyses and patient satisfaction, in which new instruments continue to be developed and ongoing reliability and validity testing are often needed.

Economic analyses carried out in an inpatient population are usually conducted from the perspective of the healthcare system and focus on the costs and clinical consequences that are immediate and primarily visible to healthcare professionals, hospital administrators, or healthcare purchasers. Inpatient studies offer an opportunity to create a well-controlled study in which all consequences related to an intervention can be measured during the course of the hospital admission. These types of studies frequently focus on acute illnesses with short-term clinical and economic outcomes and are conducted to determine the clinical impact on the patient and the cost impact on the healthcare system.

In contrast, research conducted using an outpatient population usually focuses on longer-term outcomes that are generally removed from the immediate domain of the healthcare system, but are more relevant to the individual patient. The ability to account for variance within this population becomes less precise since an observer cannot report and verify all patient behavior. Instead, there is increased reliance on patient self-report for measurements that focus on outcomes such as health-related quality of life or functional ability (return to work or increased mobility). These studies are usually viewed from the patient or societal perspective.

As with any other research project, pharmacoeconomic analyses should be carefully planned evaluations designed to test a specific research hypothesis. These analyses may be complex projects using prospective data collection or they may be simple cost analyses using existing data. If time or budgetary constraints dictate that a less in-depth analysis be conducted, the researcher must be cognizant of the caveats and limitations that will apply to the interpretation of the data generated. Guidelines for conducting good economic evaluations should be followed to help ensure that the results obtained are valid and free from unintentional bias.[7,8] In conducting pharmacoeconomic analyses, specific attention should be given to the points outlined in Table 1.

Table 1. Recommended Steps for Pharmacoeconomic Analyses

Research question or hypothesis is well defined
Viewpoint or perspective for the analysis is specified
Comparative or alternative therapies are identified
Clinical effectiveness is evaluated
Revelant costs and consequences are identified
Appropriate study methodology is used
All costs and consequences are measured accurately
Study results are appropriately interpreted and well communicated

---

Prospective Data Collection

The data collection method used will depend on the research question and perspective, as well as the time and resources available for the project. In general, prospective analyses are likely to require more resources and take longer to complete than retrospective data analyses. Prospective studies do, however, offer the greatest opportunity to randomize patients to different treatments and to control variables in the study. Investigators may find opportunities to collect pharmacoeconomic data in conjunction with randomized clinical trials conducted in the medical center, thus allowing the investigator to evaluate pharmacoeconomic data early in the development of a drug. This provides the medical center and the pharmaceutical company with early economic information about the new drug. However, because the protocols followed in a clinical trial may differ from how a drug is used in routine clinical practice, the relevance of the alternative therapies being compared and the protocol-driven medical costs must be considered.[9] Investigators may find it advantageous to use modeling techniques to extrapolate the data from clinical trials and simulate settings more consistent with practice at the medical center.[10]

Retrospective Data Collection

Depending on the sophistication of the medical center's information system, investigators may find that existing databases offer one of the most efficient ways to collect clinical and economic data. Financial decision support systems and electronic medical records can serve as comprehensive retrospective data sources, providing the investigator with both clinical and financial data. Some information systems can extract data from existing departmental databases such as pharmacy, laboratory, medical records, and billing systems and automatically merge the data into one integrated database (or data warehouse), creating a rich source of information that can be used for pharmacoeconomic analyses.[11] Ideally, key data elements in such a system would include information of sufficiently high quality and of such detail that minimal chart review would be required for validation or to obtain supplemental information. Some of the key data elements likely to be available in an integrated database are listed in Table 2. Clearly, it is advantageous to have access to a database that combines both clinical and financial data in an interactive mode.

One example is the sophisticated system developed by the VA that integrates existing inpatient, outpatient, and administrative databases into a single, national patient-care database. This database is housed in a central location where subsets of data (sometimes called data marts) can be extracted for investigators to conduct outcome studies and health economic analyses.[12] Another powerful resource is the VA's nationwide pharmacy benefits management database that contains all inpatient and outpatient medications dispensed to veterans, as well as relevant laboratory tests for monitoring drug therapy—a valuable data source for pharmacoeconomic investigations.[13]

Table 2. Key Database Elements

Unique patient identifier	Drug therapies and doses administered
Date of encounter or service	Length of hospitalizations
Primary and secondary diagnoses	Total cost for each encounter
Procedures performed	Medical service or physician specialty
Severity of illness measures	

Limitations associated with using databases for economic analyses include several factors. Administrative databases usually contain only summarized patient encounter data, resulting in a loss of clinical detail due to the limitations associated with computerized coding of medical diagnoses and procedures. In addition, pharmacy databases usually do not contain the indication (or contraindications) for drug therapy, so this must either be inferred or relevant diagnosis data merged with the pharmacy data or chart reviews conducted to verify the information. Hospital information systems often only store detailed data for certain cost centers or certain types of encounters, such as inpatient admissions. Drugs or resources used in other areas, such as emergency departments or operating rooms, may not even be recorded in the database. For specific cost components not adequately recorded in a database (eg, adverse events or nursing time to administer a drug), investigators can prospectively collect these data, such as with time and motion studies to determine the number of events or amount of nursing time, and then apply standard labor costs to determine a cost value.

Since databases do not allow investigators to randomize patients to different treatment groups, the clinical homogeneity of patients being compared must be evaluated to ensure that the presence of confounding variables such as age, gender, comorbid conditions, or severity of illness do not create an unintentional bias in patient outcomes. In cases where computer diagnosis codes are inadequate to determine patients' severity of illness, algorithms or alternative measures, such as the Charlson Comorbidity Index, which has been adapted for use with diagnosis and procedure codes found in claims databases,[14] may be needed to create matched groups of patients or adjust for existing differences between groups. Because of these limitations, it is imperative that investigators acquire a thorough understanding of the origin and limitations of the data in the system before designing and conducting the study. Most systems were designed for record keeping and billing purposes, so additional work may be required to accurately characterize the clinical parameters and economic outcomes of interest when using this source of data for pharmacoeconomic analyses.

Example Projects

Two example studies are described below to highlight some of the practical applications, issues, and potential compromises faced when conducting pharmacoeconomic studies in a medical center. The framework used to compare and contrast each study is based on the methods for evaluating economic analyses proposed by Drummond et al.[15]

EXAMPLE 1: MEASURING THE CLINICAL AND ECONOMIC IMPACT OF NOVEL THERAPY ON HOSPITAL COSTS

The first example is an evaluation to determine the overall clinical and economic impact that a novel drug product had on the use of hospital resources for postoperative surgery patients. This drug product was selected for evaluation because it was supposed to offer clinical advantages and reduce the length of postoperative hospital stay compared with traditional drug therapy; however, the acquisition cost was considerably higher than that of the comparator drug.

Perspective of the Study

Since the primary research question was to evaluate the cost impact on the hospital, the study used the hospital's perspective and was conducted from the viewpoint of a hospital administrator. Therefore, total costs to the hospital were considered.

Evidence of Clinical Effectiveness

Several randomized clinical trials had already confirmed the efficacy of the new product for postoperative patients; however, these trials were conducted using clinical protocols under carefully controlled conditions and did not evaluate the effectiveness in routine practice. As such, the pharmacoeconomic study also included a prospective evaluation to document the clinical effectiveness of the product relative to traditional therapy within this real-world hospital setting.

Study Methodology

The study was a prospective, observational design that used primary data collected after surgery to document clinical outcomes and adverse events for patients who received either the new drug or traditional therapy. Patients were selected so that the two groups were equally matched with regard to age, gender, comorbid conditions, surgical risk, and procedure performed. A time and motion study was conducted to determine the cost of treating patients who experienced adverse drug events. Resource utilization and costs for time in the intensive care unit (ICU), ventilator time, and postoperative length of stay were obtained from the hospital's financial database.

Results

Analysis of the data showed that postoperative ICU time and ventilator costs were significantly lower for patients who received the new drug compared with those who received traditional therapy.

Interpretation and Use of Results

The investigators found that the reductions in ICU and ventilator costs were statistically significant and large enough to offset the acquisition cost of the new drug. As a result, the new drug was adopted as standard therapy for wider use throughout the hospital's network. Study limitations included a small sample size from one hospital and the fact that patients were not randomized to different treatment groups. Since cause and effect could not be established without randomization, the reduction in costs were said to be associated with, rather than caused by, the new drug. The study took time and resources to complete that were only partially offset by an unrestricted grant from the manufacturer of the new product.

EXAMPLE 2: PREDICTING COST-EFFECTIVENESS OF CLINICAL GUIDELINES IN A HEALTHCARE SYSTEM

The second example illustrates how a decision analysis model can be used to predict the clinical and financial impact of implementing clinical guidelines for using a new drug. This project was conducted for a new biotechnology drug shown to reduce mortality in a subgroup of critically ill patients. The drug had not been widely evaluated in different types of patients, and it seemed likely that physicians would employ less stringent criteria than used in the clinical trial once the drug was available, resulting in great additional expense to the institution, with potentially limited benefit for some patients. A decision was made to implement drug policy guidelines that would ensure appropriate utilization and to conduct a pharmacoeconomic analysis to predict the clinical and cost impact of these guidelines.

Perspective of the Study

The analysis used the health system's perspective and considered patient response rates, as well as overall cost to the institution including the cost to develop, implement, and monitor use of the guidelines.

Evidence of Clinical Effectiveness

The analysis used efficacy and safety data from a single published, randomized, controlled clinical trial.

Study Methodology

A decision tree was constructed to evaluate the outcomes of 100 percent compliance with the guidelines compared with not implementing any guidelines. Outcomes were defined as the number of lives saved with the new treatment and total hospital costs. The potential clinical benefits were based on the treatment effect observed in the clinical trial and extrapolated to a similar group of critically ill patients identified from the hospital's database who would have been candidates for the new therapy (ie, they met the proposed guideline criteria). Potential candidates were identified based on review of key data elements in patients' electronic medical records. The basic model required a set of assumptions, including the

1. percent of patients who would receive the drug and meet the guideline criteria for treatment with the new drug,
2. percent of patients who would benefit from the new drug (based on the published trial),
3. percent of patients who would experience an adverse event related to the new drug (based on the published trial),
4. cost for patients who experienced adverse events with the new drug,

5. cost for patients who were successfully treated and those who failed treatment,
6. cost of implementing and monitoring guidelines.

Results

The decision analysis model showed that the marginal cost for each additional life saved with the new drug would be significantly lower if the guidelines were followed.

Interpretation and Use of Results

Restricting use of the new drug to patients most likely to benefit by using the clinical guidelines was deemed the most cost-effective option. By calculating the potential benefits of using the guidelines, the medical center evaluated whether the benefits of the guidelines offset the cost of implementing and monitoring their use. This analysis provided the medical center with a rational basis for making a decision as to whether it was beneficial to implement guidelines for an expensive new technology.

Challenges

FINDING SUPPORT FOR PROJECTS

One of the primary challenges facing investigators in medical centers is finding the time and resources necessary to conduct full-scale pharmacoeconomic analyses. Large medical centers may find it useful to create a separate, full-time group dedicated to conducting these types of analyses. This allows high-priority, time-consuming projects identified by hospital committees or administrators to be channeled to the appropriate staff and facilitates completion of the analysis in a timely fashion with results specific to the institution. Some organizations, including the Cleveland Clinic and many VA hospitals, have funded full-time positions for pharmacoeconomic and cost analyses, allowing internal analyses to be conducted using the organizations' own data.

Most major pharmaceutical and biotechnology companies in the United States have health economics and outcomes research departments that conduct analyses to support products already on the market and for drugs still in the development process.[16]

Many of these companies also provide funding to healthcare providers to conduct investigator-initiated outcome studies. Collaboration between researchers in pharmaceutical companies, academia, and healthcare organizations has the potential to facilitate research endeavors by bringing together funding sources, research expertise, and data sources.[17] Ethical standards and guidelines to help minimize the potential for bias in economic analyses funded by the pharmaceutical industry have been published.[18]

The federal government has supported pharmacoeconomic research since 1992 by funding grants for the Pharmaceutical Outcomes Research Program. The impetus for funding studies that evaluate the impact of pharmaceuticals on patient outcomes may date back to the Omnibus Budget Reconciliation Act of 1986, which mandated analysis of the cost-effectiveness of medical treatments. Findings from these pharmaceutical outcomes studies have yielded important insights into "which medicines work best for which patients and at what costs."[19] The Agency for Healthcare Research and Quality (AHRQ) continues to fund studies and programs to evaluate clinical and economic outcomes and guide the appropriate, cost-effective treatment of patients. The agency has designated a number of evidence-based practice centers, each of which has a specific technology assessment assignment and many that involve evaluations of drug therapy.

SELECTING OUTCOME MEASURES

Selection of the appropriate outcome measures is key to successfully completing a pharmacoeconomic study. The outcomes must be (1) representative of the drug or program's impact, (2) feasible to measure, and (3) consistent with the timeline and perspective for the study. Direct medical costs are the easiest to measure since these data are typically stored in a cost accounting or financial system. If cost data are not available, hospital charges may be converted to costs by applying the appropriate departmental cost-to-charge ratio for each cost center. Departmental ratios should be used since overall hospital cost-to-charge ratios do not adequately reflect individual costs for different areas of the hospital.[20]

Short-term clinical outcomes, such as acute responses to treatment, are other outcomes that are relatively easy to measure, particularly if the data can be accessed through an online electronic medical record. Clinical outcomes (morbidity and mortality) that occur after hospital discharge are not always feasible to measure since patients may see a physician outside the healthcare system for follow-up care. In a closed setting, return visits or hospital readmissions can be used to identify treatment failures. Patient-focused, humanistic outcomes, such as quality of life, pose the greatest challenge for investigators because questionnaires can be time-consuming to administer and additional follow-up may be required for patients outside the hospital setting.

COMMUNICATING STUDY RESULTS

Once the study data have been collected, analyzed, and interpreted, investigators need to effectively communicate the results within the institution. Key internal personnel who should receive the results of economic analyses include the chair of the P&T committee, the director of the pharmacy, and others involved with setting policies for formulary drug use. These people should have immediate access to the detailed methods and results of the pharmacoeconomic analyses, and summary results should be prepared, along with tables and graphs, for presentation to medical staff leaders and administrative staff. If the results will be published or presented to anyone external to the healthcare organization, appropriate procedures should have been followed to obtain approval from the organization's institutional review board or research committee.

If the organization already has a task force or committee designated to receive and act on the results of pharmacoeconomic analyses, the acceptance and use of such information will be greatly simplified. For organizations without this avenue, economic analyses may represent new concepts requiring additional education about the methodology used and how the results can be incorporated in the decision-making process. Presenting examples of how pharmacoeconomic results have been utilized to benefit patient care or improve financial status in similar institutions is a good way to begin the education process. Interest in the results of economic analyses can be fostered through newsletter briefings, presentations at research and education meetings, and discussions at departmental meetings. The publication of study results in peer-reviewed journals and presentations at national symposiums can also foster greater interest and respect for economic analyses.

EXTERNAL VALIDITY OF RESULTS

Caution should be exercised before extrapolating the results of a pharmacoeconomic analysis conducted as part of a clinical trial to a different type of setting since costs and practice patterns may be quite different.[21] If costs are different, the study results may be incorporated into a model and recalculated by applying internally derived cost data to the data reported for patients in the study.[10] For example, if a published study reported the average length of ICU stay for surgical patients who received a new drug, the cost of the ICU time could be recalculated using another hospital's internal ICU costs. However, if practice patterns were significantly different from those in the study and postoperative patients did not stay in the ICU, the study results would less likely be directly applicable. When the patient population, clinical practice patterns, or financing methods of a healthcare organization are quite disparate, many cost analyses will have little relevance to decision-makers in different settings (eg, the VA system compared with networks of private physician practices).

Quality-of-life evaluations across different organizations may be more consistent and can be enhanced by providing thorough descriptions of the study population, including factors that may influence quality-of-life scores such as demographics (eg, age, sex, comorbidities). The external validity of study results may be further enhanced by including sufficiently large numbers of patients in the analyses or by conducting multicenter studies with a mix of different practice sites.

Future Directions

Pharmacy managers, healthcare administrators, insurers, and government payers have become sufficiently concerned about increasing pharmaceutical expenditures to dedicate resources to programs that encourage the appropriate utilization of new drugs and minimize their economic impact. Some medical centers have joined networks or associations that routinely conduct evidence-based economic evaluations. For example, more than 80 academic health centers belong to the University HealthSystem Consortium (UHC), a not-for-profit membership organization headquartered in Chicago. The UHC has a special technology assessment group that prepares reports about the costs and benefits of high-cost or controversial pharmaceutical and medical technologies and procedures. The information group works with clinical experts in the membership to produce approximately 20 drug monographs each year. In-house technology assessment specialists produce one to two drug-related technology assessments per year.[5]

Not every healthcare organization in the United States has resources for these memberships or can afford a full-time pharmacoeconomics position to conduct economic analyses. As such, the full value of some products may be inadequately evaluated in some settings. To facilitate the economic evaluation process, the Academy of Managed Care Pharmacy produced a guidance document in 2001 for pharmaceutical manufacturers to follow for the preparation and submission of economic information to managed care formulary committees.[22] This document encourages pharmaceutical manufacturers to conduct a full range of pharmacoeconomic analyses and create comprehensive economic models using the healthcare system's perspective and then submit the requisite supporting documentation to the formulary committee for full evaluation. Time will tell how well this system works and whether it is suitable for adoption in other healthcare settings.

Debate still exists as to who should be responsible for conducting scientifically sound economic analyses for new pharmaceuticals. Leading health economists suggest that independent third parties, rather than those who have a vested interest in the results of the economic analyses, should be responsible for conducting these analyses. Dr. Uwe Reinhardt, health economics professor at Princeton University, advocates the creation of not-for-profit pharmacoeconomic research institutes that are completely independent of third-party payers and pharmaceutical companies.[23]

One independent nonprofit organization, RxIntelligence, was created in 2000 by the Blue Cross and Blue Shield Association to provide "independent, credible, and objective pharmaceutical information to healthcare providers, consumers, medical communities and health plans."[5] It has an in-house staff of physicians, pharmacists, and a pharmacoeconomist who work with external clinical experts and consultants to promote rational, appropriate, and cost-effective use of pharmaceutical products by evaluating the effectiveness and cost-benefit of new prescription drugs. An annual subscription provides member organizations with several such reports each year.

Access to relevant pharmacoeconomic analyses conducted by independent centralized sources may be particularly valuable to medical centers in the United States as emerging pharmaceutical technologies continue to consume ever-increasing portions of pharmacy budgets. The availability of new drugs with better efficacy or side effect profiles is likely to increase utilization rates, since these products are readily embraced by prescribers. Thus, patients receive the newer, more expensive drugs rather than older, often generic medications.[24] New drug therapy strategies, such as the use of pharmacogenomics, to predict a patient's response to drug therapy have the potential to significantly improve patient outcomes. However, these benefits must be weighed against the cost of using gene testing strategy—something best answered through scientifically sound pharmacoeconomic analyses.[25-27] Advanced technologies, along with limited resources in United States medical centers, may require increased reliance on published analyses conducted by independent, highly trained pharmacoeconomic experts.

Summary

The use of pharmacoeconomic information in medical centers has grown and is likely to play an important role in future drug policy decisions as a result of increased concern by consumers about drug costs and the increased purchasing power of integrated healthcare systems, as well as challenges presented to manufacturers to produce timely, credible economic information.[28] Pharmacoeconomic data generated internally by trained staff in medical centers are being used for decisions on how to best use products and services in the clinical setting. Decision analysis models are also used to help identify areas where treatment is cost-effective and to predict and evaluate the impact of guidelines or drug-use policies on health outcomes and health system costs.

Sophisticated information systems and trained personnel greatly facilitate the collection, analysis, and use of pharmacoeconomic data for important clinical and purchasing decisions. By conducting well-designed economic evaluations, investigators can produce projects of sufficient quality for publication in peer-reviewed journals. Publication of the studies increases interest in the results and provides information to other healthcare organizations about the overall clinical, economic, and humanistic impact of pharmaceutical products, services, and programs. Pharmacoeconomic analyses are important tools that can help rationalize the selection and guide the appropriate use of pharmaceutical agents in the medical center setting, especially in an era of cost constraints, combined with release of breakthrough pharmaceutical technologies.

References

1. Drummond M, Brown R, Fendrick AM, Fullerton P, Neumann P, Taylor R. ISPOR Task Force on Use of Pharmacoeconomic/Health Economic Information in Health Care Decision Making. Princeton, NJ: International Society for Pharmacoeconomics and Outcomes Research. November 20, 2001.
2. Mather DB, Sullivan SD, Augenstein D, Fullerton DS, Atherly D. Incorporating clinical outcomes and economic consequences into drug formulary decisions: a practical approach. Am J Manag Care 1999;5:277-85.
3. Committee on the Role of Institutional Review Boards in Health Services Research Data Privacy Protection. Protecting data privacy in health services research: a workshop summary. Institute of Medicine, Division of Health Care Services. Washington, DC: National Academy Press, 2000.
4. Ervin KC, Skledar S, Hess MM, Ryan M. Data analyst technician: an innovative role for the pharmacy technician. Am J Health Syst Pharm 2001;58:1815-8.
5. Johnson NE. Creating an outcomes-based formulary: resources to assist in determining a drug's value. Formulary 2001;36:807-10.
6. VA Office of Research & Development. New HSR&D Research Enhancement Award Program. HSR&D Res Briefs 2001(1);1:7-8.
7. Drummond MF, Jefferson TO. Guidelines for authors and peer reviewers of economic submissions to the BMJ. The BMJ Economic Evaluation Working Party. BMJ 1996;313:275-83.

8. Jolicoeur LM, Jones-Grizzle AJ, Boyer JG. Guidelines for performing a pharmacoeconomic analysis. Am J Hosp Pharm 1992;49:1741-7.

9. Ramsey SD, McIntosh M, Sullivan SD. Design issues for conducting cost-effectiveness analyses alongside clinical trials. Annu Rev Public Health 2001;22:129-41.

10. Sanchez LA, Lee JT. Applied pharmacoeconomics: modeling data from internal and external sources. Am J Health Syst Pharm 2000;15:146-55.

11. Wyderka KC. Data warehouse techniques for outcomes management. Health Manag Technol 1999;20:16-7.

12. Cowper DC, Hynes DM, Kubal JD, Murphy PA. Using administrative databases for outcomes research: select examples from VA Health Services Research and Development. J Med Syst 1999;23:249-59.

13. Cunningham F, Sales M, Valentino M. The Pharmacy Benefits Management (PBM) database: a primary resource for nation-wide VA medication data. Hines, IL: VA Information Resource Center. VIReC Insights 2001;2(2):1-8.

14. Deyo RA, Cherkin DC, Ciol MA. Adapting a clinical comorbidity index for use with ICD-9-CM administrative databases. J Clin Epidemiol 1992;45:613-9.

15. Drummond MF, O'Brien BJ, Stoddart GL, Torrence GW. Methods for the economic evaluation of health care programmes. 2nd ed. Oxford: Oxford University Press, 1997.

16. DiMasi JA, Caglarcan E, Wood-Armany M. Emerging role of pharmacoeconomics in the research and development decision-making process. Pharmacoeconomics 2001;19:753-66.

17. Kong SX, Wertheimer AI. Outcomes research: collaboration among academic researchers, managed care organizations, and pharmaceutical manufacturers. Am J Manag Care 1998;4:28-34.

18. Hillman AL, Eisenberg JM, Pauly MV, Bloom BS, Glick H, Kinosian B, et al. Avoiding bias in the conduct and reporting of cost-effectiveness research sponsored by pharmaceutical companies. N Engl J Med 1991;324:1362-5.

19. Gigin M, Awwad R. Final report: the impact of studies funded under Outcomes of Pharmaceutical Outcomes Research. Rockville, MD: US Department of Health and Human Services. Agency for Healthcare Research and Quality, October 2001.

20. Shwartz M, Young DW, Siegrist R. The ratio of costs to charges: how good a basis for estimating costs? Inquiry 1995–1996;32(4):476-81.

21. Drummond M. Economic analysis alongside clinical trials: problems and potential. J Rheumatol 1995;22:1403-7.

22. Sullivan SD, Lyles A, Luce B, Gricar J. AMCP guidance for submission of clinical and economic evaluation data to support formulary listings in United States health plans and pharmacy benefits management organizations. J Manage Care Pharm 2001;7:272-82.

23. Reinhardt UE. Perspectives on the pharmaceutical industry. Health Aff 2001;20:136-49.

24. Dubois RW. Explaining drug spending trends: does perception match reality? Health Affairs 2000;19:231-9.

25. Phillips KA, Veenstra DL, Eyal O, Lee JK, Sadee W. Potential role of pharmacogenomics in reducing adverse drug reactions. JAMA 2001;286:2270-9.

26. Veenstra DL, Higashi MK, Phillips KA. Assessing the cost-effectiveness of pharmacogenomics. AAPS PharmSci 2000;2:E29.

27. Danzon P, Towse A. The economics of gene therapy and of pharmacogenetics. Value Health 2002;5(1):5-13.

28. Greenberg PE, Arcelus A, Birnbaum HG, Cremieux PY, LeLorier J, Ouellett P, et al. Pharmacoeconomics and health policy. Current applications and prospects for the future. Pharmacoeconomics 1999;16:425-32.

Pharmacoeconomics and Community Practice

CHAPTER

13

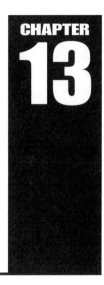

Gene Reeder,
Jean Paul Gagnon,
and W Mark Moore

Pharmacoeconomics is an emerging and dynamic discipline. As with most emerging disciplines, the pharmacoeconomic literature has been conceptual in nature, defining terminology and developing guidelines necessary for conducting quality research. Few articles detail how pharmacists can use the principles of pharmacoeconomics within their practice settings, especially pharmacists practicing in a community environment. It is possible that some community pharmacists will design or conduct cost-minimization, cost-benefit, cost-effectiveness, cost-utility, or cost-consequence analyses. However, trends in health care indicate that community pharmacists are more likely to be participating in these studies and using the data generated through pharmacoeconomic analyses to evaluate manufacturers, products, and services.

The profession of pharmacy has begun to espouse the concept of pharmaceutical care. With the adoption of this concept comes increased responsibilities for measuring the value of products and services. *Value* is the trade-off of costs versus clinical and humanistic outcomes.[1] A new phrase, *patient-reported outcomes,* is beginning to appear in the literature to refer to a variety of humanistic outcomes that can only be provided by the patient such as symptom severity, perception of daily functions, feelings of well-being, and health-related quality of life.[2] Through the provision of pharmaceutical care, pharmacists must be concerned not only with providing patients with the highest quality of care (ie, ensuring the best outcomes), but also with providing this quality to a cost-conscious patient. The combination of quality and cost is the underlying principle of pharmacoeconomics and suggests that community pharmacists have an important role to play in these analyses.

Recent trends in health care, such as the movement toward a system of defined contribution plans and an increased emphasis on cost containment, indicate that quality and cost containment are concerns not only at the individual level, but also at the state and national levels. Ensuring that quality care is provided at the least cost is not a role relegated only to third-party administrators or government agencies; other healthcare practitioners, including the community pharmacist, also are involved. If community pharmacists are to assume this important role, they must understand the principles of pharmacoeconomics and be able to apply them in their practices. Finally, community pharmacists must be prepared to document the value of their professional services in terms of costs versus clinical and humanistic outcomes.

Sometimes the pressures of daily routines restrict our ability to recognize changes taking place in society. Few of us take the time to think of our profession as it might be in the not too distant future. As Levitt[3] pointed out in his classic article, "Marketing Myopia," many businesses fail because they define themselves too narrowly and do not adapt as technology advances. Levitt's example of the railroad industry provides an interesting comparison for the state of community pharmacy practice.

The railroads did not stop growing because the need for passenger and freight transportation declined. The railroads are in trouble today not because the need was filled by others, but because it was not filled by the railroads themselves. They let others take customers away from them because they assumed themselves to be in the railroad business rather than in the transportation business. The reason they defined their industry wrongly was because they were railroad-oriented instead of transportation-oriented; they were product-oriented instead of customer-oriented.[3]

The lesson for community pharmacy is clear: in order to continue to grow and be a viable part of the future healthcare system, pharmacy must recognize and act on customer wants and needs and not be satisfied with the status quo. Pharmacists must realize that they are not in the pharmacy business, but rather in the "patient therapy management" business. Community pharmacy must not limit itself by focusing on the short term; it must look into the future to determine whether changes in the way pharmacists practice will make pharmacoeconomics and outcomes management an important part of what community pharmacists will do.

The fact that nearly all major pharmaceutical associations have embraced pharmaceutical care as a practice philosophy certainly portends a future of change for the profession. Smith,[4] in his teaching of leadership, uses the concept of the "Merlin factor." This approach refers to the legendary wizard who lived backward in time (Merlin was born in the future and aged as he proceeded into the past). He influenced the behaviors of kings by drawing on his foreknowledge of their destinies. In other words, Merlin had the amazing ability to assess the potential of the present moment from the perspective of a clearly envisioned point in the future. Because he knew what was going to happen, he could instill direction and knowledge into persons whose actions could achieve the future that he had envisioned.

Although the application of pharmacoeconomics and outcomes management within community pharmacy practice may not seem feasible at present, the future holds endless possibilities. What is needed is the Merlin approach, a look into the future to envision the practice of community pharmacy and how pharmacists will use pharmacoeconomic data. Once we see the future, we can think and plan backward from that vision to generate effective action in the present. Moreover, by practicing the Merlin approach, the profession can dedicate itself to a future that is strategically alluring, but very improbable if evaluated solely from a historical perspective.

The Future of Community Pharmacy Practice

The realm of pharmacy has evolved from the days of compounding and dispensing through a period of distribution and "insurance clerking" to the embracement of pharmaceutical care and the management of disease. Pharmacognosy was superceded by medicinal chemistry and the development of powerful synthetic analogs, but not to be overshadowed by the resurgence of herbal therapies. The challenges and opportunities for community pharmacies have expanded past the traditional dispensing functions to more educational and clinical roles. A number of pharmacies have risen to the challenge by operating patient clinics that employ disease-state management monitoring and even include prescribing via protocols in certain states.

Pharmacy practice has also been greatly affected by many changes in the environment. The Information Age and the advent of super computers with powerful software systems allow researchers to store, retrieve, and analyze data. These resources also provide access for savvy consumers to empower themselves with information extracted from the World Wide Web, as well as providing a mechanism for ordering medications that bypasses normal distribution channels. In an effort to facilitate self-medication by patients for routine conditions, many medications have been shifted from legend to over-the-counter status. As a result, the future of community pharmacy will continue to be dynamic and will require all participants to acquire better personal, clinical, and analytical skills to ride the paradigm shift from the distribution function to playing an integral role in the continuum of cost-effective health care.

One way to determine what community pharmacy will look like decades from now is to examine current trends in our society. Popcorn,[5] the founder of Brain Reserve, continually examines general consumer trends and their unique relationships to the future marketplace. In a more recent analysis, Popcorn has identified a trend she calls "Give me back my Saturday!" Consumers find that they spend many Saturdays going to the cleaners, getting their prescriptions filled, and running other errands. By the time they are finished, their Saturday is over and they have not had time to relax and enjoy themselves. Ordering their prescriptions from an online pharmacy and having them delivered by mail frees up time on Saturdays. Pharmacists must identify ways to accommodate their patients who lead very busy lives. In addition to becoming efficient in the distribution of pharmaceuticals, pharmacists must also provide prescription drug therapy management to patients at moderate to high risk with their disease. Thus, the future role of pharmacists will center around two functions: (1) using the Internet, robotics, technicians, automation, and other emerging technologies to better deliver pharmaceuticals and (2) providing quality prescription drug therapy management to their patients.

COMPETITION IN THE EMERGING HEALTHCARE SYSTEM

As the United States grapples with soaring healthcare costs, important environmental changes are focused on the healthcare delivery system. These modifications have players jostling for position to take advantage of the market of the future. Because of the growth of managed care, interest in healthcare reform, and ever-rising costs, the scope, role, and structure of payers, providers, and suppliers are changing. A scan of the healthcare environment reveals that networks or alliances of hospitals and providers, fueled by the concept of managed competition, are proliferating at a rapid rate. Hospitals and other healthcare providers are banding together to achieve economies of scale. In the very near future, instead of 10 to 15 hospitals and a number of primary care practices in a city, there will be two or three systems or integrated networks comprised of hospitals and providers. To further this concept, the Federal Trade Commission has published guidelines that allow networks to form without violating antitrust laws.[6] An example of this type of health system alliance is the merger of two Columbia, South Carolina, hospitals—Baptist Medical Center and Richland Memorial Hospital—in the formation of the Palmetto Health Alliance. The South Carolina Health Care Cooperation Act provides immunity to healthcare providers who participate in such state-supervised arrangements from state and federal antitrust legislation.[7] Formation of networks like the Palmetto Health Alliance is part of an overall trend toward integration of the healthcare system. This process of integration and consolidation is being accelerated by coalitions of employees who are leveraging the healthcare distribution system.

After hospitals are united into systems, they strive to improve or maintain the quality of patient care by offering a seamless provision of services; in addition, they seek to fulfill their goal of cost containment through the elimination of fragmentation and duplication of services. Favorite redundancies targeted for elimination include multiple formularies and segregated pharmacy systems. Obviously, costs can be saved by having one formulary among the hospitals with one pharmacy and therapeutics committee. One of the goals of such systems will be to develop a formulary that provides cost-effective pharmaceuticals. Mergers also continue within the drug distribution system. Acquisitions and mergers within community pharmacy chains, drug wholesalers, and manufacturers are occurring at a rapid pace. These mergers seek to achieve economies of scale in operations as well as research and development. As the healthcare market becomes even more competitive, mergers are likely to continue in sectors where economies can be gained.

At the community pharmacy level, pharmacists should explore opportunities in "niche" markets in which a smaller scale of operation is efficient. Examples include customized medicines such as home infusion therapy, compounded specialty therapies, pediatric and geriatric specialties, and the emerging area of biotechnology-derived regimens. While hospitals and other providers are networking to form more efficient health system alliances, suppliers are responding to these market changes by forming vertical market systems, which may adapt more easily in fulfilling the product and service needs of the dynamic healthcare market. These alliances will probably be composed of a number of pharmaceutical companies, wholesalers, and networks of pharmacies that will ultimately offer a formulary to the integrated health system. Also, suppliers may integrate with a pharmacy benefit management organization that provides the outside management of prescription drug benefits including claims processing, formulary management, drug utilization review, observation and influence of physician prescribing patterns, database collection and analysis, and education to provider and patient. It is quite conceivable that, in the future, four or five vertically integrated networks of manufacturers, wholesalers, and retailers will be selling formularies and pharmacy services instead of products. This amalgamation has spawned concerns about the ability of these alliances to remain unbiased and objective in providing services, benefits, and formulary products.[8] Under this scenario, pharmacists will need the skills to build a cost-effective formulary, select a vertically integrated group, evaluate the quality/cost of a formulary, and change prescriber behavior using drug utilization evaluations, practice policies, and clinical guidelines. All of these skills require extensive training in pharmacoeconomics and outcomes management.

In summary, using the Merlin approach to envision the future of community pharmacy practice reveals that future pharmacists will be held accountable for managing drug use through compliance programs, drug utilization review and drug protocol management, monitoring and assessing pharmaceutical outcomes, determining the value of the pharmaceuticals dispensed and the pharmaceutical care services rendered, and selecting suppliers. New roles and niches for monitoring cost-effectiveness and outcomes will arise as payers begin to compensate pharmacists on the basis of their services, what they have done to improve the quality of health care, and how well they evaluate, monitor, and manage the demand for the products and services they deliver.

Future Uses of Pharmacoeconomic Principles by Community Practitioners

As Weinstein and Fineberry[9] have stated, it is not the results of a pharmacoeconomic analysis that will impact a decision, it is the process of structuring information in a systematic framework that brings to light the key uncertainties and the most important value trade-offs. Given the review of important trends in society and where community pharmacy might be in the future, the remainder of this chapter focuses on how pharmacists will apply pharmacoeconomic principles and data in their practices to allow them to meet the wants and needs of their patients.

HEALTH STATUS MONITORING

Patient-reported outcomes will have an important role in optimal patient treatment in the future. As the most accessible health professional, community pharmacists are in an ideal position to collect health status data from their patients. A number of general- and disease-specific instruments discussed in Chapter 7 will be perfected and readily available for use by pharmacists. The Sickness Impact Profile[10] and Quality of Well-Being Scale[11] are examples of the type of instruments that provide an easy and valid measure of a patient's functional and social well-being. The Medical Outcomes Study SF-36, a general measure of a patient's health-related quality of life, provides a profile of the patient's quality of life along eight dimensions.[12] Changes in a patient's health status and quality-of-life profile are important indicators of how well the patient is responding to medications and will be used to manage and improve patient therapy. Such information will be used routinely in patient counseling and physician communications. Coupled with traditional physiologic measures, such as blood pressure, and serum glucose or lipid concentrations, these measures of health status will provide a clearer picture of the patient's overall health and progress.

Consider, for example, the patient who receives an antihypertensive medication. The drug is successful in lowering the patient's blood pressure, but has the undesirable effect of persistent sedation. As a result of sedation, the patient becomes nonadherent and blood pressure increases. The use of a patient-reported outcome metric could have assisted the pharmacist in identifying the decline in the patient's well-being and social functioning. The patient could have been counseled and the physician contacted, if necessary, to consider alternative treatments or dosage adjustments. To survive and prosper, pharmacists must become responsible for proactively monitoring patient drug use and outcomes. Identification of under- and overuse of medications and their consequences for therapeutic, economic, and quality-of-life outcomes will be an integral part of the future pharmacist's role.

Technologic advances will allow the pharmacist to automate data collection and management tasks associated with health and quality-of-life assessments, thus allowing the pharmacist to conduct prospective drug-utilization review. Pharmacy computer systems will be enhanced to read optical scan forms, store patient data, and print patient health and quality-of-life profiles. This information can be linked to a physician database to keep the patient's physician informed of treatment outcomes and problems with therapy. In addition, pharmacists will be responsible for collecting economic data on the indirect costs and consequences for pharmaceutical therapies and services using handheld equipment. Documentation of costs related to lost productivity and caregiver opportunity costs represent significant aspects of patient outcomes from pharmaceuticals and pharmaceutical services. An important role for the pharmacist will be therapy management. Success in this capacity will depend on the pharmacist's ability to collect and maintain comprehensive databases on patient outcomes and use this information to improve decisions about appropriate therapy.

Great opportunities will exist for pharmacists to use health status and quality-of-life indices to improve patient care, enhance the image of their pharmacies, and increase interprofessional communication. With increasing interest in patient health outcomes, it will be important for pharmacists to demonstrate the value of their services to the healthcare system.

EVALUATING PHARMACY SERVICES

Another area in which community pharmacists will apply the principles and tools of pharmacoeconomics is in justifying the value of their professional services. This will be accomplished by documenting the effects of pharmaceutical care on patient health outcomes. In consequence to a continual rise of healthcare spending as a significant percentage of the gross domestic product, cost-effectiveness impact statements for new services will be increasingly desired by individuals, governments, and third-party payers. In allocating scarce resources, everyone will be cognizant of where the most benefit can be gained for each dollar spent. For pharmacy, the major question will be: What difference do pharmacists, pharmaceuticals, and pharmaceutical services make in patient health outcomes? Several societal trends identified earlier point to the consumer's desire for valued services. To justify future existence, community pharmacists must be prepared to answer this question on an ongoing basis. Pharmacists will create and maintain patient databases that relate their functions to positive, cost-effective patient outcomes.

Efforts are underway to evaluate the impact of pharmaceutical care on patient health and well-being. This represents the initial step in the broader quest to establish the added value of pharmacists. Third-party and government payers will refuse to reimburse for any functions that do not offer benefits in excess of costs. Compensation for increases in cost associated with providing cognitive services will need to be justified. Justification will hinge upon the value of the service provided relative to the cost to the healthcare system. Some industrious pharmaceutical clinicians have utilized this portal of opportunity to make a difference by demonstrating benefit and value, resulting in reimbursement for their cognitive services. An example of such financial remuneration in the community setting was shown by the Washington State Cognitive Activities and Reimbursement (CARE) Project's successful implementation of a system of documentation and payment for cognitive services delivered by pharmacists.[13] Community pharmacists must think in terms of costs and consequences as they enhance their practices through the new millennium. Although making these justifications may appear to be onerous, if not impossible, tasks, pharmacists can team with researchers at local schools of pharmacy to conduct pharmacoeconomic analyses of pharmaceutical services. A good example of such collaboration is the Asheville Project, which demonstrated that pharmacists can have a positive impact on patients with diabetes that is associated with a decline in direct medical costs for these patients.[14] Such cooperation and mutual interests should facilitate the development of the requisite database.

POSTMARKETING SURVEILLANCE

Another potentially productive and rewarding area of pharmacoeconomics that community pharmacists might consider is participation in Phase IV postmarketing surveillance studies. These studies are typically sponsored by pharmaceutical companies as part of the drug approval and marketing process. Experience has shown that, while clinical testing of drugs under controlled conditions is important, the real value of a new drug or device is its effectiveness in general patient populations. Numerous examples exist of drugs completing the elaborate and time-consuming premarket drug approval process only to be recalled shortly after marketing because of untoward effects not detected during clinical trials.

Community pharmacists will be involved in and compensated for participation in postmarketing studies. To do so typically will require collaboration with a sponsoring pharmaceutical firm and working with researchers in a school of pharmacy that might coordinate study conduct, data collection, and analysis. Postmarketing studies follow the consequences of using a therapy in general practice. Community pharmacists are in an ideal position to identify patients who are receiving a medication and to collect pertinent information regarding patient status and therapeutic outcomes. Because postmarketing studies are conducted under specified research protocols, the major functions of the pharmacist in these types of studies are to identify patients, discuss the use of the medicine, and document consequences of therapy. Community pharmacists have an advantage in this regard in that they not only can identify a patient receiving a drug for the first time, but also can perform follow-up surveys to determine adherence, side effects, adverse reactions, and ultimately, therapeutic and quality-of-life outcomes. Networks of research-oriented community pharmacies are likely to evolve to accommodate the need for large-scale postmarketing studies of pharmaceutical products and services.

Participation in postmarketing studies meshes nicely with monitoring patient health outcomes in that the structure necessary to perform either activity is similar. Pharmacy computer systems can be modified or adapted to identify potential subjects and alert pharmacists to collect the appropriate information. Moreover, pharmacists can use the system to follow scheduled refill dates and collect data on medication use at some point after the medication is prescribed. Postmarketing studies can become a routine part of a pharmacy's medication and health status monitoring program.

Determining the Value of Pharmaceuticals

Most major pharmaceutical firms are establishing medical outcome or pharmacoeconomic research units within the company. Health insurance companies, benefits managers, and government agencies are demanding evidence that their premium dollars are well spent. Other countries, including Germany, Canada, the United Kingdom, France, and Australia, have already begun to require pharmacoeconomic analyses for reimbursement of new products. The United States is certain to follow in questioning the value of all components of the healthcare delivery system. As a consequence, more emphasis will be placed on conducting studies on cost-effectiveness and therapeutic outcomes to justify the acceptance of and payment for new pharmaceutical therapies.

To survive in the marketplace, a pharmaceutical manufacturer must demonstrate the superiority of its products over existing therapies. The development and introduction of drugs with little or incremental therapeutic benefit will become increasingly difficult to justify, whereas products that offer therapeutic advantages or improvement in patient outcomes will find success. It will be important for community pharmacists to scientifically evaluate new treatment modalities and make recommendations on their value and cost to patients, prescribers, and payers. Moreover, pharmacists must prepare themselves to assume additional responsibility for pharmaceutical therapy selection. This role goes beyond the traditional concept of drug product selection in which the pharmacist simply chooses a reliable generically and therapeutically equivalent drug product. In this expanded role, pharmacists will need to tailor pharmaceutical therapy to a specific patient's clinical, economic, and quality-of-life needs.

Formularies

In the not-too-distant future, pharmacists will not only be responsible for evaluating specific pharmaceutical entities, but also formularies of drugs offered by integrated systems. It is conceivable that, instead of offering products, networks of suppliers and retailers will be selling formularies or drug management systems. The pharmacy and therapeutics (P&T) committee as we know it today will resemble technology assessment committees that consider the cost of a new treatment in addition to efficacy, safety, and quality. Teams of pharmacists will be responsible for evaluating the cost-effectiveness of formulary offerings and claims purported by these groups. These formularies will have to be cost-effective and produce positive quality-of-life effects on patients. Food and Drug Administration (FDA) regulations control the traditional pharmaceutical promotional claims regarding safety, efficacy, and cost; however, they only regulate cost-effectiveness claims made by pharmaceutical companies to P&T committees in managed care organizations under Section 114 of the FDA Modernization Act of 1997. Sophisticated cost-effective analysis models and computer software will be available for use in evaluating these formularies utilizing hand-held technology.

Pharmacists will have to be educated in decision analytic and database management, as well as traditional pharmacoeconomic skills. Serving on these evaluation teams will require considerable analytic and decision-making skills because the effects of the choice of a formulary will dramatically impact the operation of the health partnership and its network of hospitals. These same skills will be required as pharmacists participate in the development and implementation of treatment guidelines, protocols, and disease-state management programs.

Pharmaceutical Care Services

Community pharmacists can use the knowledge of pharmacoeconomics and patient outcomes to their advantage, but to do so will require creativity and a proactive posture. Community pharmacists are accustomed to receiving contracts from third parties that, at best, offer to pay part of the pharmacy's usual prescription charge. Why have these contracts been so arbitrary and unprofitable? Possibly because third-party administrators see little added value in the services and care pharmacists provide. Not recognizing quality differences among therapies and services, much less the consequences of inappropriate therapy, the primary cost-containment strategy of third-party payers has been to reimburse for the lowest-cost product. Most of the evidence offered in support of higher professional fees and charges has been anecdotal or self-anointed without sufficient justification for the value of the pharmaceutical services provided.

Rather than having a third-party administrator dictate a formulary or fee schedule, community pharmacists will work with other healthcare providers or third-party administrators to develop a pharmaceutical care package that can be marketed to benefit managers, employers, managed care plans, and insurers in their local area. This coalition will develop, in conjunction with local physicians, its own formulary based on the most cost-effective therapies. Group buying will then be practiced to secure the lowest product cost for members. The pharmacy group will market itself on the outcomes it can offer the patients it serves.

Such an endeavor will require pharmacists to evaluate products based on clinical, economic, and humanistic outcomes and decide which bundle of services will optimize therapeutic outcomes. As part of a buying group or managed competition network, pharmacists will be in the position of evaluating pharmaceutical manufacturers not only on the quality of their products, but also on the value of the services they supply to pharmacists and patients.

Pharmacists must position themselves to manage not only their business, but also their patients' health outcomes. The impact of prospective and retrospective drug utilization review and drug protocol management on patient well-being, use of medical sources, and cost must be documented at the community pharmacy level. Do we have all the information needed to do this? Not at the present; however, community pharmacists do have the background, ability, and resources to perform these new functions and apply pharmacoeconomic principles to evaluate and document pharmaceutical outcomes.

Skills Needed to Compete in the Emerging Healthcare System

What skills do community pharmacists need to successfully integrate these new opportunities into their current practice? Certainly, pharmacists must be able to interpret and evaluate findings from pharmacoeconomic studies. A major portion of this book is devoted to helping the reader critically evaluate the quality and applicability of this literature. As part of their future practice, community pharmacists using published guidelines will be required to evaluate studies provided by pharmaceutical manufacturers or published in the medical literature regarding the cost-effectiveness, cost-benefit, or cost-utility of pharmaceuticals. Likewise, community pharmacists will work with researchers who are interested in conducting pharmacoeconomic evaluations and pharmaceutical outcome studies. Pharmacists also will be responsible for selecting manufacturers using a number of important variables including policies regarding returned goods, reputation, and liability protection.

Pharmaceutical outcomes manager will become an apt descriptor for a contemporary pharmacist. Therapeutic success will be measured not only in clinical terms, but also in terms of the ability of pharmacists to balance the cost and consequences of therapy. Perhaps the most important duty that pharmacists will assume will be managing humanistic outcomes, ensuring that the patient's quality of life, the most important outcome, is the focus of therapy. They will accomplish this by using the results of patient-reported outcomes to evaluate and adjust drug therapies. Lastly, community pharmacists must market their value and contributions for patient well-being to the public, healthcare payers, and other decision-makers. This means developing a proactive marketing campaign based on sound pharmacoeconomic studies and a cooperative effort among all community pharmacists to establish their cost-effectiveness to the healthcare system. Demonstrating and reporting the outcomes of their work will be key elements of the pharmacist's value story. Controls on utilization and costs are essential components of a well-managed healthcare system and will not be abolished simply because community pharmacists demonstrate their value to the healthcare system. The real challenge of the future will be to convince healthcare payers and decision-makers to consider the full impact of pharmaceuticals and pharmaceutical care on patient outcomes and the total cost of care.

References

1. Kozma CM, Reeder CE, Schulz RS. Economic, clinical, and humanistic outcomes: a planning model for pharmacoeconomic research. Clin Ther 1993;15:1121-32.
2. Patient-Reported Outcomes 'PRO' Symposium: Conceptual and Methodological Issues. Presented at: International Society for Pharmacoeconomics and Outcomes Research 7th International Meeting, May 19, 2002, Arlington, VA.
3. Levitt T. Marketing myopia. Harvard Bus Rev 1960;38(4):45-56.
4. Smith CE. The Merlin factor. Washington, DC: Leadership and Strategic Intent, 1991.
5. Popcorn F. In: The 21st century: hospital pharmacy in a changing health care delivery system. Orlando, FL: Lederle Laboratories, December 1992.
6. Federal Trade Commission, Justice Department announce joint policies for health care antitrust enforcement. FTC News, September 15, 1993.
7. McKnew NM, Miller SL. The Health Care Cooperation Act: panacea or peril? South Carolina Law Review 1996;47:615-28.
8. Thomas M, Larson LN, Bell NN. Pharmacy benefits management. Brookfield, WI: International Foundation of Employee Benefit Plans, 1996:117.

9. Weinstein MC, Fineberry HV, eds. Clinical decision analysis. Philadelphia: WB Saunders, 1980.

10. Bergner M, Bobitt RA, Pollard WE, Martin DP, Gilson BS. The sickness impact profile: validation of a health status measure. Med Care 1976;14:57-67.

11. Kaplan RM, Bush JW, Berry CC. Health status: types of validity and the index of well-being. Health Serv Res 1976;11:478-507.

12. Ware JE, Sherbourne CD. The MOS 36-item short-form health survey (SF-36) I. Conceptual framework and item selection. Med Care 1992;30:473-83.

13. Christensen DB, Holmes G, Fassett WE, Neil N, Andrilla CH, Smith DH, et al. Influence of a financial incentive on cognitive services: CARE Project design/implementation. J Am Pharm Assoc (Wash) 1999;39:629-39.

14. Cranor CW, Bunting BA, Christensen DB. The Asheville Project: long-term clinical and economic outcomes of a community pharmacy diabetes program. J Am Pharm Assoc (Wash) 2003;43:173-84.

The Application of Pharmacoeconomics in Managed Healthcare Settings

CHAPTER 14

Andy S Stergachis PhD,
Dell B Mather PharmD,
Deborah E Atherly MHA,
and Sean D Sullivan PhD

Managed care organizations (MCOs) face the challenge of balancing access, cost, and quality to provide appropriate, effective, and efficient health care to enrolled populations. MCOs attempt to achieve numerous goals, such as improve member satisfaction and retention, control healthcare costs and utilization, and provide high-quality patient care and outcomes. To fulfill these responsibilities, MCOs need to make proper decisions regarding the appropriate use of pharmaceuticals and the design of prescription drug benefits. These decisions are strengthened through the conduct and application of credible, relevant pharmacoeconomic research. Findings from pharmacoeconomic studies can provide the basis to better judge the value of pharmaceuticals and pharmaceutical services in achieving desired outcomes for managed care plans. This chapter describes the current and future role of pharmacoeconomics in the management of pharmaceuticals, pharmaceutical services, and drug policies in MCOs. In addition, the Academy of Managed Care Pharmacy *Format for Formulary Submissions* is described as a tool for use in the pharmacy and therapeutics (P&T) committee process.

.

Managed Health Care

The majority of employed Americans are covered by some type of managed healthcare plan. The term *managed health care* is used to characterize health plans that use mechanisms to monitor and control the cost, quality, and use of health services generally delivered by a specified network of healthcare providers. Managed care also involves the delivery of a predetermined level of healthcare benefits to a defined population on a prepaid basis. MCOs primarily consist of health maintenance organizations (HMOs) and preferred provider organizations (PPOs). In addition to these predominant forms of MCOs, other types of healthcare delivery and/or financing organizations share some characteristics with MCOs, but have less restrictive controls over choice of providers and utilization of services. These include network models, exclusive provider organizations, triple option plans, and fee-for-service insurance programs with active utilization quality management programs, such as managed indemnity programs.

A total of 625 HMO plans operated in 2000, down from 820 plans in 1999. Enrollment in HMOs was 99 million persons in 2000 or 36 percent of the United States population versus 105 million in 1999.[1,2] In 2000, approximately 20 million persons were enrolled in *point-of-service* (POS) HMO plans. POS plans give enrollees the option of obtaining their care from the provider of their choice and being reimbursed for a portion of the cost. That same year, some 6.7 million Medicare and 11.5 million Medicaid beneficiaries were enrolled in HMOs. HMOs are characterized by their requirement for enrollees to use the services of designated physicians and other providers, except in a medical emergency. In general, HMOs have greater control of utilization and use a capitation payment system with providers. One type of HMO, the *staff-model HMO*, employs physicians and may own clinics, hospitals, and pharmacies for the exclusive use of their enrollees. In an *independent practice association* (IPA) model, the HMO contracts with independent physicians throughout a community. The majority of HMOs are organized as IPAs, whereby physicians are reimbursed by the HMO on the basis of a discounted fee-for-service, or capitation payment.

A *preferred provider organization* is a managed care arrangement consisting of a network of hospitals, physicians, and other providers who have contracts with an insurer, employer, third-party administrator, or other sponsoring group to provide healthcare services to covered persons. There were 988 operating PPOs in 2000, down slightly from 1,127 in 1998.[1,2] However, the number of persons enrolled in PPOs increased over that time period from 98 million to 111 million. PPOs generally offer a reduced fee-for-service rate in return for the channeling of subscribers to network providers. PPOs are characterized by the presence of financial incentives for patients to use a network of providers on a preferred basis. PPO network providers commit to accepting reduced or fixed reimbursement and observing an appropriate, effective, and cost-efficient practice style. POS plans combine several of the features of the HMO and PPO. Subscribers under this plan choose how they will receive services at the time they need them. They can choose to use network providers or go out-of-plan for services but pay a higher amount of the cost. It is common for IPA and PPO providers to be involved with several managed care plans simultaneously.

MCOs are characterized by their use of strategies for controlling healthcare costs and utilization. They also have been leaders in attempts to assess and ensure the quality of care, including patient outcomes, and in the application of evidence-based medicine. For most MCOs, key dimensions of performance are tracked in accordance with the Health Plan Employer Data and Information Set measures of the National Committee for Quality Assurance and/or other indicators of care. Overall strategies used by MCOs include the use of prepaid financing arrangements for a full range of covered services, a focus on primary care and prevention, and the use of information technologies and other managerial approaches to optimize the utilization of services.

Prepaid financing arrangements place the organization and its providers at financial risk because a capitation amount is actuarially computed to cover the expected cost of care for the average enrollee over a defined period of time, typically one year. Such a risk-based method of payment provides incentives for providers to control utilization of services. Additionally, MCOs have monitoring mechanisms to assess underutilization by providers as well. The General Accounting Office summarized that most managed care plans include the following cost control features: use of provider networks, with explicit criteria for selection of providers; alternative payment methods and rates that often shift some financial risk to providers; and utilization controls over hospital services and specialist physician services.[3]

MCOs often turn to pharmacy benefit management companies to perform some or all of the management of prescription drug benefits. Approximately 80 percent of HMOs utilize pharmacy benefits managements.[4] Pharmacy benefit managers are organizations that apply managed care principles, such as administrative and clinical functions, to prescription drug programs to promote optimal, cost-effective drug use for a positive impact on the total cost of health care. While there are approximately 100 pharmacy benefit management companies in the United States, the industry is highly concentrated, with the top three companies accounting for over 80 percent of the prescriptions dispensed by pharmacy benefit managements. HMOs rely on pharmacy benefit managements for services such as pharmacy network management, drug utilization review, formulary management, and disease management services.

Managed Care Pharmacy Benefits Programs

Virtually all HMOs offer a prescription drug benefit to their enrolled members. In a survey of HMOs completed in 2000, over 90 percent of HMOs that responded offered a prescription drug benefit.[4] Prescription drug expenditures for HMOs are rising, paralleling national trends. Nationally, Americans spent over $121 billion on prescription drugs in 2000, an increase of 17.3 percent compared with 1999.[5,6] The rise in spending on prescription drugs in 2000 represents the sixth straight year that the percentage increase in spending on prescriptions was in double digits. The number of retail prescriptions per capita was 10.5 per person in 2000, up from 8.3 in 1995.[4] HMOs spent an average of $300 per member annually on prescription drugs for an average of 12 prescriptions per member per year.

Rapid growth in prescription drug spending has been attributed to a variety of factors, such as greater utilization, driven in part by the aging population, price inflation, provision of drug benefit coverage with low copayments, heightened demand fueled by direct-to-consumer advertising, and increased use of newer, more expensive therapies.[7,8] Over $2.4 billion was spent by pharmaceutical companies to reach consumers via direct-to-consumer advertising in 2000 alone.[8] Some recent studies examining the factors involved in increased prescription drug expenditures identified different primary causes for the spending trend increases. Dubois et al.[9] examined seven diseases/drug categories in which spending increases ranging from 43 percent to 219 percent were observed from 1994 to 1997. Volume factors contributed at least 70 percent of total growth in each of the categories that were analyzed. In a separate analysis conducted for the National Institute of Healthcare Management (NIHCM) Research and Educational Foundation, higher prices represented 64 percent of total drug spending increases from 1993 to 1998. Much of the increase in the average price per prescription was linked to the use of newer, more expensive drugs.[10] Another NIHCM report examined the growth in spending on outpatient prescription drugs in retail stores from 2000 to 2001. The 17 percent increase in spending was attributed to the following factors: increase in number of prescriptions (39 percent), price increases (37 percent), and shift to higher-cost drugs (24 percent). Important reasons identified included increasing incidence and prevalence of chronic conditions, increasing diagnosis and treatment of chronic conditions, managed care lowering of patients' financial burden for buying prescription drugs, increased marketing of new drugs to physicians and patients, and efforts by manufacturers to extend the franchise on their best-selling products.[11]

Individual MCOs can conduct their own analyses to better understand the specific factors that play a role in their organizations. The contribution of prescription price inflation to drug expense can be determined by analyzing contractually determined price increases, rebate programs, and the availability of generic alternatives to drugs losing patent protection. An analysis of the contribution of drug utilization to increases in drug expenses should take into account major drugs likely to be released by the Food and Drug Administration (FDA) or added to the drug formulary. For example, in 2000, 27 new drugs and six new biologicals were approved by the FDA.[12] The availability of sophisticated information systems enables the assessment and projection of changes in drug use patterns. By breaking down drug expenditure increases into their component parts, a managed healthcare organization should be better able to focus its efforts at managing its drug budget.

Strategies Used to Manage Drug Benefits: Implications for Pharmacoeconomics

MCOs use a variety of strategies to manage the cost, quality, and access to pharmaceuticals. The basic elements of MCO pharmacy programs include a P&T committee, a drug formulary, generic and therapeutic interchange, the use of special controls for high-cost drugs, treatment guidelines, and a variety of pharmaceutical care interventions including drug utilization review, disease management programs, and academic detailing. Other characteristics of pharmaceutical benefits include member cost-sharing, some degree of financial risk-sharing with prescribers, and, in many cases, contracting with specialty, mail-service, and community-based pharmacies to provide pharmaceuticals and pharmaceutical care services to members. Managed care plans also effectively use contracting with pharmaceutical manufacturers to achieve rebates and price discounts, including solicitation of bids from manufacturers of drugs designated as therapeutically equivalent by health plans.

To better select and evaluate the specific strategies for managing pharmaceutical benefits, managed care plans frequently access and analyze primary and secondary data about the care received by their enrollees. Relatively new methods, such as decision analysis and outcomes modeling, have emerged as contributors to improved medical decision-making in managed health care. As more fully described in the remainder of this chapter, managed care plans are beginning to use the methodologies of pharmacoeconomics to improve decision-making. Illustration of the application of pharmacoeconomics to managed care is categorized into three general areas: formulary policy, appropriate drug use by prescribers and pharmacists, and drug benefit design.

DRUG FORMULARY POLICY

At the center of most managed care plans' pharmacy benefits programs is the P&T committee, the committee charged with maintaining the drug formulary system. Approximately 90 percent of HMOs use a drug formulary. A drug formulary is a continually updated list of prescription drugs that represents the current clinical judgment of providers and experts in the diagnosis and treatment of disease. Functions of effective P&T committees are

1. operate by monitoring the ongoing research and development activities of the pharmaceutical industry;
2. determine which drugs should be added, deleted, or restricted in the formulary based on uniformly applied criteria;
3. define criteria and/or restrictions for use of drugs within the managed care plan;
4. take necessary organizational and educational steps to implement committee action;
5. evaluate and measure drug utilization and outcomes, taking appropriate actions when opportunities for improvement are identified.

Formulary systems play a major role in facilitating appropriate drug usage, decreasing costs, and improving quality. Although formularies can be an important educational tool, they are primarily designed to promote the cost-effective use of safe and effective pharmaceutical products. Formularies provide access to clinically proven treatments while providing savings in pharmaceutical product expenses by facilitating the purchase of drug products at lower prices, reducing drug inventories, and increasing the use of clinically similar but less expensive drugs. Successful formularies restrict access to or discourage the use of drugs for which appropriate lower-cost substitutes are available, thereby encouraging more efficient use of medications. Although there is considerable debate as to whether formularies result in overall cost savings, there is evidence that the use of generic products is increasing and savings are realized for particular drug categories.[13-16]

When compiling and revising formularies, frequently used criteria for selecting among alternative drugs include clinical efficacy, risk of adverse effects, and daily cost of drugs. Too often, cost analyses focus on a search for the least costly alternative without an explicit analysis of overall cost-effectiveness within the healthcare system. In fact, cost-minimization analysis is the most frequently applied pharmacoeconomic method in formulary decision-making. For example, if a drug is determined to be therapeutically similar to existing drugs on the formulary, then the daily cost of drug therapy is weighed heavily by the P&T committee. Additional factors, including quality of life, patient preference, and outcomes, are often not routinely considered as part of the formulary decision-making process.

In recent years, many health plans have expressed interest in using pharmacoeconomic data, but numerous barriers exist.[17-19] Methodologic issues, organizational incentives, and concern about public perception have somewhat limited the use of pharmacoeconomics by MCOs. Despite these challenges, some P&T committees are beginning to examine cost information on a broader basis, taking patient outcomes into account. This is being done with the conviction that the goal of formulary management should not be to decrease the drug budget alone, but rather to improve the efficiency of healthcare delivery and optimize patients' health status in an environment of limited resources.

In an attempt to improve the quality and relevance of information available for P&T committee decisions, the Academy of Managed Care Pharmacy (AMCP) released its *Format for Formulary Submissions* in October 2000.[20] A revision of the *Format* was released in October 2002.[21] This template for MCOs and pharmacy benefits managements details a formalized submission process through which manufacturers present a detailed package of clinical and economic data, along with a disease-based economic model (Table 1). Through the *Format*, AMCP hopes to address several key limitations in the traditional process of obtaining information for formulary decisions, such as:

1. sufficient data are often not available at the time of formulary review;

2. unpublished data and information on unapproved indications are difficult to obtain;

3. pharmacoeconomic data are not routinely supplied by manufacturers;

4. the time required by pharmacy staff to obtain and summarize important information can be excessive.

By requiring submission of an AMCP *Format* dossier, a health plan places a greater burden on manufacturers to provide data supporting the use of their products and demonstrate the value of those products through budget impact or cost-effectiveness analyses.

Since 1998, Regence BlueShield, a 1.1-million member health plan in Seattle that is part of The Regence Group, has required pharmaceutical manufacturers to submit information in a manner very similar to that detailed in the AMCP *Format*.[22,23] In addition to critically appraising trial results, Regence staff uses

Table 1. Components of a Drug Formulary Dossier[21]	
Product description	generic name, brand name, therapeutic class
	all dosage forms, National Drug Codes
	copy of official product labeling/literature
	average wholesale price and wholesale acquisition cost per-unit size and plan contract price, if available
	FDA approved and other studied indication(s)
	AHFS or other drug classification
	pharmacology
	pharmacokinetics/pharmacodynamics
	contraindications
	warnings/precautions
	adverse effects
	interactions
	dosing and administration
	access (eg, restrictions on distribution, supply limits)
	coprescribed/concomitant therapies
	comparison with the profiles of other agents in the therapeutic area
Place of product in therapy	epidemiology and relevant risk factors
	pathophysiology
	clinical presentation
	approaches to treatment
	alternative treatment options including non-drug therapies
	place of proposed therapy
	expected outcomes of therapy
Supporting clinical and economic information	name of clinical trial or study, location and study date
	trial design, randomization, and blinding procedures
	washout, inclusion/exclusion criteria
	characteristics of study sample
	patient follow-up procedures
	treatment and dosage regimens
	clinical outcome(s) measures
	other outcome measures (eg, quality of life)
	statistical significance of outcomes and power calculations
	validation of measures, if applicable
	adherence behavior
FDA = Food and Drug Administration.	

(continued on page 324)

disease-based and budget impact models to help estimate the impact of introducing each product to its formulary. Overall, Regence reports that their process has been accepted. They have received over 100 submissions from manufacturers and have improved the quality, relevance, and timeliness of the information that is available for their P&T committee, leading to improved decision-making. Submission of a dossier, presentation of quality models and projections, and effective communication with the manufacturer are all factors that have been correlated with an above-average formulary acceptance rate.

The AMCP *Format* for standard request of product information is part of a larger trend seen among reimbursement authorities throughout the world. Notable examples include Australia,[24-26] Canada,[27-29] the United Kingdom,[30] and many other European states.[31] In the United States, the Blue Cross & Blue Shield Association launched RxIntelligence, a company intended to provide various groups with information needed to evaluate new products and compare existing drugs.[32] The first areas of research included generic substitution of levothyroxine, a therapeutic comparison of proton-pump inhibitors, and a thera-

Table 1. Components of a Drug Formulary Dossier[21] (continued)

Clinical and disease management intervention strategies	generalizability publication citation
Outcomes studies and economic evaluation supporting data	
Modeling report	disease-based analytic model that is tailored to the plan
Product value and overall cost	summary of information presented within the value argument presented by the manufacturer
Supporting information	spreadsheet models, copies of clinical and pharmacoeconomic references made in dossier

peutic comparison of the cyclooxygenase-2 inhibitors and non-steroidal antiinflammatory drugs.

Not surprisingly, pharmaceutical companies have expanded their activities to generate data in an attempt to estimate the value of their products. Virtually all major pharmaceutical and biotechnology companies have pharmacoeconomics departments with staff who perform and/or contract for economic appraisals as well as quality-of-life studies. Pharmaceutical companies report that pharmacoeconomic analyses have been increasingly initiated early in drug development and decision-making during the drug development process.[33] Most managed care pharmacy directors would agree that valid outcomes and cost-effectiveness data can lead to more effective formulary decisions regardless of the source of funding. However, concerns are growing about variability in the quality of such studies, leading to the development of standards for conducting and reporting pharmacoeconomic evaluations.[34-38] The FDA recently became more involved in the cost-effectiveness field by accelerating the development of principles for substantiation and disclosure necessary to support promotional claims.[39] The FDA Modernization Act of 1997 (FDAMA) was intended to increase the flow of health economic information from pharmaceutical manufacturers to managed care decision-makers attempting to protect consumers from misleading claims and keeping incentives for manufacturers to conduct rigorous studies.[40]

While MCOs typically base their drug formulary decisions on clinical parameters and drug acquisition costs, pharmacoeconomic issues are increasingly being considered as well.[41] Healthcare plans themselves have performed pharmacoeconomic studies in support of formulary decision-making. They can frequently access either primary or secondary health, utilization, and cost data to support pharmacoeconomic analyses. There are examples of data that have been used for cost-of-illness, cost-minimization, and cost-effectiveness studies in managed care settings. Clouse and Osterhaus[42] conducted a cost-of-illness study using United HealthCare Corporation databases. The investigators compared healthcare use and associated costs in patients with and without migraine headache to determine the cost incurred by the health plan for the care of each of these groups. Glauber and Brown[43] conducted another example of a cost-of-illness study.

Using data from the Northwest Region of Kaiser Permanente, a group practice HMO, they evaluated the use and cost of drugs among patients with diabetes and found that those patients use a greater variety of drugs in larger quantities and at greater cost than people without diabetes. Pharmacy expenditures accounted for 17 percent of the total cost of caring for that population of patients with diabetes.

In yet another example, data from a staff-model HMO were used to assess the medical outcomes and costs associated with the pharmacologic treatment of patients with peripheral arterial disease.[44] Among the outcomes assessed were the incidence of invasive diagnostic and therapeutic procedures, hospitalizations, and the cost of care related to peripheral arterial disease. Other economic evaluations of drug utilization following formulary decisions have been reported.[45,46]

Another strategy for making or evaluating formulary policy is decision analysis. Decision analysis offers a framework for evaluating a wide variety of decisions: to select a drug for addition to a formulary, to determine a treatment strategy, to improve clinical decision-making, and to make better policy decisions.[47] As an example, Ofman et al.[48] used decision analysis to estimate the clinical and economic outcomes of using rabeprazole versus ranitidine in the acute and maintenance therapy of erosive esophagitis. Investigators used results from clinical trials and estimates from the literature to model the cost-effectiveness of preventing the symptomatic recurrence of erosive esophagitis. Results were reported as average and incremental cost-effectiveness ratios. Other examples of pharmacy-related decision analysis can be found in the literature.[49,50]

There have been other economic appraisals of various components of formulary management, including the effects of therapeutic interchange. Therapeutic interchange, within the context of a formulary, allows the pharmacist to substitute drug products that are deemed therapeutically equivalent, although not chemically equivalent. Managed care programs are increasingly allowing the interchange of one drug with another of the same pharmacologic or therapeutic class when deemed appropriate. This decision is usually made by the P&T committee and enables the organization to stock only one of these drugs based on the best contract terms it can negotiate. There have been a few formal assessments of cost savings associated with therapeutic interchange. McDonough et al.[51] reported the total direct cost and savings associated with a voluntary program that switched enalapril to lisinopril in patients with benign essential hypertension who were enrolled in Harvard Community Health Plan, a staff-model HMO. Direct costs included drug acquisition, office visits, laboratory monitoring, management of adverse effects, pharmacy administrative costs, and the time value of money. Using computerized pharmacy records and a review of patient medical records for a random sample of enalapril- and lisinopril-treated patients, the authors demonstrated a net savings in less than 12 months following initiation of the voluntary therapeutic interchange program. More recently, Baluch et al.[52] reported on the experience of one HMO in substituting esterified for conjugated estrogens. Cost savings were estimated and patient acceptance of the conversion was assessed. The HMO avoided $653,119 of an expected $750,000 cost increase for oral estrogren therapy during the first year of the program.

APPROPRIATE DRUG USAGE

Ensuring appropriate drug use (ie, prescribing, dispensing, patient adherence) can maximize the benefit that enrollees receive from their medications and associated medical care services. Table 2 depicts the major therapeutic categories of drugs for managed care plans.[4] One of the reasons that clinical pharmacy practice has been successful in many managed care settings is the availability of a formal structure and communication network among healthcare professionals.[53] Managed healthcare plans use a variety of approaches for improving drug prescribing and achieving improved patient outcomes including the use of practice guidelines, pharmaceutical care services, drug utilization review programs, and academic detailing. There has been a continuing and growing effort to use economic models to evaluate the effects of programs and policies designed to influence the practice of prescribers and pharmacists. Pharmacists also are one of the most effective resources for influencing physician and patient compliance with formulary policy. The effectiveness of pharmacists in a variety of clinical roles has been demonstrated in HMO settings.[54,55]

Table 2. Top Therapeutic Drug Classes Reported by HMOs in 2000[4]

Rank ($)	Drug Class	Per Member per Year ($)	Utilization per 1000 Enrollees
1	antidepressants	29.62	475.2
2	cholesterol reducers	29.00	388.8
3	proton-pump inhibitors	20.44	167.3
4	antihistamines	12.98	237.7
5	ACE inhibitors	12.51	395.3
6	calcium-channel blockers	11.73	284.3
7	antidiabetic agents	10.98	268.2
8	anticonvulsants	7.96	136.3
9	estrogen products	7.51	356.1
10	oral contraceptives	6.38	228.0
11	bronchial steroids	5.70	96.2
12	intranasal steroids	5.43	126.5
13	macrolides	5.37	152.5
14	antipsychotics	5.15	31.8
15	penicillins	5.11	247.8
16	COX-2 inhibitors	5.08	69.2
17	NSAIDs	4.80	256.4
18	fluoroquinolones	4.42	68.3
19	beta-agonists	4.30	195.3
20	beta-blockers	4.24	305.8
21	antimigraine agents	4.11	33.1
22	H_2-antagonists	3.76	133.3
23	osteoporosis products	3.75	60.9
24	cephalosporins	3.60	132.7
25	alpha-blockers	3.41	85.7

ACE = angiotensin-converting enzyme; COX = cyclooxygenase; H_2 = histamine$_2$; HMO = health maintenance organization; NSAIDs = nonsteroidal antiinflammatory drugs.

Managed healthcare plans commonly use prescribing guidelines to promote the quality of drug therapy, while minimizing unnecessary expenditures. Often developed by the P&T committee as a component of formulary review, *prescribing guidelines* also are referred to as clinical guidelines, algorithms, clinical road maps, stepped care protocols, and drug usage criteria.[56] Preprinted prescription order forms, if structured in a preferred order-of-prescribing, also can be considered as tools to promote fomulary compliance. As noted by Schrogie and Nash,[57] the presence of a recommended guideline may have remarkable effects on pharmacotherapy. For example, by mentioning selected drugs as candidates for use, other competing and therapeutically equivalent drugs may be excluded. Stuart et al.[58] described an educational program that featured a clinical algorithm to encourage the rational use of lipid-lowering drugs at Group Health Cooperative of Puget Sound. A preliminary analysis suggested that the program was associated with a $1 million cost-avoidance in this drug category in 1990 $US. To be most effective, the development and evaluation of practice guidelines should be augmented with a pharmacoeconomic and outcomes analysis to provide more specific direction.

Poor adherence to prescribed medications can significantly reduce the effectiveness of drug therapy, resulting in suboptimal health and economic outcomes. Numerous studies have shown that patients who have good persistence with their medication regimens have better health outcomes with lower healthcare costs than patients with a pattern of poor persistence. The major difference between persistence and adherence is that a patient may be taking a medication and is therefore persistent, but may be taking the medication in a manner not consistent or adherent with the doctor's prescribed regimen. Nonadherence with medications for cardiovascular disease is approximately 50 percent, contributing to poor health for the patient, decreased productivity for employers, increased total medical expenses for insurance companies and MCOs, and lost sales to the drug manufacturer and the pharmacy. One study reported that two-thirds of people taking widely prescribed cholesterol-lowering drugs do not get as much benefit from these medications because they are not taken properly, even though they contribute to improved health and economic outcomes when used effectively.[59]

In one study of a Medicaid population by McCombs et al.,[60] only 14 percent of patients with hypertension obtained their antihypertensive drugs continuously for one year. Rates of persistence varied from 33 percent for patients whose drug regimen began with angiotensin-converting enzyme inhibitors to as low as 5 percent among those started on diuretics. More recently, Caro et al.[61] examined outpatient prescriptions for antihypertensive therapy filled in Saskatchewan between 1989 and 1994 by approximately 80,000 patients with hypertension. Persistence with therapy decreased in the first 6 months after treatment was started and continued to decline. Among newly diagnosed hypertensive patients, only 78 percent persisted with therapy at the end of one year. Studies of patients in randomized trials show that those who adhere to cardiovascular drug therapy have improved outcomes compared with nonadherent persons. For example, the Beta-Blocker Heart Attack Trial (BHAT) showed lower one-year mortality rates among patients who ingested more than 75 percent of their medication.[62] Nonadherence to drug therapy diminishes the effectiveness of medications as reported in most pharmacoeconomic evaluations.[63]

DRUG BENEFIT DESIGN

Managed healthcare plans have considerable flexibility in determining the specific features of their drug benefits programs. The pharmacy benefit design of an intensively managed plan usually includes a drug formulary, a preferred pharmacy network (and/or in-house pharmacies), provider financial risk-sharing, member cost-sharing, coverage for FDA- or compendium-approved indications only, and prescription volume limitations. As part of the drug formulary provision, plans may implement prior authorization to manage high-cost pharmaceuticals (eg, drugs for catastrophic diseases, various products of biotechnology), exclude or restrict entire categories of drugs (eg, over-the-counter products, nonoral contraceptives, fertility drugs, smoking cessation products, weight loss products, cosmetic drugs, drugs for impotence), and implement provisions for member cost-sharing.

Cost-sharing can be in the form of copayments, coinsurance, deductibles, benefit caps, tiered payment schemes, and/or some combination of these approaches. Tiered prescription plans provide incentives for consumers to choose lower-cost products by offering different cost-sharing formulas based on formulary status and whether the product is a generic or a brand-name drug. Most MCOs require generic substitution. As innovator products lose patent protection, cost-savings from increased use of generic drugs will grow. Cost-minimization is the pharmacoeconomic method most frequently used to support formulary decisions pertaining to generic substitution.

Soumerai et al.[64,65] have called attention to the need to evaluate the intended and unintended impacts of drug policies. Based on their experience with Medicaid and other state drug benefit programs, the authors argue for more rigorous evaluation of several popular cost-sharing and other intervention programs. Using a historical cohort design, Harris et al.[66] analyzed how the use and cost of pharmaceuticals varied by level of drug co-payment in a staff-model HMO. Based on an analysis of 19,982 enrollees aged less than 65 years, they determined that the implementation of progressively greater levels of copayments continued to have a marked effect on drug utilization, prescription unit costs, and per capita drug costs. There is a need for greater research into the effects of cost-sharing provisions on total drug costs, patient satisfaction, and patient outcomes.

Methodologic Challenges

There are a variety of methodologic challenges facing investigators who wish to perform pharmacoeconomic studies to meet the needs of managed care plans.[19,67] One of the most important considerations is adoption of the viewpoint of the managed care plan in the design and analysis of pharmacoeconomic studies. This perspective would influence numerous design features including selection of the specific comparator drug(s), selection of meaningful clinical outcomes, use of cost versus charge data, and relative importance (or unimportance) of indirect consequences such as worker productivity. As managed care plans continue to use large automated databases, there is a need to be attentive to the development of variables such as indications for use, severity of illness, comorbidities, and other potential confounding factors.[68]

When affordable and appropriate, randomized prospective trials of the cost-effectiveness of pharmacologic interventions contribute valuable information for managed care plans. In addition, controlled postmarketing observational studies provide valuable information on the effectiveness of medications under customary use conditions. Factors reported to impede the use of pharmacoeconomic data by MCOs include departmental budgetary constraints, untimely publications, limited reliability of available studies, and lack of knowledge by MCO personnel to evaluate such studies.[41]

Summary

Prescription drugs and their associated costs have become a major issue for MCOs, causing plan administrators to become even more aggressive managers of the cost and utilization of pharmaceuticals. While MCOs have generally been more successful than traditional fee-for-service plans in controlling drug costs, recent double-digit annual increases in the cost of providing prescriptions for enrollees have resulted in MCOs taking an even closer look at pharmacy benefits. Even though the term *pharmacoeconomics* is relatively new, managed care plans have historically scrutinized the economic value of their pharmacy benefit programs (pharmaceuticals, pharmaceutical services, drug policies). There is little doubt that managed care plans are increasingly demanding and using pharmacoeconomic data to manage drug benefit programs. In interviews with MCOs that have formulary committees, medical and pharmacy directors considered cost-effectiveness to be an important type of information to be considered in formulary decisions. It ranked above cost of treatment and just below safety and efficacy in importance.[67] However, many managed care pharmacy directors and employer benefit managers continue to make coverage decisions largely from a drug price perspective.

MCOs need to continue to incorporate pharmacoeconomics into their formulary decision-making process and design of drug benefits. Pharmaceutical companies have responded to MCOs' demand for pharmacoeconomic data by expanding their activities in pharmacoeconomics, including quality-of-life studies. Moreover, MCOs are increasingly performing outcomes research studies, including pharmacoeconomic evaluations. However, pharmaceutical companies cannot provide complete information on the clinical and economic outcomes of drug therapy based on premarketing studies alone. Collaborative efforts between managed care, academia, government agencies, and the pharmaceutical industry can facilitate the design and conduct of valid, objective, and timely pharmacoeconomic evaluations.

References

1. Managed care digest, 2001. Bridgewater, NJ: Aventis Pharmaceuticals, 2001.

2. Eichenholz J. Trends in managed care pharmacy: responding to changing environments. J Managed Care Pharm 2002;8:102-7.

3. Managed health care: effect on employers' costs difficult to measure. Washington, DC: General Accounting Office, GAO/HRD-94-3, October 1993.

4. Pharmacy benefit report. Facts & figures. East Hanover, NJ: Novartis, 2001.

5. Centers for Medicare and Medicaid Services, Office of the Actuary, National Health Statistics Group. www.hcfa.gov (accessed 2002 Jan 14).

6. Levit K, Smith C, Cowan C, Lazenby H, Martin A. Inflation spurs health spending in 2000. Health Affairs 2002;21:172-81.

7. Heffler S, Levit K, Smith S, Smith C, Cowan C, Lazenby H, et al. Health spending growth up in 1999; faster growth expected in the future. Health Affairs 2001;20:193-203.

8. Sonderegger Research Center. Prescription drug trends: a chartbook update. Menlo Park, CA: The Kaiser Family Foundation, November 2001.

9. Dubois RW, Chawla AJ, Neslusan CA, Smith MW, Wade S. Explaining drug spending trends: does perception match reality? Health Affairs 2000.

10. Factors affecting the growth of prescription drug expenditures. Washington, DC: National Institute of Healthcare Management Foundation, July 1999.

11. Prescription drug expenditures in 2001: another year of escalating costs. Washington, DC: National Institute of Healthcare Management Foundation, April 2002.

12. Pal S. 364 drugs marketed between 1990–2000. US Pharmacist 2002; 27(1):1-3.

13. Motheral BR, Delate TA, Shaw J, Henderson R. The effect of a closed formulary in the face of real-life enrollment and disenrollment patterns. J Managed Care Pharm 2000;6:293-7.

14. Hazlet TK, Hu TW. Association between formulary strategies and hospital drug expenditures. Am J Hosp Pharm 1992;49:2207-10.

15. Sloan FA, Gordon GS, Cocks DL. Hospital drug formularies and use of hospital services. Med Care 1993;31:851-67.

16. Gabrowski HG, Schweitzer SO, Shiota SR. The effect of Medicaid formularies on the availability of new drugs. Pharmacoeconomics 1992;1(suppl 1):32-40.

17. Schumacher GE. Multiattribute evaluation in formulary decision making as applied to calcium-channel blockers. Am J Hosp Pharm 1991;48:301-8.

18. Evans C, Dukes EM, Crawford B. The role of pharmacoeconomic information in the formulary decision-making process. J Managed Care Pharm 2000;6:108-21.

19. Prosser LA, Koplan JP, Neumann PJ, Weinstein MC. Barriers to using cost-effectiveness analysis in managed care decision making. Am J Managed Care 1999;6:173-9.

20. Gricar JA, Langley PC, Luce B, Lyles A, Sullivan SD. Format for formulary submissions. Alexandria, VA: Academy of Managed Care Pharmacy, October 2000.

21. Format for formulary submissions. Version 2.0. Alexandria, VA: Academy of Managed Care Pharmacy, October 2002.

22. Fullerton DSP, Sullivan SD. Regence BlueShield's mandatory data submission requirement for manufacturers: a progress report. Formulary 2000;35:514-31.

23. Mather DB, Sullivan SD, Augenstein D, Fullerton DSP, Atherly D. Incorporating clinical outcomes and economic consequences into drug formulary decisions: a practical approach. Am J Managed Care 1999;5:277-85.

24. Hill SR, Mitchell AS, Henry DA. Problems with the interpretation of pharmacoeconomic analyses. A review of submissions to the Australian Pharmaceutical Benefits Scheme. JAMA 2000;283:2116-21.

25. www.health.gov.au/hfs/haf/docs/pharmpac/gusubpac.htm (accessed 2002 Jan 14).

26. Commonwealth Department of Human Services and Health. Guidelines for the pharmaceutical industry on preparation of submissions to the pharmaceutical benefits advisory committee including major submissions involving economic analyses. Canberra: Australian Government Publishing Service, 1995.

27. Rennie D, Luft HS. Pharmacoeconomic analyses: making them transparent, making them credible. JAMA 2000;283:2158-60.

28. Canadian Coordinating Office for Health Technology Assessment. www.ccohta.ca/pubs/index.htm (accessed 2002 Jan 14).

29. Baladi JF, Menon D, Otten N. Use of economic evaluation guidelines: 2 years' experience in Canada. Health Econ 1998;7:221-7.

30. National Institute for Clinical Excellence. www.nice.org.uk (accessed 2002 Jan 14).

31. Drummond M, Dubois D, Garattini L, Horisberger B, Jonsson B, Kristiansen IS, et al. Current trends in the use of pharmacoeconomics and outcomes research in Europe. Value Health 1999;2:323-32.

32. RxIntelligence announces fall research agenda. October 12, 2000. www.rxintelligence.com (accessed 2002 May 6).

33. DiMasi JA, Caglarcan E, Wood-Armany M. Emerging role of pharmacoeconomics in the research and development decision-making process. Pharmacoeconomics 2001;19:753-66.

34. Hillman AL, Eisenberg JM, Pauly MV, Bloom BS, Citick H, Kinosian B, et al. Avoiding bias in the conduct and reporting of cost-effectiveness research sponsored by pharmaceutical companies. N Engl J Med 1991;324:1362-5.

35. Task Force on Principles for Economic Analysis of Health Care Technology. Economic analysis of health care technology: a report on principles. Ann Intern Med 1995;122:61-70.

36. Udvarhelyi IS, Colditz GA, Rai A, Epstein AM. Cost-effectiveness and cost-benefit analyses in the medical literature. Are the methods being used correctly? Ann Intern Med 1992;116:238-44.

37. Agro KE, Bradley CA, Mittmann N, Iskedjian M, Ilersich AL, Einarson TR. Sensitivity analysis in health economic and pharmacoeconomic studies: an appraisal of the literature. Pharmacoeconomics 1997;11:75-88.

38. Drummond MF, Jefferson TO. Guidelines for authors and peer reviewers of economic submissions to the BMJ. The BMJ Economic Evaluation Working Party. BMJ 1996;313:275-83.

39. Division of Drug Marketing, Advertising and Communications, Food and Drug Administration. Principles for the review of pharmacoeconomic pro-

motion. Presented at: Center for Pharmaceutical Outcomes Research Meeting, Chapel Hill, NC, 1995.

40. Neumann PJ, Claxton K, Weinstein MC. The FDA's regulation of health economic information. Health Affairs 2000;19:129-37.

41. Suh DC, Okpara IR, Agnese WB, Toscani M. Application of pharmacoeconomics to formulary decision making in managed care organizations. Am J Managed Care 2002;8:161-9.

42. Clouse JC, Osterhaus JT. Healthcare resource use and costs associated with migraine in a managed healthcare setting. Ann Pharmacother 1994; 28:659-64.

43. Glauber HS, Brown JB. Use of health maintenance organization data bases to study pharmacy resource usage in diabetes mellitus. Diabetes Care 1992;15:870-6.

44. Stergachis A, Sheingold S, Luce BR, Psaty BM, Revicki DA. Medical care and cost outcomes after pentoxifylline treatment for peripheral arterial disease. Arch Intern Med 1992;152:1220-4.

45. Goldfarb SD, Duncan BS, Dans PE, Sloan AS. HMO direct costs and health care resources use after implementation of a monthly limit on sumatriptan. Am J Health Syst Pharm 1999;56:2206-10.

46. Lofland JH, Kim SS, Batenhorst AS, Johnson NE, Chatterton ML, Cady RK, et al. Cost-effectiveness and cost-benefit of sumatriptan in patients with migraine. Mayo Clin Proc 2001;7:1093-101.

47. Barr JT, Schumacher GE. Applying decision analysis to pharmacy management and practice decisions. Top Hosp Pharm Manage 1994;13:60-71.

48. Ofman JJ, Yamashita BD, Siddique RM, Larson LR, Willian MK. Cost-effectiveness of rabeprazole versus generic ranitidine for symptom resolution in patients with erosive esophagitis. Am J Managed Care 2000;6:905-16.

49. Mohle-Boetani JC, Lieu TA, Ray GT, Escobar G. Preventing neonatal group B streptococcal disease: cost-effectiveness in a health maintenance organization and the impact of delayed hospital discharge for newborns who received intrapartum antibiotics. Pediatrics 1999;103:703-10.

50. Revicki DA, Brown RE, Keller MB, Gonzales J, Culpepper L, Hales RE. Cost-effectiveness of newer antidepressants compared with tricyclic antidepressants in managed care settings. J Clin Psychiatry 1997;58:47-58.

51. McDonough KP, Weaver RH, Viall GD. Enalapril to lisinopril: economic impact of a voluntary angiotensin-converting enzyme-inhibitor substitution program in a staff-model health maintenance organization. Ann Pharmacother 1992;26:399-404.

52. Baluch WM, Gardner JS, Krauss RH, Scholes D. Therapeutic interchange of conjugated and esterified estrogens in a managed care organization. Am J Health Syst Pharm 1999;56:537-42.

53. Stergachis A, Campbell WH, Penna PM. Clinical pharmacy and managed healthcare systems. Top Hosp Pharm Manage 1988;8:78-88.

54. Okamoto MP, Nakahiro RK. Pharmacoeconomic evaluation of a pharmacist-managed hypertension clinic. Pharmacotherapy 2001;21:1337-44.

55. The ACCP Clinical Practice Affairs Committee. Clinical pharmacy in the noninstitutional setting: a white paper from the American College of Clinical Pharmacy. Pharmacotherapy 1992;12:359-64.

56. Field MJ, Lohr KN, eds. Clinical practice guidelines. Washington, DC: National Academy Press, Institute of Medicine, 1990.

57. Schrogie JJ, Nash DB. Relationship between practice guidelines, formulary management, and pharmacoeconomic studies. Top Hosp Pharm Manage 1994;13:38-46.

58. Stuart ME, Handley MR, Chamberlain MC, Wallach R, Penna P, Stergachis A. A successful HMO education program to encourage rational use of lipid lowering drugs. HMO Pract 1991;5:198-204.

59. How effective are cholesterol drugs? Study: many are less beneficial in real world than in studies. Nov 12, 2001, www.msnbc.com/news/656411.asp (accessed 2002 Jan 14).

60. McCombs JS, Nichol MB, Newman CM, Sclar DA. The costs of interrupting antihypertensive drug therapy in a Medicaid population. Med Care 1994;32:214-26.

61. Caro JJ, Salas M, Speckman JL, Raggio G, Jackson JD. Persistence with treatment for hypertension in actual practice. Can Med Assoc J 1999; 160:31-7.

62. Horwitz RI, Viscoli CM, Berkman L, Donaldson RM, Horowitz SM, Murray CJ, et al. Treatment adherence and risk of death after a myocardial infarction. Lancet 1990;336:542-5.

63. Hughes DA, Bagust A, Haycox A, Walley T. The impact of non-compliance on the cost-effectiveness of pharmaceuticals: a review of the literature. Health Econ 2001;10:601-10.

64. Soumerai SB, Ross-Degnan D. Experience of state drug benefit programs. Health Affairs 1990;9:36-54.

65. Soumerai SB, Ross-Degnan D, Avorn J, McLaughlin TJ, Choodnovskiy I. Effects of Medicaid drug-payment limits on admission to hospitals and nursing homes. N Engl J Med 1991;325:1072-7.

66. Harris BL, Stergachis A, Ried LD. The effect of drug co-payments on utilization and cost of pharmaceuticals in a health care maintenance organization. Med Care 1990;28:907-17.

67. Luce BR, Brown RE. The use of technology assessment by hospitals, health maintenance organizations, and third-party payers in the United States. Int J Technol Assess Health Care 1995;11:79-92.

68. Von Korff M, Wagner EH, Saunders K. A chronic disease score from automated pharmacy data. J Clin Epidemiol 1992;45:197-203.

Pharmacoeconomics and Clinical Practice: A Physician's View

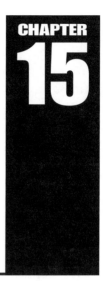

CHAPTER

15

Kevin A Schulman

C hanges in health policy around the world are focusing on the goal of ensuring that the provision of medical care occurs in a fiscally rational manner. The development of pharmacoeconomics as an assessment tool is one means of developing coherent data surrounding the outcomes of pharmaceutical therapy.[1-9] Although many authors have developed metrics we can use to assess the economic impact of pharmaceutical therapies, all too few have described how these data can be understood and interpreted to improve the efficiency of clinical practice.

This chapter discusses this implementation issue in a clinical context, both on a national and regional health services level. In addition, this chapter reviews pharmacoeconomic issues as they relate to the interpretation of published economic analyses, discusses two case examples of interpretation of pharmacoeconomic data, and discusses the state of the art in implementation of pharmacoeconomics in clinical practice, highlighting the possible next directions in the evolution of this clinical management tool.

Economic Issues in Clinical Practice

Pharmacoeconomic analyses supply practitioners with several different types of important clinical data. Properly designed studies include an assessment of current medical practice, an assessment of the clinical efficacy of a new pharmaceutical product, and an economic analysis evaluating the impact of the product on clinical practice.

Economic analyses can report results in four different economic categories for the treatment under investigation compared with a control treatment (either placebo or an established therapy). Two of these categories are for new therapies with improved clinical outcomes, and two are for new therapies with worsened clinical outcomes. These categories are:

1. the new therapy is cost saving with improved clinical outcomes,
2. the new therapy is cost additive with improved clinical outcomes,
3. the new therapy is cost saving with worse clinical outcomes, and
4. the new therapy is cost additive with worse clinical outcomes.

A therapy that falls into the first category is said to be dominant in that it is always the treatment of choice. A new therapy that falls into the fourth category is dominated by the control therapy and is never the treatment of choice. Selection of therapies in categories 2 and 3 will depend on the relationship of the costs of the therapies and outcomes achieved with the therapy. For category 2 and potentially for category 3, cost-effectiveness ratios can be calculated to allow economic assessment of these agents relative to other funded therapies.

Although pharmacoeconomic data are always interesting and sometimes compelling, they need to be interpreted in terms of the specific clinical context being addressed before they can be used to influence the clinical decision-making process. Interpretation of these data involves several specific issues:

1. translation of treatment efficacy results to treatment efficiency results,
2. comparison of the clinical trial population with the population under consideration for treatment with the therapy,

3. translation of the costs reported to costs relevant to the perspective of the decision-maker, and
4. translation of the clinical outcome measures to outcomes relevant to the length of treatment being proposed by the practitioner.

Each of these issues is addressed separately.

EFFICIENCY

Phase III clinical trials are designed to measure the efficacy of new therapeutic products. Efficacy is the effect of an agent in the "idealized" setting of a randomized, controlled clinical trial. Efficiency of a therapy is the effect of a therapy as observed in actual clinical practice, outside a clinical protocol. Efficacy may differ greatly from efficiency.

Factors that may lead to pharmacoeconomic efficacy being greater than pharmacoeconomic efficiency include:

1. specific criteria for patient selection,
2. protocol-induced benefits for patients receiving the new medication,
3. optimization of medication dosage and monitoring of patients receiving treatment,
4. physician experience with the new medication, and
5. patient motivation and adherence with the new treatment.

Factors that may lead to efficiency being greater than efficacy include:

1. a large placebo benefit to therapy (the efficacy benefit would be the benefit of therapy on an incremental basis and would not include this placebo effect; the efficiency benefit would be the total benefit observed in patients and would include this effect),
2. identification of a superior population for the therapy compared with the population selected for the Phase III trial,
3. increased comfort with the use of the agent, resulting in reduced intensity of the new treatment in clinical practice compared with that for patients receiving the new treatment in the Phase III trial protocol, and
4. decreased efficiency of control treatment in clinical practice compared with that in the clinical trial (eg, if physicians underdose a particular control medication in clinical

practice, but its use is optimized in a clinical trial, the difference in effectiveness between a new treatment and the control treatment will be greater in clinical practice than that observed in the clinical trial).

Beyond these issues, one must assess whether inefficiencies in clinical practice may affect the use of the agent once it is available. To the extent that misuse of controlled therapies in clinical practice is responsible for the economic advantage of a new agent, these benefits may be achievable through less costly programs such as educational interventions. At the same time, to the extent that the demand for medical care services is not related to the clinical condition of the patient, the potential economic advantage afforded by the new therapy may not be achieved. For example, physicians can loosen their criteria for therapeutic procedures in an attempt to maintain service volume when patients experience a decrease in severity of illness with a new medication. In this case, one would not see the expected reduction in procedure volume after the therapy is introduced.

In most cases, efficacy is expected to be greater than efficiency of new therapeutic modalities. However, each therapy must be assessed individually to determine whether this maxim holds.

GENERALIZABILITY

Clinical trial populations can be very specific, as discussed above. Understanding the generalizability of a pharmacoeconomic study involves two processes: understanding the generalizability from the clinical population being treated to the population for which treatment is being considered, and understanding the economic system being assessed in the study. The generalizability of the results from the clinical population under study is relatively straightforward to most clinicians. The generalizability of the economic system under consideration is a much newer activity for clinicians and policy-makers (generalizability does not include perspective, which will be discussed separately).

In the United States alone, a tremendous change has occurred in the provision of healthcare services over the last decade because of changes in health insurance and government payment policies for physicians and hospitals. A pharmacoeconomic study conducted before the implementation of the Medicare Prospective Payment System may have reported significant reduction in length of stay for patients receiving a particular treatment. This finding may no longer be relevant, however, given the reduction in length of stay observed since the Prospective Payment System was implemented. Similarly, a study that reported on the reduction of inpatient costs for a disease that is now treated on an outpatient basis would have limited generalizability.

The healthcare system also can affect the intensity of services. Length of stay is much greater in Germany than in the United States at the present time. Thus, one must review the quantity of resources used to care for both treatment and control patients to see if the intensity of resource consumption in the pharmacoeconomic study matches that expected in the system of concern to the decision-makers.

PERSPECTIVE

Perspective is the point of view from which costs and benefits are assessed for a study. The most commonly reported perspectives are patient, provider, payer, and society. Most published studies have a specific perspective. Thus, the reported costs and benefits from an economic analysis need to be translated into costs and benefits relevant to the perspective of the decision-maker for the clinical question being addressed. For example, pharmaceutical and laboratory costs can be adjusted to reflect a provider's perspective (eg, health maintenance organization [HMO] or Veterans Affairs Hospital) rather than a societal perspective. Similarly, treatment benefits can be translated from a societal perspective to a patient perspective (eg, rather than reporting the number of physician visits for gastrointestinal adverse effects, the study can report number of days of stomach upset for patients).

OUTCOMES

Outcomes assessment is the most difficult task associated with the analysis of pharmacoeconomic data. Clinical trials are usually of short duration compared with the expected period of treatment, especially when assessing treatments for chronic disease. Although forecasting the future efficacy of therapy with certainty is impossible, one can readily identify reasonable bounds for the lifetime impact of therapy either from clinical trial data[10] or through the use of a computer model.[11-15] As the methodology of outcomes research advances, we may also need to consider patients' treatment preferences on a disease-specific basis.[16]

For therapies expected to provide an improvement over current treatments, pharmacoeconomic analysis can focus on both the short- and long-term costs and benefits of therapy. Most agents do not have identical treatment efficacy, so a lifetime perspective should be maintained wherever possible for economic analysis.

Interpretation Cases

Two analyses reported in the medical literature will be reviewed in this section. These reports are analyzed using the four interpretation issues highlighted in the previous section: efficiency, generalizability, perspective, and outcomes.

CASE 1: COST-EFFECTIVENESS OF PHARMACEUTICAL MANAGEMENT OF HIGH BLOOD CHOLESTEROL

The treatment of high blood cholesterol was first established as a national health priority by the National Cholesterol Education Program (NCEP) in 1987.[17] This program recommended that all American adults be screened for high blood cholesterol and that patients with elevated levels of low-density lipoprotein cholesterol (LDL-C) be treated. Treatment recommendations included two stages of diet therapy, with pharmaceutical management reserved for patients in whom diet therapy failed. The NCEP stipulates first- and second-line therapeutic agents for patients who require pharmacologic therapy. Nevertheless, these recommendations do not include any economic assessment of the different therapies or the cost-effectiveness of the treatment recommendations.

Schulman et al.[18] reported a cost-effectiveness analysis of the pharmacologic treatment of high blood cholesterol for patients in whom diet therapy failed. This analysis was conducted from a societal perspective and included only the direct medical costs of pharmacologic therapy. Benefits were reported as changes in total blood cholesterol, LDL-C, and high-density lipoprotein cholesterol (HDL-C) concentrations, as well as changes in an LDL-C/HDL-C index representing total reduction in cardiovascular risk resulting from treatment (including changes in both HDL-C and LDL-C concentrations). Direct medical costs included pharmaceuticals, physician and laboratory monitoring, comedication (required to reduce adverse effects of specific agents), and adverse effects. Resource consumption for the use of these agents was based on expert opinion and literature review.

Some of the findings of this analysis are reported in Figure 1. This figure represents the costs of five years of therapy for the treatment of high blood cholesterol and the benefits of therapy in terms of LDL-C reduction. The closer the agents are positioned toward the upper left portion of the curve, the more efficient they are in terms of the cost-per-percent reduction in LDL-C.[18]

The most efficient agents in this figure represent an efficiency frontier. Nonfrontier agents (ie, those above the efficiency frontier) for a given treatment effect have higher costs than frontier agents. Alternatively, relative to agents on the frontier, nonfrontier agents, for a given cost, have less clinical benefit. Agents that lie below the frontier offer less clinical benefit than agents on the frontier with the same cost or the same clinical benefit as agents on the frontier but for greater cost. The efficiency frontier allows physicians to select from a range of therapeutic agents, acknowledging that different clinical indications and adverse effect profiles exist for different therapeutic agents and that physicians may consider these factors in making a treatment decision.

One obvious result of analysis of this figure is that, while the efficiency of the agent plays an important role in clinical decision-making, other criteria are required to determine the optimal therapy for patients. This curve lends itself to three different treatment decision criteria: effect, budget, and cost-effectiveness. For patients who require a 20% reduction in LDL-C, lovastatin 20 mg/day achieves this clinical endpoint at the lowest cost. If it is desired to use the most effective agent that costs no more than $3,500 over five years, then colestipol 20 mg/day is the agent of choice. If it is desired to use the most cost-effective agent for the reduction of LDL-C concentrations, then niacin ($139 per percent reduction in LDL-C) and lovastatin 20 mg/day ($177 per percent reduction in LDL-C) are the agents of choice.[18]

Data Interpretation

In assessing the information provided in this study, we should review the four major analytic issues outlined in this chapter.

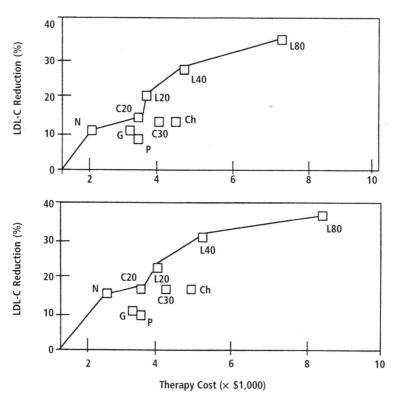

Figure 1. Cost (on x-axis) and effect (on y-axis) of reduction of low-density lipoprotein cholesterol (LDL-C) concentrations for the clinical trial model (top) and the primary care model (bottom). The points that are higher and to the left in each figure describe an efficiency frontier, defined as those points that produce a given effect at the least cost. These points dominate those that are lower and rightward. An agent is dominated if it can be replaced by at least one other agent that produces either the same or greater effect for less cost or more effect for the same cost. Costs are in terms of the present value of five years of therapy; effects are in nominal terms. N = niacin; G = gemfibrozil; P = probucol; C20 = colestipol 20 g; C30 = colestipol 30 g; Ch = cholestyramine; L20 = lovastatin 20 mg; L40 = lovastatin 40 mg; and L80 = lovastatin 80 mg. Reprinted with permission.[18]

Efficiency

The first assessment was to determine whether this analysis reported efficacy measures or efficiency measures. In this article, the authors presented an analysis of both efficacy and efficiency. Efficacy was represented by a clinical trial model, which is based on an intent-to-treat analysis of the clinical and economic data. In this analysis, patients who were nonadherent did not receive the cost or benefit of therapy other than the therapy initiation cost. Patients who were nonresponders continued to receive the cost of therapy while they may have had little clinical benefit from treatment.[18]

The authors also presented a primary care model, where the agent in patients who were nonadherent or nonresponders was changed to a second or third agent until 98% of patients were taking a medication they tolerated (Figure 1). This primary care model assessed the efficiency of the use of these agents in practice and resembles clinical practice more closely than the clinical trial model. Patients were to be followed by their physician until they were taking a drug that they tolerated and their blood cholesterol concentration was reduced. Nonadherent patients were to be given second and third agents to achieve their treatment goal.[18]

Compared with the clinical trial model, the primary care model may report higher costs for drugs that may be difficult for patients to tolerate. In this study, these included niacin, colestipol, and cholestyramine, with the cost of niacin increasing 60% in the primary care model compared with the clinical trial model. The clinical benefit also increased, however, because more patients were receiving therapy to which they responded in the primary care model compared with the clinical trial model. In this analysis, the authors reported that the agents on the efficiency frontier remained unchanged in either analysis.[18]

Generalizability

This analysis was based on the results of a survey of 115 studies reported in the medical literature on the treatment of patients with high blood cholesterol. Efficacy results were reported to be for patients with type II hyperlipidemia, with total cholesterol concentrations of 251 mg/dL or greater. Although gender was not an inclusion or exclusion criterion for the literature review, women were greatly underrepresented in the clinical studies. Further, women had a lower relative risk of heart disease than did men of the same age.[18] Thus, these results may not be generalizable to women or to patients with disease other than type II hyperlipidemia.

Perspective

The costs reported in the article were derived from several different sources. Resource consumption was based both on the practice patterns of a panel of medical experts in a specific geographic region and on their impressions of the intensity of resources required to treat patients before some of the treatments were widely available. Pharmaceutical costs were based on wholesale prices, and laboratory costs were based on laboratory costs in Maryland.[18] Thus, both intensity of treatment and costs of resources need to be reviewed before implementing treatment recommendations based on this analysis.

Outcomes

The authors based their analysis on five years of treatment costs and effects.[18] While this may be a reasonable time frame for analysis, patients probably will receive lifetime treatment with these agents. Glick et al.[19] reported lifetime treatment analyses that support the results of this five-year treatment model.

CASE 2: COST-EFFECTIVENESS OF NEBACUMAB FOR GRAM-NEGATIVE SEPSIS—ECONOMIC ANALYSIS OF A NEW THERAPEUTIC AGENT

Despite the availability of appropriate antibiotic therapy for the treatment of patients with sepsis, this clinical syndrome still has a substantial mortality rate that may be due to the ability of a bacterial infection to overstimulate the host's immune response, a process that continues despite the presence of antibiotic therapy. A new class of therapeutic agents was developed to treat this disease by tempering the host's immune response. Nebacumab was the first of this class of agents that neared approval for use in the United States; it was marketed in several countries in Europe. (The agent was withdrawn from the market in Europe and from clinical trials in the United States in 1993.) In the original clinical trial,[20] nebacumab demonstrated efficacy in patients with gram-negative bacterial infections. However, this infection was found in only 36 percent of patients with sepsis in the trial. Even though this drug was never marketed in the United States, the case of nebacumab provides an excellent example of a pharmacoeconomic analysis of this class of therapeutic agents. Subsequent research has shown an unexplained increase in mortality for patients with gram-positive bacteremia who received this therapy.[21]

An economic analysis of this drug was performed to understand its potential use in clinical practice[22] and to assess whether it would meet funding guidelines for new therapeutic agents.[23-25] Since nebacumab was not available in the United States, the base price was set at the cost of the agent in one of the European countries where it was marketed (in the Netherlands, the price was $3,750 per dose[22]).

The economic analysis of nebacumab was based on the mortality of patients who received the drug versus those who received placebo, the proportion of treated patients with gram-negative infections, the cost of the agent, the cost of treating its adverse effects, and the costs resulting from use of the agent.[22] Since nebacumab is only effective in the treatment of patients with gram-negative bacterial infections, its clinical effect would be a product of the expected reduction in mortality in patients with gram-negative bacterial infections and the prevalence of patients with gram-negative infections in the treated population. The data used to construct this analysis are presented in Table 1.

The effectiveness of this intervention is dependent on the long-term outcome of the patients treated with this medication. The average age of patients in this trial was 58 years, meaning the patients who benefit from this therapy would be expected to have an additional 20 years of survival based on their actuarial life expectancy. The majority of patients in this trial, however, had substantial comorbidities including cancer, liver or kidney disease, diabetes, and alcoholism. In this analysis, it was estimated that patients would survive an average of 5 years beyond hospital discharge. This estimate was examined extensively using sensitivity analysis.[22]

An analysis of the economic impact of a diagnostic test for gram-negative infection also was constructed. In this analysis, only patients who tested positive for gram-negative infection were treated with nebacumab therapy (the test strategy compared with the treat strategy where all patients are treated, as in this trial). The net effect of the test strategy was to reduce the number of patients with gram-positive infection treated with nebacumab, while providing patients with gram-negative infection and positive tests the benefit of therapy. This strategy reduced costs while maintaining efficacy (although efficacy is dependent on the sensitivity of the test). The results of this analysis and the sensitivity analysis are presented in Table 2 and Figure 2. The results of the test analysis are presented in Table 3 and Figure 3.[22]

Data Interpretation

Again, in assessing the information provided in this article, we reviewed the four major analysis issues outlined in this chapter.

Table 1. Economic Analysis of Nebacumab Therapy in the Treatment of Gram-Negative Sepsis[22]

Parameter		95% CI
Observed mortality in patients with gram-negative infection receiving placebo (%)	0.52	0.41 to 0.62
Observed mortality in treated patients with gram-negative infection (%)	0.37	0.28 to 0.47
Proportion of patients with gram-negative infection (%)	0.36	0.32 to 0.41
Reduction in mortality in patients with gram-negative infection (%)	0.29	
Cost of therapy ($)	3,750	
Cost of adverse effects ($)	0	
Induced costs per patient ($)	1,900[a]	

CI = confidence interval.
[a]Induced costs of therapy include increased use of hospital resources for patients who would have died without nebacumab therapy, increased use of hospital resources for patients who died despite therapy, and decreased use of resources for patients who would have survived without therapy.

Efficiency

This article reported treatment efficacy in the primary analysis. The authors recognized, however, that in clinical practice, the patient population being treated with nebacumab may be very different from the clinical trial population. Efficiency issues in this analysis included an assessment of the proportion of patients with gram-negative bacteremia in the treatment population and the life expectancy of treated patients.[22] The first of these two issues is discussed in this section. The second is discussed in the generalizability section.

The authors presented an analysis of the efficiency of nebacumab therapy. As shown in Table 3, the cost-effectiveness ratio for this therapy can vary almost threefold under the treat strategy if patient selection varied greatly from that seen in the clinical trial.[22] Since the clinical indications for treatment with this therapy

Table 2. Sensitivity Analysis[a]

Input	Test Strategy ($)	Treat Strategy ($)
Cost of base case	14,900	24,100
Cost of nebacumab therapy ($)		
2,500	12,800	18,800
5,000	17,000	29,500
Cost of acute-care hospital stay		
reduced by 50%	10,800	20,100
increased by 50%	19,000	28,200
Additional survivors only[b]	11,200	20,500
Test cost ($)		
50	14,700	24,100
200	15,300	24,100
2,160	24,100	24,100
Years of life gained		
1	67,900	110,200
20	5,200	8,400
Cost of worst-case scenario[c]	851,700	1,227,600

[a]Reprinted with permission.[22]
[b]Patients who would have died without nebacumab therapy, but are expected to survive with it.
[c]Uses the most pessimistic assumptions from the analysis.

are relatively nonspecific, the efficiency of nebacumab therapy in clinical practice may differ from the treatment efficacy observed in the clinical trial. In this case, patient selection may increase the cost per treated patient. However, since the clinical benefit is limited to patients with gram-negative sepsis, this additional cost was not expected to confer any additional clinical benefit.

Similarly, different hospitals may have different rates of gram-negative infection as a cause of sepsis. From the perspective of an economic analysis, a decrease in the rate of gram-negative infection among patients with sepsis from 36 percent to a lesser percentage is equivalent to a change in prevalence of gram-negative infection from any other cause.

Generalizability

The major issue in discussing the generalizability of these findings was that of patient selection and the life expectancy of treated patients. Ideally, this agent would be used in otherwise

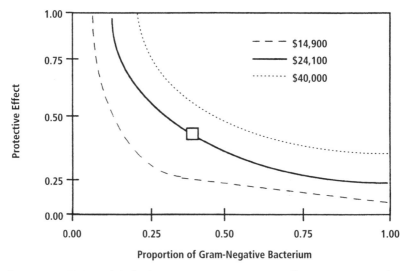

Figure 2. Sensitivity analysis for the treat strategy, reporting cost-effectiveness ratios resulting when estimates of the proportion of gram-negative bacteremia in the treated population and the protective effect of nebacumab therapy among patients with gram-negative bacteremia are varied. The curves represent combinations of these variables that have the same ratios of cost per year of life saved. The square on the middle curve represents the proportion of patients with gram-negative bacteremia and the protective effect used in the principal analysis. Other points represented by this curve all have cost-effectiveness ratios that are identical to the one for the principal analysis. Reprinted with permission.[22]

healthy patients, such as those who developed infection as a complication of surgery. These patients would be expected to return to full health and to live out their full life expectancy. In fact, the cost-effectiveness of therapy in otherwise healthy patients would be far greater than that reported in the primary analysis presented in Table 2.

As discussed previously, however, most patients in the nebacumab clinical trial had substantial underlying illnesses; we do not know much about their expected mortality.[22] While life expectancy for patients such as these may be as long as five years, the patients receiving nebacumab therapy may be substantially more ill than those previously studied (since the patients with gram-negative infection surviving as a result of this treatment would have died without nebacumab therapy). If nebacumab therapy lengthens the dying process for these patients by only a short time, then this therapy will have a much reduced clinical benefit compared with that seen in the primary analysis presented in Table 2. This would result in a substantial decrease in the efficiency of therapy and, potentially, an increase in suffering of patients and their families.

While this discussion suggests that we may wish to limit the use of nebacumab therapy to only patients without underlying illnesses, the reality is that most patients with sepsis probably have some comorbidity and that patients with sepsis will clini-

Table 3. Cost and Cost-Effectiveness of Therapy in Clinical Practice[a]

| Prevalence[b] | Total Annual Costs (in Millions of $) | | | Cost per Year of Life Gained ($) | |
	Test Strategy	Treat Strategy	Savings	Test Strategy	Treat Strategy
0.10	1,622	6,160	4,538	18,300	65,900
0.20	1,415	3,460	2,045	15,900	37,000
0.30	1,346	2,560	1,214	15,200	27,400
0.36	1,323	2,260	937	14,900	24,100

[a]Reprinted with permission.[22]
[b]Proportion of patients with gram-negative bacteremia in the treated population, assuming relaxation of the criteria used to determine candidates for nebacumab therapy.

cally resemble those enrolled in the nebacumab trial. Further, as this discussion suggests, implementation of this therapy would require substantial discussion and education to ensure its best possible use. The generalizability of the results of this analysis is contingent on the success of this process and on the degree to which the therapy is used in a fashion similar to that seen in the clinical trial.

Perspective

As in the study of cholesterol treatment, the costs reported in the nebacumab article were derived from several sources.[22] Pharmaceutical costs were based on the price of the agent in the Netherlands, and hospital costs were based on patients treated for sepsis at the Hospital of the University of Pennsylvania in Philadelphia. Induced costs of therapy, in terms of changes in length of stay for patients treated with nebacumab, were based on a series of assumptions discussed in the article. Thus, the as-

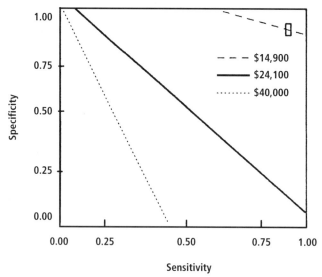

Figure 3. Sensitivity analysis of the test strategy, assessing cost-effectiveness ratios with varying combinations of test sensitivity and test specificity. The lines represent combinations of these variables that have the same ratios of cost per year of life saved. The square on the line at top right represents the sensitivity and specificity used in the principal analysis. Other points represented by this line all have cost-effectiveness ratios that are identical to the one for the principal analysis. Reprinted with permission.[22]

sumptions regarding resource costs and treatment intensity need to be reviewed before implementing treatment recommendations based on this analysis.

Outcomes

In this analysis, the authors assessed the impact of therapy over a patient's lifetime.[22] Quality of life was not incorporated into this analysis. Much of the discussion in the generalizability section also holds true for a discussion of an economic analysis of nebacumab therapy adjusted for quality of life.

Implementation

Both of these case examples provide means of interpreting published economic data for use in making clinical treatment decisions. Discussions based on these data are now commonly heard at formulary committee meetings on both a national (Canada,[26] Australia,[27] the Netherlands,[28] the United Kingdom[29]) or a local population basis (such as an HMO). Four different types of implementation strategies are discussed in this section: treatment efficiency thresholds, formulary committee discussions, treatment decision rules, and timing of the economic evaluation.

THRESHOLDS

Treatment efficiency thresholds have been suggested for inclusion of new therapeutic products on a national formulary.[26] Although efficiency criteria are never published by decisionmakers, inclusion of new pharmaceutical agents on the national formulary would be based on five grades of recommendation in one Canadian proposal using strict pharmacoeconomic criteria for reimbursement (currency values are in Canadian dollars).

1. Compelling evidence for adoption and appropriate utilization. The new therapy has equal or improved clinical efficacy and reduced cost.

2. Strong evidence for adoption and appropriate utilization. The new therapy has increased clinical benefit and costs less than $20,000 per quality-adjusted life-year (QALY) gained, or the new therapy has decreased clinical benefit but its use would save more than $100,000 per QALY gained.

3. Moderate evidence for adoption and appropriate utilization. The new therapy has increased clinical benefit and costs between $20,000 and $100,000 per QALY gained, or the new therapy has decreased clinical benefit but its use would save between $20,000 and $100,000 per QALY gained.

4. Weak evidence for adoption and appropriate utilization. The new therapy has increased clinical benefit and costs more than $100,000 per QALY gained, or the new therapy has decreased clinical benefit but its use would save less than $20,000 per QALY gained.

5. Compelling evidence for rejection. The therapy has equal or decreased clinical benefit at increased cost.

These guidelines offer a clear and consistent means of evaluating the new therapeutic products, yet they are not perfect. The confidence intervals surrounding cost-effectiveness estimates for new therapeutic products are generally large and may cross these thresholds.[30] Small differences in utilization of resources associated with the use of new agents may alter the economic analysis of the therapy as physicians become more proficient with the use of the product. Finally, the results of the economic analysis are dependent on our ability to generalize from the patient population studied in the clinical trial to the population that will eventually receive the drug.

FORMULARY COMMITTEE DISCUSSIONS

Formulary management committees now exist in most settings where physicians practice in an organized fashion. Pharmacoeconomic data are an important part of an informed discussion about the adoption of a new therapeutic agent by the group. Pharmacoeconomic data allow discussion of comparative efficacy and cost of specific products, as well as explicit discussion of the clinical and ethical issues surrounding implementation of new agents by physicians and pharmacists. More than a discussion of the cost of the product itself, pharmacoeconomic evaluation is concerned with assessment of all resources used in the care of patients including hospital treatment, outpatient medical visits, and monitoring of patients. Also, these assessments include a detailed discussion of the outcomes of therapies. From the patient's perspective, these same analyses can be used to evaluate the adverse effects and cost of the therapy to the patient.

Before adopting recommendations based on these discussions, published and other pharmacoeconomic data need to be evaluated in light of the interpretation issues reviewed previously and adapted to the practice setting under consideration. When comprehensive reanalysis of the data is not possible, interpretation and analysis can occur in a descriptive fashion by members of the formulary committee.

TREATMENT DECISION RULES

National pharmaceutical treatment guidelines, such as those used for the NCEP, need to incorporate pharmacoeconomic data into their treatment recommendations. Pharmacoeconomic analysis can help ensure that we achieve the greatest possible efficiency in the treatment of patients through these national public health programs.

Pharmacoeconomic analysis also can include an assessment of patient selection criteria for inclusion in a treatment program. For example, the NCEP proposed different sets of treatment recommendations based on the risk status of a patient (eg, threshold levels of LDL-C at which treatment should be initiated). However, these recommendations are not consistent regarding the cost-effectiveness of treating individual groups of patients.

As shown in Figure 4,[19] treating men aged 45–49 years with cholesterol-lowering agents who have no risk factors for heart disease and a total cholesterol concentration of 260 mg/dL results in a decrease in cardiac events at a cost-effectiveness ratio of $74,200 per year of life saved. Consistent guidelines from an economic perspective would recommend therapy for all patients who can be treated at or below this cost-effectiveness threshold. From Figure 4, that would include men who smoke and have a cholesterol concentration of 220 mg/dL, men with hypertension who have a cholesterol concentration of 220 mg/dL, and men with hypertension who also smoke and have a cholesterol concentration of less than 200 mg/dL.[31] Yet patients with total cholesterol concentrations of less than 240 mg/dL may not meet the NCEP treatment guidelines for initiation of cholesterol-lowering therapy. Some researchers have suggested that the ratio of to-tal cholesterol to HDL-C may be a better measure of risk for coro-nary heart disease than either total cholesterol level or LDL-C.[32]

TIMING OF ECONOMIC EVALUATION

Pharmacoeconomic studies are currently being conducted as substudies in Phase III efficacy trials to allow decision-makers access to economic data at the time of product introduction. However, as discussed previously, clinical trials may not mirror clinical practice. Projection from efficacy to efficiency can occur as part of the evaluation of the Phase III trial economic data and as part of the treatment guideline development process on a formulary level. Phase III pharmacoeconomic evaluations are the only opportunity to collect economic information prior to the introduction of a new therapeutic agent so that decision-makers can include pharmacoeconomic assessments in their initial deci-sion about whether to adopt the new therapy. Phase III trials also are often the only opportunity to assess economic and quali-ty-of-life impact of the therapy in a controlled setting. It is still important to remember, though, that pharmacoeconomic evalu-ation is intended as a management tool for decision-makers. Thus, pharmacoeconomic analysis will need to be revisited after

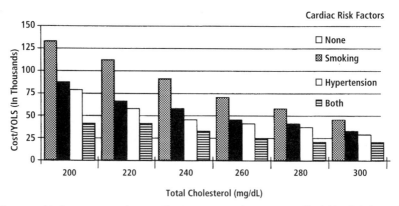

Figure 4. This figure presents the cost-effectiveness ratios for treatment of high blood cholesterol for men aged 45–49 years in whom diet therapy has failed. Pharmacologic therapy in this exam-ple is niacin. Results are presented for patients with no cardiac risk factors (other than male gen-der), smoking as a single risk factor, hypertension as a single risk factor, and both smoking and hypertension.[19] YOLS = years of life saved.

the therapy is introduced into clinical practice, usually through postmarketing studies. This is especially true when the Phase III trial was designed to restrict the use of the agent to high-benefit populations in a manner that may not be implementable in clinical practice. For example, the nebacumab clinical trial excluded patients "with a rapidly fatal course."[20] Without a clinical trial as a mechanism for selecting patients for this therapy, clinicians may be uncomfortable in making this distinction in practice.

In one of the largest concurrent pharmacoeconomic evaluations ever conducted in a postmarketing setting, the Health Care Financing Administration (HCFA; now the Centers for Medicare and Medicaid Services) of the Department of Health and Human Services has monitored the costs and effects of epoetin in the treatment of patients with end-stage renal disease.[33] The Medicare program, insures more than 90 percent of patients with end-stage renal disease. For reimbursement, the HCFA requires providers to record patients' epoetin doses and their hemoglobin concentrations at each visit in which epoetin is administered. In an assessment of the program after 10 months of data collection, the HCFA found that, among patients who had received epoetin for six months or longer, fewer than 45 percent had ever reached a hematocrit concentration over 30 percent. Dosing of epoetin also was lower than expected in the first year of Medicare coverage.[34] These data suggested that the efficiency of epoetin therapy is less than the clinical trial efficacy. The potential reasons for this difference include the following: (1) physicians were under-dosing epoetin in practice during this period due to the Medicare payment policy for the medication, (2) physicians were not titrating the dose appropriately when patients did not respond significantly to initial doses of therapy, or (3) the clinical trial patient population was not generalizable to the Medicare dialysis population. Later research showed that the efficiency of epoetin dosing was associated with provider organizational status, with for-profit providers realizing greater profits by prescribing epoetin more often but in smaller doses than not-for-profit and government providers.[35] When Medicare payment policy for epoetin changed to variable payment based on dosing amount per treatment, mean dose per treatment increased nearly 15 percent in the first six months after the policy shift.[36]

This type of concurrent economic evaluation is becoming more common in European countries as well as in the United States. Further, these assessments can include studies of appropriateness of patient selection in clinical practice compared with selection for the clinical trial or clinical practice guidelines.

The Future

With the increasing worldwide focus on assessing relative value of new technologies and therapies, pharmacoeconomic analysis is taking on a new importance in the pharmaceutical development process. Pharmacoeconomic data are now being developed during Phase III investigations of most new therapeutic products that are thought to have substantial market potential. Further, the quality of the pharmacoeconomic data available to decision-makers is rapidly improving, as data collection becomes more comprehensive and assessments are routinely conducted on a prospective basis. Most pharmaceutical manufacturers now hold their pharmacoeconomic assessments to the same research standards that they have developed for the treatment of clinical data, and most users of these data are now educated to the need for this level of rigor for these assessments.[37-39]

In the United States, we now see the integration of pharmacoeconomics into clinical trials sponsored by the National Institutes of Health[40] and into the guideline development process sponsored by the Agency for Healthcare Research and Quality (formerly the Agency for Health Care Policy and Research).[41] One major shortcoming of the NCEP study[17] is that it did not include pharmacoeconomic data in its initial treatment recommendations.[31]

Summary

This chapter reviewed the interpretation of pharmacoeconomic analysis from a clinical perspective and discussed the implementation of pharmacoeconomic analysis in clinical practice. Interpretation of clinical economics studies is based on four issues: (1) translation of treatment efficacy results to treatment efficiency results, (2) comparison of the clinical trial population with the population under consideration for treatment, (3) translation of the costs reported to costs relevant to the perspective of the decision-maker, and (4) translation of the clinical outcome measures to outcomes relevant to the length of treatment being proposed by the practitioner. Implementation issues include treatment efficiency thresholds, formulary committee discussions, treatment decision rules, and timing of the economic evaluation.

I would like to thank Bruce Kinosian MD for recalculating the data for Figure 4, Henry Glick PhD for his ideas and suggestions, and Zeses Roulidis MD for his editorial comments.

References

1. Detsky AS, Naglie IG. A clinician's guide to cost-effectiveness analysis. Ann Intern Med 1990;113:147-54.
2. Gold MR, Siegel JE, Russell LB, Weinstein MC, eds. Cost-effectiveness in health and medicine. New York: Oxford University Press, 1996.
3. Brown M, Glick HA, Harrell F, Herndon J, McCabe M, Moinpour C, et al. Integrating economic analysis into cancer clinical trials: the National Cancer Institute–American Society of Clinical Oncology economics workbook. J Natl Cancer Inst Monogr 1998;24:1-28.
4. Drummond MF, ed. Methods for the economic evaluation of health care programmes. 2nd ed. New York: Oxford University Press, 1997.
5. Coyle D, Davies L, Drummond MF. Trials and tribulations: emerging issues in designing economic evaluations alongside clinical trials. Int J Technol Assess Health Care 1998;14:135-44.
6. Eddy DM. Cost-effectiveness analysis: is it up to the task? JAMA 1992; 267:3342-8.
7. Eisenberg JM. Clinical economics: a guide to the economic analysis of clinical practices. JAMA 1989;262:2879-86.
8. Warner KE, Luce BR. Cost-benefit and cost-effectiveness analysis in health care: principles, practice and potential. Ann Arbor, MI: Health Administration Press, 1982.
9. Weinstein MC. Principles of cost-effective resource allocation in health care organizations. Int J Technol Assess Health Care 1990;6:93-103.
10. Schulman KA, Lynn LA, Glick HA, Eisenberg JM. Cost effectiveness of low-dose zidovudine therapy for asymptomatic patients with human immunodeficiency virus (HIV) infection. Ann Intern Med 1991;114:798-802.
11. Glick H, Heyse JF, Thompson D, Epstein RS, Smith ME, Oster G. A model for evaluating the cost-effectiveness of cholesterol-lowering treatment. Int J Technol Assess Health Care 1992;8:719-34.
12. Grover SA, Coupal L, Zowall H, Dorais M. Cost-effectiveness of treating hyperlipidemia in the presence of diabetes: who should be treated? Circulation 2000;102:722-7.
13. Prosser LA, Stinnett AA, Goldman PA, Williams LW, Hunink MG, Goldman L, et al. Cost-effectiveness of cholesterol-lowering therapies according to selected patient characteristics. Ann Intern Med 2000;132:769-79.

14. Zethraeus N, Johannesson M, Jonsson B. A computer model to analyze the cost-effectiveness of hormone replacement therapy. Int J Technol Assess Health Care 1999;15:352-65.

15. Marchetti M, Barosi G. Cost-effectiveness of epoetin and autologous blood donation in reducing allogeneic blood transfusions in coronary artery bypass graft surgery. Transfusion 2000;40:673-81.

16. Gaskin DJ, Kong J, Meropol NJ, Yabroff KR, Weaver C, Schulman KA. Treatment choices by seriously ill patients: the Health Stock Risk Adjustment model. Med Decis Making 1998;18:84-94.

17. Adult Treatment Panel. Report of the National Cholesterol Education Program Expert Panel on detection, evaluation, and treatment of high blood cholesterol in adults. Arch Intern Med 1988;148:36-69.

18. Schulman KA, Kinosian B, Jacobson TA, Glick H, William MK, Koffer H, et al. Reducing high blood cholesterol level with drugs: cost-effectiveness of pharmacologic management. JAMA 1990;264:3025-33.

19. Glick H, Kinosian BP, Juhn P, Schulman KA, Jacobson TA, Eisenberg JM. Cost-effectiveness of drug treatment for high blood cholesterol (abstract). Med Decis Making 1991;11:326.

20. Ziegler EJ, Fisher CJ Jr, Sprung CL, Straube RC, Sadoff JC, Foulke GE, et al. Treatment of gram-negative bacteremia and septic shock with HA-1A human monoclonal antibody against endotoxin: a randomized, placebo-controlled trial. N Engl J Med 1991;324:429-36.

21. McCloskey RV, Straube RC, Sanders C, Smith SM, Smith CR. Treatment of septic shock with human monoclonal antibody HA-1A: a randomized, double-blind, placebo-controlled trial. CHESS Trial Study Group. Ann Intern Med 1994;121:1-5.

22. Schulman KA, Glick HA, Rubin H, Eisenberg JM. Cost-effectiveness of HA-1A monoclonal antibody for gram-negative sepsis: economic analysis of a new therapeutic agent. JAMA 1991;266:3466-71.

23. Health Care Financing Administration, Department of Health and Human Services. Medicare program: criteria and procedures for making medical service coverage decisions that relate to medical technology. Fed Register 1989;54(Jan 30):4302-18.

24. Leaf A. Cost effectiveness as a criterion for Medicare coverage. N Engl J Med 1989;321:898-900.

25. Pear R. Medicare to weight cost as a factor in reimbursement. New York Times 1991;(April 22):A-1, A-26.

26. Glennie JL, Torrance GW, Baladi JF, Berka C, Hubbard E, Menon D, et al. The revised Canadian Guidelines for the Economic Evaluation of Pharmaceuticals. Pharmacoeconomics 1999;15:459-68.

27. Hill S, Henry D, Pekarsky B, Mitchell A. Economic evaluation of pharmaceuticals: what are reasonable standards for clinical evidence—the Australian experience. Br J Clin Pharmacol 1997;44:421-5.

28. Postma MJ, Bos JM, van Gennep M, Jager JC, Baltussen R, Sprenger MJ. Economic evaluation of influenza vaccination: assessment for the Netherlands. Pharmacoeconomics 1999;16(suppl):33-40.

29. Rawlins M. In pursuit of quality: the National Institute for Clinical Excellence. Lancet 1999;353:1079-82.

30. Polsky D, Glick HA, Willke R, Schulman K. Confidence intervals for cost-

effectiveness ratios: a comparison of four methods. Health Econ 1997; 6:243-52.

31. Kinosian BP, Glick HA, Juhn P, Jacobson T, Schulman KA, Eisenberg JM. Inconsistent guidelines: is the National Cholesterol Education Program soft on cholesterol? (abstract). Clin Res 1991;39:579A.

32. Kinosian B, Glick H, Garland G. Cholesterol and coronary heart disease: predicting risks by levels and ratios. Ann Intern Med 1994;121:641-7.

33. Sisk JE, Gianfrancesco FD, Coster JM. Recombinant erythropoietin and Medicare payment. JAMA 1991;266:247-52.

34. Griffiths RI, Powe NR, Greer J, de Lissovoy G, Anderson GF, Whelton PK, et al. A review of the first year of Medicare coverage of erythropoietin. Health Care Financ Rev 1994;15:83-102.

35. de Lissovoy G, Powe NR, Griffiths RI, Watson AJ, Anderson GF, Greer JW, et al. The relationship of provider organizational status and erythropoietin dosing in end stage renal disease patients. Med Care 1994;32:130-40.

36. Powe NR, Griffiths RI, Anderson GF, de Lissovoy G, Watson AJ, Greer JW, et al. Medicare payment policy and recombinant erythropoietin prescribing for dialysis patients. Am J Kidney Dis 1993;22:557-67.

37. Adams ME, McCall NT, Gray DT, Orza MJ, Chalmers TC. Economic analysis in randomized controlled trials. Med Care 1992;30:231-43.

38. Hillman AL, Eisenberg JM, Pauly MV, Bloom BS, Glick H, Kinosian B, et al. Avoiding bias in the conduct and reporting of cost-effectiveness research sponsored by pharmaceutical companies. N Engl J Med 1991;324:1362-5.

39. Udvarhelyi IS, Colditz GA, Ri A, Epstein AM. Cost-effectiveness and cost-benefit analysis in the medical literature: are the methods being used correctly? Ann Intern Med 1992;116:238-44.

40. The SOLVD Investigators. Effect of enalapril on survival in patients with reduced left ventricular ejection fractions and congestive heart failure. N Engl J Med 1991;325:293-302.

41. Eisenberg JM. Cost-effective medical practice. In: Kelley WN, ed. Textbook of internal medicine. Philadelphia: JB Lippincott, 1991:30-1.

Assessing Pharmacoeconomic Studies

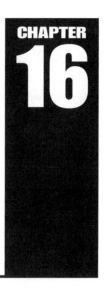

CHAPTER

16

Jacob Abarca

I n the current cost-sensitive healthcare environment, the decision to use a pharmaceutical product depends not only on the safety and efficacy of that product, but now is also influenced by the cost. For this reason, the relevance of pharmacoeconomic evaluations in decision-making has increased dramatically over the last several years and has resulted in thousands of published articles in this field. Several authors have written guides to assist healthcare practitioners in understanding and assessing economic analyses as applied to healthcare programs.[1-4] These methods have also been applied specifically to the evaluation of drug therapies.[5-8] To consider the results of pharmacoeconomic studies in decision-making, it is important that the user be able to critically read the published works in the area.

Assessing the Pharmacoeconomic Literature

Reading and applying the results from pharmacoeconomic studies is much like using the results of any research in that a critical assessment of methods, assumptions, limitations, and the like is required. Moreover, criteria specific to pharmacoeconomic evaluations, such as valuing costs and consequences, discounting, sensitivity analysis, and incremental analysis, are also important. The following criteria were assembled based on published checklists and recommendations for the conduct, evaluation, and use of pharmacoeconomic evaluations.[2,3,8-15] These criteria are not provided to make readers hypercritical and unaccepting of pharmacoeconomic evaluations; few, if any, reports would meet these criteria in total. However, as a guide, they can be useful in determining whether it is worth the reader's time to continue and, if so, whether results and conclusions are deemed valid based on the methodologies used. Some journals stipulate section headings, length, and content requirements. This may need to be considered when critiquing a published report. However, the advent of online journals and electronic communication makes it possible for authors to readily provide detailed information about the pharmacoeconomic evaluation to the reader in the form of appendices or technical reports. Users are encouraged to obtain these additional data (if possible) when assessing any pharmacoeconomic evaluation.

CRITERIA FOR EVALUATING PHARMACOECONOMIC STUDIES

I. Introduction

A. Are the problem statement and resultant study questions clearly and precisely stated?

B. Is the significance of the inquiry discussed with resultant justification of the research?

C. Whose perspective is considered (society, healthcare payer, patient, healthcare provider)? Was the study perspective clearly stated?

II. Methodology

A. Type of Analysis/Study Design

1. What type of analysis is being performed (cost-minimization, cost-effectiveness, cost-benefit, cost-utility, cost-consequence)?

2. What study design was employed (eg, prospective vs retrospective, randomized clinical trial, decision analysis, survey)? Was an experimental or quasi-experimental design used? Is the design internally valid? Is the description complete enough to allow replication?

3. What is the time horizon? Is the time horizon appropriate for the given disease state? Is the time horizon appropriate for the study perspective?

B. Subjects

1. Are the sampling frame and method described?

2. If applicable, are sources of sampling bias considered?

3. Are the salient characteristics of the patient population described in sufficient detail?

4. Is the patient population appropriate for the study question? How will the population limit the generalizability of the results?

5. Are the diagnostic criteria adequately described? Are they appropriate for the study disease state?

C. Alternatives

1. What alternatives are compared?

2. Are the options described in sufficient detail?

3. Are the appropriate alternatives compared? Does the analysis compare the new entity against a current standard? Is a "do-nothing" alternative included? Is it appropriate? Are all relevant alternatives considered?

4. Was the efficacy/effectiveness of each alternative established? What are the data used to establish efficacy/effectiveness?

D. Costs and Consequences

1. Are all relevant costs and consequences (including adverse events) identified for each alternative? Is their inclusion supported by available clinical data? If an important variable is excluded, is justification given?

2. Are the treatment alternatives described in sufficient detail?

3. Are the costs and consequences included consistent with the perspective and time horizon that were selected?

4. How are the costs and consequences measured or counted?

5. How are the costs and consequences valued?

E. Assumptions and Limitations

1. Are assumptions and limitations clearly stated?

F. Discounting

1. Are future costs and consequences occurring beyond one year discounted?

2. What is the rate of discounting?

G. Sensitivity Analysis

1. Is a sensitivity analysis conducted for variables that may not be measured with certainty?

2. Do the results change when factors are varied?

III. Results

    A. Costs and Consequences

      1. Are the results of the analysis clearly presented? Are the results presented in disaggregated form?

      2. Do the results present the total costs and consequences for each alternative, as well as the incremental results?

      3. Are the results of the sensitivity analyses presented?

    B. Is there sufficient evidence to answer the study questions?

IV. Discussion and Conclusions

    A. Are results discussed within the context of the original problem?

    B. Are the limitations of the evaluation discussed?

    C. Are generalizations appropriate?

    D. Are the results compared with published evaluations that are similar or focus on the same disease state?

    E. Are the practical and ethical implications of implementing the results of the analysis discussed?

Given the various methodologies that exist for conducting pharmacoeconomic evaluations, it is not possible to provide in-depth coverage of all the relevant issues for each. This discussion is intended to introduce issues that should be considered when evaluating a pharmacoeconomic evaluation.

All research reports should clearly state the question that is being considered. When reading a typical study, its purpose is presented in the introduction section of the article, usually as the last sentence. This practice also holds for pharmacoeconomic evaluations. The study question is very important because it sets the course for the entire evaluation and gives the reader a frame of reference from which to begin evaluating the appropriateness and usefulness of the study. Ideally, the study question should clearly state the type of pharmacoeconomic evaluation being conducted, the alternatives being considered, the outcome or disease state that is being studied, and the perspective of the study. The following are two hypothetical research questions:

The purpose of this study was to evaluate the pharmacoeconomics of aspirin.

The purpose of this study was to evaluate, from a societal perspective, the cost-effectiveness of aspirin versus no treat-

*ment in the prevention of recurrent acute myocardial infarc-
tion (AMI).*

The first example, a poorly written research question, introduces a broad topic that has implications across a number of
clinical conditions and perspectives. It does not give the reader a
practical sense of the focus of the economic evaluation. The second example, a well-written research question, specifically addresses the type of evaluation (ie, cost-effectiveness), the perspective (ie, society), the treatment alternatives being compared
(ie, aspirin vs no therapy), and the outcome that is being studied
(ie, prevention of recurrent AMI). A well-written research question also allows the reader to determine whether the pharmacoeconomic evaluation will be of interest.

Along with a well-written research question, the authors
should adequately justify the need for conducting the pharmacoeconomic evaluation by presenting the clinical and economic
data available and demonstrating a gap in the available information. There is great variation in the clinical and economic impact of therapeutic decisions and, in general, the complexity of
evaluation should be commensurate with the magnitude of the
impact. Thus, there are some questions that merit a simple
comparison of acquisition costs, whereas others demand an extensive pharmacoeconomic evaluation.[16]

The pharmacoeconomic evaluation should use a patient population that is appropriate and relevant to the disease state that
is being considered. Since the ultimate goal of the evaluation is
to aid in decision-making, the salient characteristics of the patient population should resemble those for whom these results
are targeted. In order to evelute this, the salient characteristics
of the patient population that was included in the economic
analysis should be clearly stated. These include demographic information (eg, age, sex) as well as diagnostic criteria. Information
on comorbidities or other factors that have the potential to influence the outcome of the evaluation (eg, probability of successful
treatment, risk of adverse events) should also be presented.

For prospective and retrospective studies, inclusion and exclusion criteria should be provided. For models, a clear description of each cohort that is included in each treatment arm
should be provided. Another important component to consider,
particularly for retrospective studies using claims databases, is

the patient's access to health care (eg, eligibility for medical insurance) since it can dramatically affect resource utilization. Uneven distribution of eligibility for health benefits across groups can lead to differences that are independent of any treatment alternative.

Some pharmacoeconomic evaluations list the type of analysis (ie, cost-minimization, cost-effectiveness, cost-utility, cost-benefit) and the study perspective (eg, patient, payer, society) separately from the research question. Although not preferred, this is acceptable as long as it is clearly stated. Once these parameters are established, the evaluation should remain consistent with them. This is particularly important for the perspective. The cost-effectiveness of a medication can, and often does, have a different profile depending on the perspective that is taken. For example, if a third-party payer perspective is selected, it is appropriate to include the reimbursed hospitalization costs, physician visits, and medication costs, but not productivity costs (eg, lost wages) or caregiver time. Lack of consistency with the perspective threatens the validity of the results.

The study design used also has important implications on the validity and generalizability of the results. The most familiar design is the randomized clinical trial (RCT). RCTs use protocols that limit differences among comparison groups for the treatment alternatives, increasing confidence that the results are due to the treatment alternatives and not extraneous variables. However, these strict protocols may not be representative of routine clinical practice and limit the generalizability of the results. In such cases, efficacy is established but effectiveness is unknown.

Conversely, retrospective designs try to increase generalizability by using actual data from routine clinical practice (eg, claims databases, medical records). Since these designs are neither randomized nor controlled, the possibility of confounding variables affecting the results is increased, which limits internal validity. These confounding variables can be controlled via the study design or statistical analyses (ie, multivariate analyses). However, full accounting of differences is often not possible. Models (ie, decision analysis, Markov models) are also used to integrate data from various sources to perform an evaluation. These models can be useful and are necessary when comparative data between treatment alternatives are not available. The authors should provide justification for selecting the study design.

The time horizon of the study should be clearly stated and appropriate for the disease state. For example, an evaluation of treatment alternatives for blood pressure that considers stroke and survival as consequences would appropriately use a lifetime time horizon. An evaluation of treatment alternatives for otitis media would use a shorter time horizon (eg, 3 to 6 months). The time horizon should also be consistent with the perspective. For instance, the time horizon for the payer perspective in the United States is typically 12 to 24 months due to the high turnover rate of insured patients.

Treatment alternatives should be described in sufficient detail. This includes the medication, dose, frequency of administration, route of administration, and duration of therapy. The treatment alternatives should be dosed comparably to avoid bias. Ideally, comparisons should be made against the current standard(s) of practice to be relevant to decision-making. Many clinical trials use a placebo comparison ("do-nothing" alternative) when evaluating efficacy, which may or may not be appropriate for pharmacoeconomic evaluations. If the medication is a new entity that is being used to treat a condition for which no alternative exists, then including a do-nothing alternative in the pharmacoeconomic evaluation is appropriate. However, if other treatment alternatives do exist, as is often the case, including a do-nothing alternative is inappropriate and the results will not be relevant to clinical practice. In cases where head-to-head comparison trials are not available, it will be necessary to compare the interventions using a model.

Another critically important component of all pharmacoeconomic evaluations is to establish the effectiveness of the treatment alternatives. This is often an issue of concern for pharmacoeconomic evaluations. Good pharmacoeconomic methodology cannot resolve issues concerning questionable effectiveness data. The authors should clearly state how each probability (eg, effectiveness, adverse events, adherence) was derived. If RCTs are the data source, the authors should take into account the effects of protocol-driven outcomes (eg, increased adherence, evaluation of outcomes) in their effectiveness estimates. Effectiveness measures taken from retrospective studies should be adjusted for potential confounding variables that could bias the estimate. Effectiveness measures used in models should be taken from studies that are relevant to the patient cohorts included in the model.

The costs and consequences included in a pharmacoeconomic evaluation depend heavily on the perspective of the study and so must be consistent with the perspective. Often, the outcomes of pharmacoeconomic evaluations depend on a few key variables (eg, drug acquisition cost, effectiveness, adverse events). Therefore, it is important that all relevant costs and consequences associated with the treatment alternative be included in the evaluation. These can be identified from published clinical trials, observational studies, claims databases, expert opinion, or personal knowledge of a treatment alternative or condition. For instance, obvious examples of costs and consequences (from a third-party payer perspective) include drug acquisition, disease complications, physician visits, and hospitalizations. Other important costs and consequences that should not be overlooked include adverse drug events, laboratory or clinical monitoring, administration costs (eg, intravenous infusions, supplies), and follow-up care.

It is not necessary to include every cost that is associated with each treatment alternative. In some cases, both alternatives will incur the same costs and will not impact the incremental analysis. In other cases, costs may be insignificant and will not influence the results. If costs are excluded from the analysis, the authors should provide adequate justification for their exclusion. Simple disclosure of the excluded costs does not constitute adequate justification.

Measuring/counting the costs and outcomes in an economic evaluation can take on several different forms including case reports, reviewing medical records, analyzing claims databases, or making assumptions regarding the amount of resource utilization based on published literature or expert opinion when no data are available. Consistency and validity of measurement across all the treatment alternatives is important to avoid biasing the evaluation. When the treatment alternatives are similar (eg, drugs within the same class), this is less likely to be a problem. However, in cases where the medications or the nature of the consequences (eg, adverse events) are different, the authors need to ensure that the events are being measured evenly for all treatment alternatives. Finally, the authors must state clearly how each cost and consequence was valued and present the values used in the evaluation in disaggregated form so that the reader can assess generalizability. Pharmacoeconomic evaluations should include costs (the actual amount paid), not charges (the amount that was billed). Common data sources used to value resources include government and private reimbursement schedules, proprietary price lists, and claims databases.

It is rare that all of the necessary information for a pharmacoeconomic evaluation is available. Therefore, some assumptions are always necessary. When data are not available, the authors should explicitly state all of the assumptions that are made in the evaluation and discuss how the assumptions affect the outcome of the analysis. When assumptions are made, they should be reasonable and conservative. The assumptions should also be evaluated in sensitivity analyses to determine their influence on the results of the evaluation.

With certain types of data, it is possible to calculate confidence intervals around the cost-effectiveness ratio to test the robustness of the results. More commonly, sensitivity analyses are used to evaluate uncertainty in pharmacoeconomic evaluations by varying the value of one or more variables at a time and seeing how the results change. Extensive sensitivity analyses should be performed over a plausible range of expected values to determine how the results change. Some experts recommend performing sensitivity analyses over extreme ranges. In any case, the authors should list the variables that were included in sensitivity analyses along with the ranges selected for sensitivity analyses and a justification for selecting that particular range. Conducting a threshhold analysis for the variables that have the most impact on the results can also be helpful in evaluating the robustness of the results.

Costs and consequences occurring beyond a one-year period should be discounted to account for the time preference of money and outcomes. The authors should explicitly state whether costs and consequences were discounted and, if they were, the rate that was used. The United States Panel on Cost-Effectiveness recommends a 3 percent rate as a starting point.[3] However, it is appropriate for a range of discount rates to be used to evaluate the impact of discounting on the analysis.

The authors should clearly state the results of the economic evaluation in disaggregated form along with the incremental analysis. Specifically, the costs and consequences should be broken down for each treatment alternative so that the reader can evaluate the source of any difference between them. Results should also be presented in undiscounted and discounted form. The results of the sensitivity analyses should be clearly presented with specific data on the parameters that had the most influence on the results. Most importantly, the authors should provide results that specifically answer the research question.

The authors should summarize the findings of the results in the discussion. The results of the sensitivity analyses and the impact of any assumptions in the model should be discussed. In general, the overall validity of the findings should be addressed. Limitations of the study (eg, design, data sources, assumptions, or generalizability) should also be discussed. The authors should compare their findings with those from previously published evaluations that have examined the same or similar disease states. Finally, pharmacoeconomic evaluations are intended to aid in the decision-making process regarding the use of pharmaceutical products. Therefore, the authors should address the practical and ethical issues of implementing the results in actual practice.

Economic Evaluations in the Literature

Several issues have been raised concerning the misapplication of terminology and the methodologic conduct of published pharmacoeconomic evaluations. For example, simple terms, such as *cost-effectiveness*, have been used in various contexts to mean cost savings, clinically effective, or being worth the additional cost.[17] Several studies have documented that methodologic problems are common in published economic evaluations.[18,19] Problems have included poorly defined research questions, not explicitly stating the study perspective, improper handling of costs or not explicitly stating which costs were included, not discounting costs and consequences, inadequate or no sensitivity analyses, and not adequately addressing the practical and ethical implications of the results. These studies did not detect significant improvements in the quality of published pharmacoeconomic evaluations over time.

Similar concerns have been raised about pharmacoeconomic evaluations submitted to national governments for reimbursement purposes. Hill et al.[20] found that almost half of pharmacoeconomic evaluations submitted to the Australian government used questionable comparative efficacy data and over one-fifth had problems with their models including unsubstantiated assumptions, problems with the estimation and incorporation of costs, and other technical issues.

Summary

Although several methodologies exist for conducting pharmacoeconomic evaluations, there are widely accepted principles, such as those discussed in this chapter, that apply to all evaluations. Using these principles to evaluate pharmacoeconomic literature will help the user determine whether the conclusions of these studies are valid and relevant. Adherence to these principles does not guarantee that an evaluation is useful. Conversely, pharmacoeconomic evaluations that do not strictly adhere to all of the principles presented in this chapter are not automatically invalid. Every pharmacoeconomic evaluation should be assessed based on its own merit. Empirical evidence has demonstrated that methodologic problems are common in these studies. This fact underscores the need for users to familiarize themselves with the principles of pharmacoeconomics in order to critically evaluate data and use the information wisely.

References

1. Drummond MF, Richardson WS, O'Brien BJ, Levine M, Heyland D. Users' guides to the medical literature. XIII. How to use an article on economic analysis of clinical practice. A. Are the results of the study valid? JAMA 1997;277:1552-7.
2. Drummond MF, O'Brien B, Stoddart GL, Torrance GW. Methods for the economic evaluation of health care programmes. 2nd ed. New York: Oxford Press, 1997.
3. Gold MR, Siegel JE, Russell LB, Weinstein MC. Cost-effectiveness in health and medicine. New York: Oxford Press, 1996.
4. O'Brien BJ, Heyland D, Richardson WS, Levine M, Drummond MF. Users' guides to the medical literature. XIII. How to use an article on economic analysis of clinical practice. B. What are the results and will they help me in caring for my patients? Evidence-Based Medicine Working Group. JAMA 1997;277:1802-6.

5. Vogenberg RF. Introduction to applied pharmacoeconomics. 1st ed. New York: McGraw-Hill, 2000.

6. Drummond MF, Smith GT, Wells N. Economic evaluation in the development of medicines. London: Office of Health Economics, 1988.

7. Freund DA, Dittus RS. Principles of pharmacoeconomic analysis of drug therapy. Pharmacoeconomics 1992;1:20-31.

8. Jolicoeur LM, Jones-Grizzle AJ, Boyer JG. Guidelines for performing a pharmacoeconomic analysis. Am J Hosp Pharm 1992;49:1741-7.

9. Clemens K, Townsend R, Luscombe F, Mauskopf J, Bobula J. Methodological and conduct principles for pharmacoeconomic research. Pharmacoeconomics 1995;8:169-74.

10. Sacristan JA, Soto J, Galende I. Evaluation of pharmacoeconomic studies: utilization of a checklist. Ann Pharmacother 1993;27:1126-33.

11. Siegel JE, Torrance GW, Russell LB, Luce BR, Weinstein MC, Gold MR. Guidelines for pharmacoeconomic studies. Recommendations from the Panel on Cost Effectiveness in Health and Medicine. Pharmacoeconomics 1997;11:159-68.

12. Task Force on Principles for Economic Analysis of Health Care Technology. Economic analysis of health care technology. A report on principles. Ann Intern Med 1995;123:61-70.

13. Weinstein MC, Siegel JE, Gold MR, Kamlet MS, Russell LB. Recommendations of the Panel on Cost-Effectiveness in Health and Medicine. JAMA 1996;276:1253-8.

14. Langley PC, Sullivan SD. Pharmacoeconomic evaluations: guidelines for drug purchasers. J Managed Care Pharm 1996;2:671-7.

15. Torrance GW, Blaker D, Detsky AS, Kennedy W, Schubert F, Menon D, et al. Canadian guidelines for economic evaluation of pharmaceuticals. Pharmacoeconomics 1996;9:535-59.

16. Sanchez LA. Applied pharmacoeconomics: evaluation and use of pharmacoeconomic data from the literature. Am J Health Syst Pharm 1999;56: 1630-40.

17. Doubilet P, Weinstein MC, McNeil BJ. Use and misuse of the term "cost effective" in medicine. N Engl J Med 1986;314:253-6.

18. Lee JT, Sanchez LA. Interpretation of "cost-effective" and soundness of economic evaluations in the pharmacy literature. Am J Hosp Pharm 1991;48:2622-7.

19. Bradley CA, Iskedjian M, Lanctot KL, Mittmann N, Simone C, St. Pierre E, et al. Quality assessment of economic evaluations in selected pharmacy, medical, and health economic journals. Ann Pharmacother 1995;29: 681-9.

20. Hill SR, Mitchell AS, Henry DA. Problems with the interpretation of pharmacoeconomic analyses: review of submissions to the Australian Pharmaceutical Benefits Scheme. JAMA 2000;283:2116-21.

Practical Applications of Pharmacoeconomics for the Real World

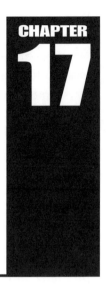

CHAPTER 17

Lisa A Sanchez

A great deal of attention has been recently paid to the discipline of pharmacoeconomics. Over the years, pharmacoeconomics has been used primarily by professionals practicing in pharmaceutical industry and academic settings. Pharmacoeconomics is used during various phases of drug development, as well as during the postmarketing phase, to assist in justifying the value of specific pharmaceutical agents within this highly competitive environment. In academia, much attention has been paid to defining pharmacoeconomic principles and theories and developing research methodologies. Unfortunately, not as much attention has been paid to how these principles, methods, and theories can be applied to traditional pharmacy practice in today's real-world settings. It is the actual application of these concepts that has been the missing link tying pharmacoeconomics to pharmacy practice.

As this text illustrates, pharmacoeconomics can be a powerful and persuasive tool to justify the value of the products and services we provide. From a pharmacy practitioner's, administrator's, or decision-maker's perspective, the real utility of pharmacoeconomics lies in its applications. *Applied pharmacoeconomics* has been defined as putting pharmacoeconomic principles, methods, and theories into practice to quantify the value of pharmacy products and pharmaceutical care services used in real-world environments.[1] Applied pharmacoeconomics may offer the most substantial benefits to pharmacists practicing in more traditional environments including hospitals and managed care organizations. Some of these benefits are summarized in Table 1.[2] How and where we apply these principles and methods to maximize their beneficial effects is precisely the challenge that many pharmacists are facing today.

To help pharmacy practitioners meet this challenge, this chapter highlights the practical applications of pharmacoeconomics in the real world. Presented are how pharmacoeconomics can be applied to inform local decision-making (for both pharmacy products and services), various strategies to put pharmacoeconomics into practice, and case studies to illustrate these applications to traditional (ie, institutional and managed care) pharmacy practice settings.

Practical Applications

From a broad perspective, the basic fundamental application of pharmacoeconomics is to inform decision-making. Pharmacoeconomic principles and methods provide practitioners with the tools necessary to make better and more complete decisions regarding pharmaceutical products and services. Specific types of decisions where pharmacoeconomics has been successfully applied in phar-

---

Table 1. Potential Benefits of Applied Pharmacoeconomics for Pharmacy Practitioners

- Pharmacoeconomic principles and methods can be applied to quantify the value of pharmacy products and services in the real world
- Pharmacoeconomics can provide the data necessary to make better and more informed medication use decisions
- Applied pharmacoeconomics can assist pharmacy decision-makers in choosing between treatment alternatives
- Pharmacoeconomics can assist pharmacy practitioners in justifying various pharmaceutical care services
- Pharmacoeconomics can allow pharmacists to balance cost with patient outcome to ensure that local decisions represent the best interest of the patient and healthcare system

macy practice range from a micro level (ie, individual patient) to a broader, macro level (ie, healthcare system).[1] For example, decisions supported by pharmacoeconomics can include those for formulary management as well as for justification of clinical pharmacy services. Examples of various decisions that can benefit from the application of pharmacoeconomics are included in Figure 1.

EVALUATION OF PHARMACY PRODUCTS

The use of pharmacoeconomics can assist institutional and managed care pharmacists in determining the most appropriate and efficient use of drugs. In fact, the primary application of pharmacoeconomics in these traditional settings has been for the evaluation of pharmacy products. These data can be a powerful tool to support various clinical and policy drug use decisions. More specifically, pharmacoeconomics can be applied to decisions regarding individual patients, formulary management, drug guideline justification and development, and disease management initiatives. For example, decisions regarding an individual patient's therapy can be enhanced with pharmacoeconomic data. Also, applying pharmacoeconomics can assist in the development and justification of drug guidelines and disease management initiatives to promote the most appropriate use of medications within a healthcare system. For formulary management decisions, pharmacoeconomics can assist in determining which agents should be included or excluded, with or without restriction, to or from a formulary.

Complete medication decisions in today's healthcare environment should include (when appropriate) an assessment of three basic types of outcomes. Figure 2 contains suggested components of contemporary clinical decisions.

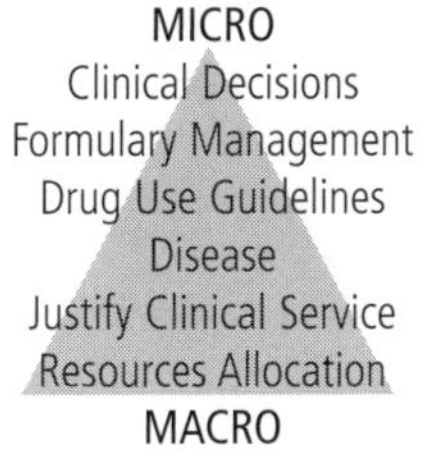

MICRO
Clinical Decisions
Formulary Management
Drug Use Guidelines
Disease
Justify Clinical Service
Resources Allocation
MACRO

Figure 1. Specific decisions for applied pharmacoeconomics.[1]

The outcomes of medical care are generally divided into three categories: clinical, economic, and humanistic.[3,4] Traditionally, most drug therapy evaluations were made primarily by assessing the clinical outcomes (eg, efficacy, safety) of drug therapy. Over the past 15 to 20 years, it has become popular and necessary to include an assessment of the economic outcomes (eg, direct, indirect, intangible costs) of drug therapy. Most recently, the trend is to bring the patient back into this decision-making equation and include an assessment of the humanistic outcomes (eg, quality-of-life effects) of drug therapy. Pharmacoeconomics provides practitioners with the tools to quantify these outcomes and make decisions that represent the best interest of both the patient and healthcare system.

EVALUATION OF PHARMACY SERVICES

Historically, most practical application of pharmacoeconomics and outcomes research has been directed toward drug therapy evaluations. As such, the benefits of clinical pharmacy services have been tightly correlated with dollars saved in drug acquisition terms. Over the past 10 to 15 years, it has become increasingly apparent that pharmacoeconomics also needs to be applied to pharmaceutical care services in the real world. Pharmacoeconomics can be useful in determining the value of an existing pharmacy service, estimating the potential worth of implementing a new service, and capturing the value of a "cognitive" pharmacy intervention. Popular clinical pharmacy inter-

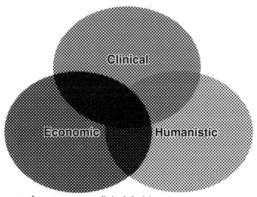

Figure 2. Components of contemporary clinical decisions.

ventions/services include therapeutic drug monitoring services (or clinical pharmacokinetic services), anticoagulation clinics, intravenous to oral switch programs, and drug information services, to name a few.

These interventions/services have an inherent value clearly understood by pharmacists; however, the value of these services has not been as widely appreciated by healthcare administrators responsible for allocating resources. Appropriate quantification and communication of the value of these services are critical to their survival. Various practice sites in the United States have been very successful in justifying these services, and some have even been reimbursed for these various cognitive services. Although it can be difficult capturing benefits such as an adverse drug reaction avoided or a treatment failure avoided, through the appropriate application of methods like cost-benefit analysis, the costs and benefits of a service can be identified, measured, and compared with other services competing for resources. In fact, it is essential that the benefits or value of pharmaceutical care be increasingly defined in terms of non-drug resources favorably affected. That is, what effect does pharmaceutical care have on resources outside the pharmacy budget? Pharmacoeconomics can assist in quantifying the return on investment or other benefits produced by a service so it can be compared with another. Practitioners and administrators can then use these data to make more informed resource allocation decisions.

Since the 1970s, there has been some documentation of the application of pharmacoeconomics to clinical pharmacy services. Many of these publications have been evaluated in review papers.[5-7] For example, McGhan and colleagues[5] evaluated 35 potential cost-benefit or cost-effectiveness studies of pharmacy services published prior to 1978. Another paper by MacKeigan and Bootman[6] reviewed 22 cost-benefit or cost-effectiveness studies published between 1978 and 1987. In 1996, Schumock et al.[7] summarized and critiqued 104 original economic evaluations of papers published between 1988 and 1995, and the clinical services reviewed in that article yielded an average cost-benefit ratio of 16:1.

Most recently, these authors updated the aforementioned review to evaluate 59 articles published from 1996 to 2000.[8] These studies were conducted primarily in hospitals (52%) and community pharmacy and clinic (41%) settings. Benefit-to-cost ratios ranged from 1.7:1 to 17.0:1 (median 4.68:1), and the reviewers noted an improvement in the overall quality of the research.

As these reviews documented, the appropriate application of pharmacoeconomics to pharmacy services has increased over the years, but there is still a need for improvement in the quality/rigor of study design.

Strategies for Applying Pharmacoeconomics to Real-World Practice

The transition from theory to practice, or the practical application of pharmacoeconomics, can be challenging. Many pharmacists are familiar with pharmacoeconomic principles and methods, but are unclear on how to best incorporate pharmacoeconomics into everyday practice. Various strategies to aid pharmacists in putting pharmacoeconomics into practice include (1) critically evaluating, interpreting, and using the results of published studies; (2) using economic modeling techniques; and (3) conducting institution- or plan-specific pharmacoeconomic studies.[9]

Although these were first introduced in 1994,[9] many of today's pharmacists are still trying to determine how best to apply pharmacoeconomics to their practice settings. Table 2 lists the advantages and disadvantages of these strategies, and each will be briefly discussed.[1]

Which strategy is most appropriate depends on the relative impact of the decision on patient quality of care and cost to the organization. Thus, prior to selecting an application strategy, practitioners need to answer the following questions: What is the potential impact of this decision on quality of care delivered? What is the potential impact of this decision on cost of care provided? Figure 3 contains a value assessment spectrum.[10]

If the potential impact of your decision on cost or quality is no to mild impact, then the application strategy employed can be a simpler, less rigorous strategy. If the impact of your decision is moderate in terms of its impact on cost or quality, then a slightly more rigorous or complex strategy may be considered. However, if the impact on cost or quality is severe, then employing a more complex and rigorous strategy, like conducting a prospective pharmacoeconomic study, may be necessary.

EVALUATE AND USE LITERATURE

The most obvious and seemingly user-friendly approach to put pharmacoeconomics into practice is to search medical, pharmacy, and health economic literature sources for any previous studies conducted on the products or services in question.[10] Over the past 20 years, many pharmacoeconomic and outcomes evaluations have been published in various journals. The abundance of data published to date makes the literature a rich source of information for pharmacists, thus making this a common and popular strategy for applying pharmacoeconomics to pharmacy practice.

When confronted with a problem, it is advisable to try this strategy first because, if rigorous studies do exist and reasonable data are available, it can provide results quickly and inex-

Table 2. Advantages and Disadvantages of Strategies to Put Pharmacoeconomics into Practice[1]

Strategy	Advantage	Disadvantage

Use published literature	inexpensive
	readily available
	provides data quickly
	subject to peer review
	results may be from a
	  large population RCT
		data may be from RCT
		  (protocol-driven)
		difficult to generalize results
		may not be comparative
		variations in quality of analyses
		  published

Build an economic model	relatively inexpensive
	provides data quickly
	can bridge efficacy
	  and effectiveness
	can be plan- or institu-
	  tion-specific
		results are dependent on
		  assumptions
		researcher bias may be
		  introduced
		controversial
		provides only a simulation

Conduct an institution-
  or plan-specific study
	usually comparative
	data will be plan- or
	  institution-specific
	designed to reflect
	  "usual care"
	can be prospective or
	  retrospective
		expensive
		time-consuming
		can be difficult to randomize
		  and control
		patient selection bias may be
		  introduced
		potential for small sample size

RCT = randomized clinical trial.

pensively. Another advantage that can be considered a disadvantage is that data published may have been generated from a randomized clinical trial (RCT). While adequate sample sizes are ensured in these trials, pharmacoeconomic data collected in this manner can be protocol driven, that is, not reflective of using a drug in a real-world setting. Also, results reported in published studies can often be difficult to generalize to other practice settings due to differences in practice patterns, patient populations, and drug acquisition costs. However, the primary disadvantage of this strategy is the documented variations in the quality of pharmacoeconomic studies published to date.[11-13] For this reason, all published studies should be critically evaluated using published guidelines and checklists[11,13-16] prior to using the results. Many of these are detailed in Chapter 16.

USE ECONOMIC MODELING

If no relevant data can be obtained from the literature or if what is in the literature is not generalizable to a specific practice setting or population, it may be appropriate to build an economic model.[17,18] The use and popularity of economic modeling as an application strategy have increased over the past few years. Modeling can be performed using a variety of popular techniques including decision analysis, Markov modeling, and MAUT models. For most local pharmacy applications, modeling employs decision analysis and decision trees to provide clinicians with a graphic framework to display treatment options, outcomes associated with treatment options, and probabilities of the outcomes occurring. Then, using a simple algebraic process, all of these variables can be reduced to a single value to ease comparison of competing treatment options.

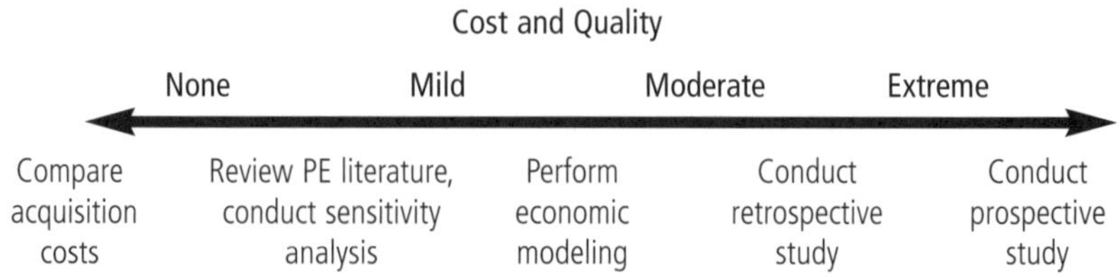

	Cost and Quality			
None	Mild	Moderate	Extreme	
Compare acquisition costs	Review PE literature, conduct sensitivity analysis	Perform economic modeling	Conduct retrospective study	Conduct prospective study

Figure 3. Value assessment spectrum.

There are many advantages of this strategy, especially the ability to forecast the impact of a decision prior to actually making it. Use of economic models can provide support for various clinical decisions, especially those that are time contingent in a relatively inexpensive and timely manner. Using economic modeling, data obtained from an RCT (eg, efficacy data) can be modeled to be more reflective of effectiveness data. Most importantly, models can be populated with institution- or plan-specific data, generating results that better reflect the usual care delivered in a practice setting. The primary disadvantage to this approach is that the results generated are highly dependent on the assumptions made when building the model; thus, some medical decision-makers may be reluctant to accept the findings generated. Any major assumptions should be tested using sensitivity analysis prior to using the results.

CONDUCT A LOCAL PHARMACOECONOMIC STUDY

Conducting an institution- or plan-specific pharmacoeconomic study is another strategy to put pharmacoeconomics into practice. Many decision-makers may find it necessary to conduct local pharmacoeconomic and/or outcomes evaluations if the previous two strategies have been exhausted (ie, no relevant data are obtained either through the literature or economic models). The decision to conduct a local study is not without its own costs. Both time and monetary resources may be consumed by these evaluations; thus, this strategy should be reserved for decisions that may have a significant impact on cost or quality of care delivered.

The primary advantage of this strategy is the flexibility it affords local researchers regarding which products and services to compare and in which patient populations. Because the evaluation is conducted locally, the results generated will be specific to that practice setting and more reflective of the real world. As it can be challenging to conduct research in the real world, there are various disadvantages, including the potential for small sample sizes and difficulty generalizing results to other hospitals or plans. Also, difficulty randomizing patients to different treatment strategies and tightly controlling the study environment can introduce the potential for patient selection bias. Various published guidelines are available for conducting and reporting pharmacoeconomic or outcomes evaluations.[19-28]

OTHER STRATEGIES

Transfer Results from Other Countries

Data from other countries may be used to inform local decision-makers. However, it can be difficult to generalize and transfer the results of a study conducted in another country due to variations in practice patterns, patient populations, and costs. Further, differences in study perspectives, data sources, and analytical styles may present a challenge for practitioners attempting to extrapolate or relate exact cost savings or cost ratios to their own practice settings. To enhance the ability to apply pharmacoeconomic results from other countries, the following must be considered: What is the technical merit (ie, quality) of the study? Are the results applicable to local decision-making? Do the results apply generally in different jurisdictions with different perspectives?[29]

Utilize Sensitivity Analysis

As a critical component of a sound pharmacoeconomic study, sensitivity analysis can also be a useful tool for pharmacy practitioners and decision-makers. When trying to apply the results of a published pharmacoeconomic study to a specific decision, using the sensitivity analyses provided by the author(s) can assist in tailoring the results of the study to a specific situation. Due to the usual differences in practice patterns and patient populations between organizations, it can be difficult to apply the exact cost ratios or cost savings to a different setting with a great degree of confidence. However, if the authors varied key variables that are most significant to the situation (ie, those that best reflect "usual care" at the organization), then recalculated results may be used in formulating a decision.

Perform a Meta-Analysis

Meta-analysis can assist readers in enhancing the applicability and generalizability of pharmacoeconomic findings extracted from published evaluations. *Meta-analysis* has been defined as an analytical method that critically reviews and statistically combines the results of previous research to increase statistical power.[30] Through the use of meta-analysis, two or more studies may be combined using a methodologically systematic approach. Pharmacy practitioners may find this a useful way to increase the power of primary endpoints and subgroups (eg, when the sample size in the original study was too small to obtain statistical significance), resolve uncertainty when studies disagree, and gain confidence in results for a specific problem where many small studies exist. However, meta-analysis is considered a legitimate form of research with its own distinct methodology, so it is important to become familiar with the methodology of meta-analysis prior to conducting a full meta-analysis of the literature.

Replicate a Benchmark or Published Study on a Smaller Scale

Another technique to apply pharmacoeconomic data obtained from another source is to replicate the study on a smaller scale. Replicating a well-done pharmacoeconomic study, conducted at another institution or published in the literature, can assist pharmacy practitioners and decision-makers in applying study results to various decisions regarding pharmaceutical products and services. Prior to undertaking a pharmacoeconomic study replication, the researcher should become familiar with the process and nuances of conducting a pharmacoeconomic evaluation that have been discussed in this chapter and other chapters within this textbook.

Regardless of which strategy is used, pharmacists who become actively involved in applying pharmacoeconomics to enhance decision-making must become "sophisticated consumers" of pharmacoeconomic research. Sophisticated consumers should have the ability to critically evaluate, interpret, and apply results of studies published in the literature and understand the essential elements of a rigorous, sound, and user-friendly pharmacoeconomic study or model.[10]

Case Studies

Presented are four case studies where pharmacoeconomics is applied in the real world to determine the value of a pharmacy product or service. In each case, the most appropriate pharmacoeconomic method (as defined in previous chapters) and application strategy (as described above) are selected and discussed.

CASE 1: INDIVIDUAL PATIENT TREATMENT DECISION

Problem

Drugs A and B are third-generation cephalosporins. Published studies have shown that they are therapeutically equivalent with respect to safety and efficacy; however, the agents do differ in a few respects.

Cost Category	Drug A	Drug B
Drug cost	$7 dose	$16 dose
Dosing regimen	4 times daily	twice daily
Pharmacist preparation time ($30/h)	9 minutes	2 minutes

As a clinical pharmacist rounding with the infectious disease team, you are asked to recommend the best treatment alternative for a particular patient on your service. Given the above information, which drug would you recommend be prescribed?

Analysis and Application Strategy

This case consists of comparing agents within the same therapeutic category, with a documented equivalency in outcome, for a treatment decision. After performing a literature search, the claims of comparable efficacy and safety are confirmed, but no published pharmacoeconomic analyses are revealed. The primary focus for this evaluation now becomes the determination of the least expensive pharmacy product.

If two agents are equal with respect to safety and efficacy, it is probably not necessary to perform cost-effectiveness or cost-utility analysis. If it was appropriate to measure and compare benefits of patient outcome in monetary terms, cost-benefit analysis might be appropriate. As there are documented claims of therapeutic equivalence, a cost-minimization analysis is the most appropriate and simple pharmacoeconomic tool to use in this case.

When determining the least expensive alternative, it is not appropriate to simply compare the acquisition costs of the agents. All relevant costs associated with the therapies must be identified, measured, and compared. The alternative with the least expensive drug acquisition cost may not always represent the least costly alternative when all utilization costs to the institution are considered. Examples of cost categories to be considered include drug acquisition, administration, and pharmacist and nursing labor, given that the therapies differ in these areas. Using organization-specific data, the three cost categories listed above are quantified. The resultant cost per day of therapy is approximately $46 and $34 for Drugs A and B, respectively, making Drug B the obvious choice for this patient.

CASE 2: FORMULARY MANAGEMENT DECISION[16]

Problem

Drugs A and B are histamine$_2$-antagonists used to treat peptic ulcer disease. The medical literature contains the following information:

	Drug A	Drug B
Drug cost (per episode)	$60	$120
Effectiveness (pain relief)	70%	90%
Adverse drug reaction	1%	2%

Drug B is an agent newly approved by the Food and Drug Administration (FDA) that is available at twice the acquisition cost of Drug A. The pharmacy and therapeutics (P&T) committee at your managed-care plan is concerned because of the higher acquisition cost of Drug B. Which drug would you recommend to the P&T committee for formulary inclusion for patients with peptic ulcer disease covered by your managed care plan?

Analysis and Application Strategy

This case also consists of comparing treatment alternatives from the same therapeutic category. However, this case differs from the first one in that the agents being compared differ in safety, efficacy, and cost. Also, the comparison is now for the purpose of a formulary management decision for a managed care plan. To appropriately compare agents that differ in these areas, the pharmacist must use a tool that weighs costs and clinical outcomes concurrently. Cost-benefit, cost-effectiveness, and cost-utility analyses may be theoretically appropriate. Since the costs of the treatment alternatives are measured in monetary units and effectiveness is measured in terms of achieving a specific clinical objective (relief of pain), then the most appropriate method to use is cost-effectiveness analysis.

A literature search reveals two published cost-effectiveness analyses comparing Drugs A and B from a managed care perspective. Prior to using these results for local decision-making, practitioners should critically evaluate the quality and rigor of the published pharmacoeconomic studies and understand where and how to apply and generalize these pharmacoeconomic results.[10] After a critical evaluation of these studies, using published guidelines,[13-16] you determine the quality of both studies to be reasonably sound. However, the methodology of one study in particular appears to be slightly more rigorous. The primary effectiveness measure was quantified in terms of patient outcome of time to healing and/or relief of peptic ulcer pain. The research question for your problem is essentially "Which drug provides the most pain relief or the quickest time to heal per dollar spent?"

The costs identified, measured, and compared in these analyses included total drug utilization costs, costs associated with the difference in effectiveness (cost of retreating a treatment failure), and costs of treating adverse effects associated with the two drugs. In the more rigorous study, the total costs also included the costs for clinic or emergency department visits, hospitalization, and diagnostic procedures (eg, barium swallow, endoscopy). The results of this cost-effectiveness analysis yield a cost-per-treatment success of $1,510 versus $870 for Drug A versus Drug B. However, a quantitative drug use evaluation conducted previously with your plan revealed effectiveness rates of approximately 75 percent and 85 percent for Drugs A and B, respectively. Fortunately, the investigators conducted a thorough sensitivity analysis varying the percent of efficacy of both agents up and down by 10 percent. Utilizing this sensitivity analysis, the recalculated cost-effectiveness ratios are $1,400 and $990 for Drugs A and B, respectively. Applying these results, it appears that Drug B is perhaps still the most cost-effective peptic ulcer disease treatment option at your organization.

On the surface, when comparing acquisition costs of Drugs A and B (ie, $60 vs $120, respectively), it appeared that the least expensive alternative was Drug A (half the acquisition cost of Drug B). However, by using a published pharmacoeconomic study and applying the results of a sensitivity analysis to better reflect the standard of care at your plan, it appears that Drug B may actually be the more cost-effective option when all costs and effects are considered. Thus, Drug B may be the best choice for inclusion to the formulary for your healthcare plan.

CASE 3: JUSTIFICATION OF A PHARMACY SERVICE FOR RESOURCE ALLOCATION

Problem

As director of pharmacy for a 750-bed teaching hospital, you want to establish a therapeutic drug monitoring service (TDMS). You believe that this program will improve the quality of patient care delivered and save money for your institution as well. After negotiations with your hospital administrator, the funding for this service is approved. However, approval is contingent for a one-year trial basis, after which you must document and justify the value of this pharmacy service to the hospital. Documenting that this service yields a high return on investment should increase the probability of your program being continuously funded by the hospital. How do you demonstrate the value of this clinical service to hospital administration at one and three years?

Analysis and Application Strategy

When available, pharmacy practitioners may be able to generalize and use the findings from previously published studies to provide support for implementing a new pharmacy intervention/service or justifying the value of an existing intervention/service. A literature review reveals various economic analyses of TDM or similar programs; however, due to differences in study perspectives and patient populations, the results are not easily generalized to your organization. As the potential impact of this decision on cost and quality of care is potentially severe, conducting a prospective pharmacoeconomic evaluation of your service may be warranted. In this case, the benefits associated with this pharmacy service will need to be measured prospectively, using the appropriate pharmacoeconomic methodology, at your practice site.

When quantifying the value of a service, it is common to employ cost-benefit analysis as a pharmacoeconomic method. This is primarily due to the need to have results expressed in a neutral dollar value so that you can compare outcomes of different services. If the potential costs and benefits of this service can be identified and measured in dollars, then cost-benefit analysis may be the most appropriate pharmacoeconomic method to use. The costs of providing this service will include the pharmacist's salary plus benefits and any additional drug, supply, and laboratory costs, all of which can be fairly easily converted into dollars and annualized. Similarly, the benefits of this service need to be identified and converted into dollars. Theoretically, the benefits will include decreased total drug costs, decreased length of stay (LOS) for patients monitored by the TDMS, reduced drug loss and waste, and perhaps decreased incidence of adverse drug reactions associated with inappropriate dosing of, for example, aminoglycosides (eg, nephrotoxicity, ototoxicity). Through a prospective data collection and a medical chart review, the following data are obtained:

Variable	Value
Average LOS for patient monitored by TDMS	7 days
Decreased LOS for patient monitored by TDMS	2.2 days
Average cost of a standard hospital day	$500
Average number of patients potentially monitored by TDMS	400
Average total cost of adverse reaction (nephrotoxicity) per patient	$7000
Incidence of nephrotoxicity in patients monitored by TDMS[a]	5%
Annual salary plus benefits for pharmacist to manage TDMS	$60,000

[a]This value was obtained from the literature.

To quantify the value of this service, the potential outcomes and consequences must be categorized into costs and benefits, annualized, and summed. The cost and benefit totals for each of the cost categories identified above are listed in this spreadsheet.

Once the total benefits and costs have been calculated, a summary measurement of efficiency should be determined. In a cost-benefit analysis, the results are often expressed as a benefit-to-cost ratio (B/C_{ratio}). To calculate a B/C_{ratio}, the total benefits are divided by the total costs.

Potential Costs	Dollars/ Year	Potential Benefits	Dollars/ Year
Salary/benefits for pharmacist to manage/ operate the TDMS annually	60,000	Decreased LOS for patients monitored	440,000
Monitoring supplies ($5/pt.)	2,000	Decreased use of antibiotics and supplies ($40/pt./day)	112,000
Serum concentration tests ($20/test, 1 test/pt./day)	56,000	Decreased incidence of adverse reaction (nephrotoxicity)	140,000
Total	118,000	Total	692,000

If all of the recommendations made by the TDMS are accepted by the medical staff, then the service yields a B/C_{ratio} of 5.86. However, in the first year, the service obtained a 75% acceptance rate, yielding a B/C_{ratio} of 4.40. Theoretically, for every dollar invested in the service, $4.40 are avoided or saved by the institution. Another way to express the results of a cost-benefit analysis is to calculate a net benefit for the service that represents an annual cost savings to the institution. To assess the net benefit of this service at years 1, 2, and 3, discounting was employed using a five percent discount rate.

Formula	100% Acceptance Rate	75% Acceptance Rate
$B/C_{ratio} = \dfrac{EB_{total}}{EC_{total}}$	$B/C_{ratio} = 5.86$	$B/C_{ratio} = 4.40$

Since it was feasible to convert the potential costs and benefits associated with this service into monetary units, cost-benefit analysis was a practical option. With careful documentation, a strong case was made that the benefits of a TDMS outweigh the costs of providing this service. As competitive pressures escalate, many centers have placed higher value on humanistic outcomes, such as patient satisfaction and improvements in patient's quality of life, and these have not been accounted for in this valuation.

Formula	100% Acceptance Rate ($)	75% Acceptance Rate ($)
Net B = EB$_{total}$ — EC$_{total}$	692,000 — 118,000 =	692,000 — 118,000 (0.75) =
(year 1)	574,000	430,500
(year 2)	574,000 — (0.05 × 574,000) = 545,300	430,500 — (0.05 × 430,500) (0.75) = 408,975
(year 3)	545,300 — (0.05 × 545,300) = 518,035	408,975 — (0.05 × 408,975) (0.75) = 388,527
Total Net Benefit	1,637,335	1,228,002

If valuation of this service needs to be performed prior to the allocation of any funds, perhaps it may be appropriate to construct an economic model using pertinent values from a meta-analysis of the literature. This could also be populated with institution-specific data to yield an estimate of the impact of this service on the hospital. Documenting that the benefit of this service yields a high return on investment should increase the probability of the program being continually funded by the institution.

CASE 4: DRUG POLICY DECISION[18]

Problem

Drug A is used for the prevention and treatment of acute chemotherapy-induced emesis in the inpatient and outpatient oncology units. Over the past two years, the use of Drug A has increased significantly throughout your healthcare system. A drug use evaluation reveals high use of this drug, with 50 percent of the doses used in the outpatient unit inappropriate. The P&T committee becomes concerned due to the higher drug acquisition cost of this agent compared with comparators and the annual pharmacy expenditures for this agent have been in excess of $300,000 since it was approved by the FDA. The P&T committee institution wants to develop and approve a policy to promote the most appropriate use of this agent to decrease total expenditures while maintaining high-quality patient care. As the oncology clinical pharmacist with P&T review responsibilities, how would you solve this problem and determine the most appropriate and cost-efficient utilization of this antiemetic agent for your healthcare system?

Analysis and Appplication Strategy

This decision, given its potential impact on quality of care and total costs, may warrant a prospective pharmacoeconomic evaluation. However, due to local time and resource constraints, this strategy is not feasible at this time. A thorough review of the pharmacy and medical oncology literature sources reveals various studies that evaluated the effectiveness of Drug A in various doses, including using lower doses of this agent. In fact, the use of lower-than-recommended doses has become common at large cancer centers, especially when customizing the dose to match the emetogenicity of the chemotherapy regimen being administered. Additionally, you locate a published pharmacoeconomic analysis that evaluates the use of various doses of Drug A for prevention of acute chemotherapy-induced emesis. The following data elements for Drug A are obtained from United States and European studies.

This case involves a comparison of different dosing regimens of the same drug for an institutional drug use policy decision. Although the drug is the same, the evidence that the two regimens are equal in effectiveness and safety is varied. However, the results of the pharmacoeconomic analysis reveals that comparable clinical effects were indeed obtained with a decreased total drug cost per patient. Initially, you believe that applying cost-effectiveness analysis is the most appropriate method to employ. Due to time constraints and your experience with clinical decision analysis, you decide to construct a model to determine the most cost-effective use of Drug A.

Parameter	Regimen 1	Regimen 2
Drug dose (intravenous)	20 mg	30 mg
Dosing schedule	once daily	once daily
Effectiveness (with 20-mg dexamethasone)	89%	85%
Safety (primary headache)	1%	1%
Drug acquisition cost per day (US$)	$90.00	$120.00
Cost-effectiveness ratios reported	$101.12	$141.76

From a small patient chart review, pharmacy database, and panel of local oncology specialists, you estimate (assume) the potential medical costs associated with the various drug regimens.

A decision tree can provide the structure for your cost-effectiveness simulation. By constructing a tree and populating it with the data from the above two tables, all of the outcomes associated with the treatment options, the probabilities of these outcomes occuring, and the costs of these outcomes can be graphically displayed. An example of this tree is contained in Figure 4. Using averaging out and folding back, all of these variables can be algebraically reduced to one value. This value represents a summary measure of effectiveness, which in this case is a cost-effectiveness ratio (CE_{ratio}). To calculate this CE_{ratio}, the following process was followed:

1. Multiply the cost of path 1 with the probability of no adverse reaction ($250 × 0.99) and repeat for path 2 ($400 × 0.01).
2. Add these numbers and multiply by the probability of success ($251.50 × 0.89 = $223.84).
3. Repeat the above steps for pathways 3 and 4 and then add the resultant values ($223.84 + $72.22 = $296.06).
4. Add the cost of the drug to this value ($296.06 + $90.00) and divide by the probability of a success with no adverse reaction (0.89 × 0.99 = 0.881), so that $386.06/0.881 = $438.20.
5. Repeat this process for regimen 2 using paths 5 to 8.

Upon modeling this decision and analyzing these data, it appears that the CE_{ratio} associated with Drug A regimens 1 and 2 are $438 and $513, respectively. These values may seem inflated relative to drug acquisition costs and CE_{ratio} calculations found in the literature; however, decision-makers must be aware that these values represent the average total medical cost per treatment success (complete or major control of chemotherapy-induced emesis) without an adverse reaction for Drug A regimens 1 and 2 over a large population. As regimen 1 appears to be the most cost-effective, obtaining the desired therapeutic effect at the least cost per patient per day, this dosing regimen can now be incorporated into institutional antiemetic treatment guidelines and brought to the P&T committee for approval. When presenting these data to the hospital staff, it may be advisable to calculate the total annual cost savings associated with promoting the use of regimen 1 (total cost per patient multiplied by the total eligible patients per year).

Option	Resources Used[a]	Cost per Patient[b] ($)
Cost of success with no adverse drug effect	Chemotherapy visit Normal laboratory values × 1	200.00 50.00
	Total	250.00
Cost of success with an adverse drug effect	Chemotherapy visit Normal laboratory values × 2 Extra therapy (physician, nurse, pharmacist time + drugs)	200.00 100.00 100.00
	Total	400.00
Cost of failure with no adverse drug effect	Chemotherapy visit Normal laboratory values × 2 Extra therapy (physician, nurse, pharmacist time + drugs) Delay in clinic (2 h)	200.00 100.00 200.00 150.00
	Total	650.00
Cost of failure with adverse drug effect	Chemotherapy visit Normal laboratory values × 3 Extra therapy (physician, nurse, pharmacist time + drugs) Delay in clinic (2 h) Hospitalization	200.00 150.00 300.00 150.00 500.00
	Total	1300.00

Adapted from reference 18.
[a]For one cycle of chemotherapy.
[b]The costs contained here were generated for the purposes of this example and are not intended to reflect actual costs.

Once the drug policy/guideline is approved, it is imperative to spend adequate time implementing the policy. To ensure success, key medical, nursing, and pharmacy staff should be targeted for a substantial educational effort. Strategies to educate staff should include face-to-face interactions (eg, inservice presentations), written materials (eg, pocket cards), and computer-

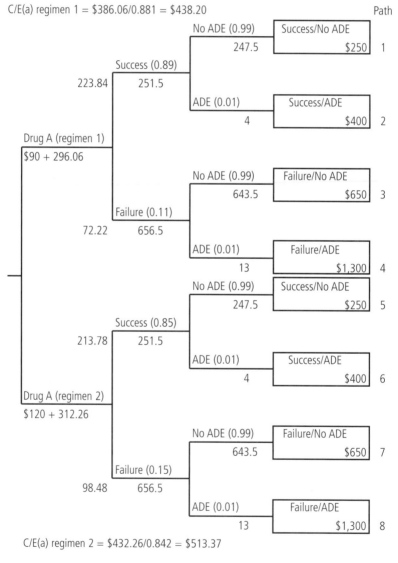

C/E(a) regimen 1 = $386.06/0.881 = $438.20

C/E(a) regimen 2 = $432.26/0.842 = $513.37

Figure 4. A decision tree to determine the cost-benefit ratio. ADE = adverse drug effect.

ized communications (online messages). Lastly, it is important to establish a system to continuously document the effect of this policy on the institution and patients. Thus, six to 12 months after policy/guideline implementation, follow-up data should be collected on a random sample of approximately 10 percent of the patients who received the drug under the policy/guidelines. Completion of this process may increase the acceptance of the drug policy by physicians, pharmacists, and nurses. Furthermore, promoting this policy as a means to provide the highest quality of patient care at a cost savings to the institution will communicate your interest in both the welfare of the patient and the healthcare organization.

Summary

Although pharmacoeconomics has been widely used by the pharmaceutical industry and academic institutions, use in real-world practice settings has been less prevalent. Applied pharmacoeconomics can offer substantial benefits to pharmacists practicing in more traditional environments, including hospitals and managed care organizations. By using the strategies described in this chapter, the real-world practitioner can realize many benefits that pharmacoeconomics offers, most importantly, the ability to make more informed and complete decisions regarding pharmaceutical products and services. With pharmacy budgets continuing to decrease while healthcare costs rise, pharmacists will be continually challenged to quantify the value of the products and services they provide. Through applied pharmacoeconomics, pharmacy practitioners can meet this challenge and provide products and services that represent the best interest of patients, healthcare systems, and society.

References

1. Sanchez LA. Pharmacoeconomics: principles, methods, and applications to pharmacotherapy. In: Dipiro JT, Talbert RL, Yee GC, Matzke GR, Posey LM, eds. Pharmacotherapy: a pathophysiologic approach. 4th ed. Stamford, CT: Appleton & Lange; 1999:1-11.
2. Sanchez LA. Expanding the role of pharmacists in pharmacoeconomics: how and why? Pharmacoeconomics 1994;5:367-75.
3. Coons SJ, Kaplan RM. Quality of life assessment: understanding its use as an outcomes measure. Hosp Formul 1995;30:412-6.

4. Kozma CM, Reeder CE, Schulz RM. Economic, clinical, and humanistic outcomes: a planning model for pharmacoeconomic research. Clin Ther 1993;15:1121-32.
5. McGhan WF, Rowland CR, Bootman JL. Cost-benefit and cost-effectiveness: methodologies for evaluating innovative pharmaceutical service. Am J Hosp Pharm 1978;35:133-40.
6. MacKeigan LD, Bootman JL. A review of cost-benefit and cost-effectiveness analyses of clinical pharmacy services. J Pharm Mark Manage 1988;2:63-84.
7. Schumock GT, Meek PD, Ploetz PA, Vermeulen LC. Economic evaluations of clinical pharmacy services—1988–1995. Pharmacotherapy 1996;16:1188-208.
8. Schumock GT, Butler MG, Meek PD, Vermeulen LC, Arondekar BV, Bauman JL. Evidence of economic benefit of clinical pharmacy services: 1996–2000. Pharmacotherapy 2003;23:113-32.
9. Sanchez LA. Pharmacoeconomic principles and methods: including pharmacoeconomics into hospital pharmacy practice. Hosp Pharm 1994;29:1035-40.
10. Sanchez LA. Applied pharmacoeconomics: evaluation and use of pharmacoeconomic data from the literature. Am J Health Syst Pharm 1999;56:1630-40.
11. Lee JT, Sanchez LA. Interpretation of 'cost-effective' and soundness of economic evaluations in the pharmacy literature. Am J Hosp Pharm 1991;48:622-7.
12. Udvarhelyi S, Colditz GA, Rai A, Epstein AM. Cost-effectiveness and cost-benefit analyses in the medical literature. Are the methods being used correctly? Ann Intern Med 1992;116:238-44.
13. Bradley CA, Iskedjian M, Lanctôt K, Mittman N, Simone C, St Pierre E, et al. Quality assessment of economic evaluations in selected pharmacy, medical, and health economics journals. Ann Pharmacother 1995;29:681-9.
14. Drummond MF, Stoddart GL, Torrance GW. Methods for the economic evaluation of health care programmes. 2nd ed. Oxford: Oxford University Press, 1997.
15. Sacristán JA, Soto J, Galende I. Evaluation of pharmacoeconomic studies: utilization of a checklist. Ann Pharmacother 1993;27:1126-33.
16. Sanchez LA. Pharmacoeconomic principles and methods: evaluating the quality of published pharmacoeconomic evaluations. Hosp Pharm 1995;30:146-52.
17. Milne RJ. Evaluation of the pharmacoeconomic literature. Pharmacoeconomics 1994;6:337-45.
18. Sanchez LA, Lee JT. Applied pharmacoeconomics: use of modeling as an external data source. Am J Health Syst Pharm 2000;57:146-58.
19. Clemens K, Townsend R, Luscombe F, Mauskopf J, Osterhaus J, Bobula J. Methodological and conduct principles for pharmacoeconomic research. Pharmacoeconomics 1995;8:169-74.
20. Jolicoeur LM, Jones-Grizzle AJ, Boyer JG. Guidelines for performing a pharmacoeconomic analysis. Am J Hosp Pharm 1992;49:1741-7.
21. Task Force on Principles for Economic Analysis of Healthcare Technology. Economic analysis of healthcare technology: a report on principles. Ann Intern Med 1995;122:61-70.

22. Sanchez LA. Pharmacoeconomic principles and methods: conducting pharmacoeconomic evaluations in a hospital setting. Hosp Pharm 1995;30:412, 415-16, 428.

23. Eisenberg JM. Clinical economics. A guide to economic analysis of clinical practices. JAMA 1989;262:2879-86.

24. Siegel JE, Torrance GW, Russell LB, Luce BR, Weinstein MC, Gold MR. Guidelines for pharmacoeconomic studies: recommendations from the Panel on Cost Effectiveness in Health and Medicine. Pharmacoeconomics 1997;11:159-68.

25. Russell LB, Gold MR, Siegel JE, Daniels N, Weinstein MC. The role of cost-effectiveness analysis in health and medicine. JAMA 1996;276:1172-7.

26. Weinstein MC, Siegel JE, Gold MR, Kamlet MS, Russell LB. Recommendations of the Panel on Cost-Effectiveness in Health and Medicine. JAMA 1996;276:1253-8.

27. Siegel JE, Weinstein MC, Russell LB, Gold MR. Recommendations for reporting cost-effectiveness analyses. JAMA 1996;276:1339-41.

28. Torrance GW, Blaker D, Detsky A, Kennedy W, Schubert F, Menon D, et al. Canadian guidelines for economic evaluation of pharmaceuticals. Pharmacoeconomics 1996;9:535-59.

29. Mason J. The generalisability of pharmacoeconomic studies. Pharmacoeconomics 1997;11:503-14.

30. Einarson TR. Meta-analysis of the pharmacotherapy literature. In: Hartzema AG, Porta MS, Tilson HH, eds. Pharmacoepidemiology: an introduction. 2nd ed. Cincinnati, OH: Harvey Whitney Books, 1991:236-69.

Pharmacoeconomics, Health Policy, and Limited Resources

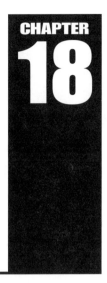

CHAPTER

18

William F McGhan
and J Lyle Bootman

Pharmacoeconomics can be a powerful tool for comprehensively examining the economic impact of alternative therapies and other medical interventions. Pharmacoeconomics is increasingly being applied to identify, measure, and compare the costs and consequences of pharmaceutical products and services. As we move through this new millennium, healthcare systems around the globe are facing a multitude of clinical and economic challenges. Health ministries and policy-makers are well aware of limited resources, and many countries are attempting to apply health economic and pharmacoeconomic principles in examining the costs and benefits of both proposed and existing drugs and health services. Both public and private sectors are experiencing tremendous pressure, and there is increasing expectation that all patient care interventions be evaluated in terms of clinical, social, and economic outcomes related to costs incurred. The World Bank's Internet site has some very interesting and useful health economic information that elaborates on many issues and approaches.[1]

A complicating factor is that different sectors have different agendas, and it is important in cost-effectiveness evaluations to consider these various perspectives. Most economists agree that the most important perspective to include in all pharmacoeconomic evaluations is that of society as a whole. Some of the various pharmacoeconomic perspectives include:

1. government
2. taxpayers
3. patients
4. practitioners
5. employers
6. hospitals
7. insurers

In considering the above points of view, it is, of course, important to consider who pays the cost of the intervention and who receives the benefits. For example, a patient may be very interested in a new therapy for treating migraine that increases his or her quality of life, but from a government perspective, a government without an integrated medical database may be concerned only about an increase in its drug budget. Few health systems include quality-of-life or outcomes data, and many people have expressed concern that national governments continually allow short-term budgetary considerations to override patients' desires for improved quality of life and long-term health outcomes. *Cost-consequence analysis*, which includes costs for the inputs against several different types of outputs, may be a method for including more perspectives in healthcare decisions.

Patients should ideally be covered for a basic roster of therapies. The World Health Organization maintains an Essential Drug List and has developed "cost-effectiveness" formulary and ranking tools that are available on the organization's Web site.[2] The essential drug list for a population can be decided in a number of ways; every health system certainly has its own method of determining what drugs are made available. In addition to debating what drugs should be covered, there is also the question of who should pay for experimental therapies. Instead of the insurance company denying payment for any part of experimental drug therapy, some policy analysts have recommended that, if patients want to pay for experimental drugs, the insurance program should at least pay the equivalent of the cost of the approved medication and the patient pays the difference for the experimental agent.

Multiple Paths Toward Cost-Effective Pharmaceutical Interventions

There are numerous methods stimulating the use of more cost-effective pharmaceuticals and services for patients. These include increasing use of drug selection and care protocols, patient education and self care, and health outcomes management. An elaboration of a longer list of methods includes activities related to:

1. Prospective approaches
   (a) protocols (therapy guidelines)
   (b) prior authorization
   (c) prospective review (pharmacy computer linkage in prescribers' offices)
   (d) decision support services
2. Retrospective approaches
   (a) drug use review/evaluation (DUR/DUE)
   (b) continuous quality improvement (CQI)
   (c) postmarketing surveillance
   (d) outcomes research
3. Financial approaches
   (a) copayment (single and multi-tiered)
   (b) coinsurance
   (c) deductibles

All of the above approaches have their strengths and limitations, and any of them could be considered with pharmacoeconomic analysis.

Considering Comprehensive Costing in Population Budgeting

From a broad health economics point of view, one could go beyond the methods that countries usually use to report health expenditures. For example, in the United States, over $1.5 trillion for health was spent in 2002. This figure represents direct costs only. Studies indicate that direct and indirect costs average about 50 percent each of the total cost of illness. Therefore, the total cost of illness in the United States is as much as $3 trillion per year. Figure 1 illustrates this point. If we could more broadly use pharmacoeconomic approaches in setting health policy priorities, we may be able to justify spending more on appropri-

ate health interventions and stimulate research on new therapies. Increased expenditure for curative and preventive therapies would probably increase the total direct costs. However, if
properly chosen, therapies could decrease the indirect costs (productivity losses) and thus potentially decrease the total cost of
illness. This figure also illustrates a concept in cost-benefit analysis, that if an intervention is cost saving to society, then there
are no budget limitations. On a national scale, the expenditures
for the intervention are ideally offset by the increase in gross domestic product of the country.

Cost-Effectiveness Rankings

It is difficult to convert outcomes to monetary terms. Table 1 illustrates another approach to policy decision-making and suggests how society could make more explicit decisions about what
medical and pharmaceutical interventions should be covered in
health plans. In developing such a table, one must try to estimate
how many people would be positively affected by each program in
the list, and this would be translated into life-years gained (LYG)
or quality-adjusted life-years (QALYs) gained as in column 2.

One must also estimate how much it will cost to treat each
target population, as listed in column 3. Programs are then
ranked by their cost-effectiveness ratio. Therefore, when a bud-

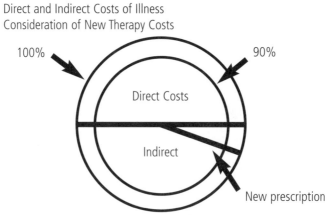

Figure 1. Global budgets and the total cost of illness. An increase in direct costs with new therapy may decrease both indirect and total costs.

get for a defined population with, for example, $400,000 is being established, based on this technique, only programs A, B, and C could be initiated. This approach is somewhat similar to what the World Health Organization is exploring and what the state of Oregon attempted for its Medicaid program for indigent patients. Oregon shifted its health policy for coverage from "who is covered" toward "what is covered."[3]

Quadrants and Cost per QALY

Another approach uses quadrants and cost-per-QALY slopes to assist in decision-making. Figure 2 has an x and y axis for effectiveness and cost, respectively. The center intercept represents the current or standard therapy (eg, Drug A) for comparison, and the angled slopes represent where a new therapy (eg, Drug B) may lie. One slope represents therapies having an incremental cost of $50,000 per QALY and the other slope represents therapies with an incremental cost of $100,000 per QALY. Depending on what cost per QALY is considered socially acceptable, any therapy falling below these slopes or in the "Encourage

Table 1. Pharmacoeconomic Selections with Fixed Budgets[a]

Therapy or Program	Effect[b] (QALYs)	Cost[c] ($Thousand)	CE Ratio[d] ($Thousand)
A	50	100	2
B	50	200	4
C	20	120	6
D	25	200	8
E	10	120	12
F	5	80	16
G	10	180	18
H	10	220	22
I	15	450	30

CE = cost-effectiveness; QALY = quality-adjusted life-year.
[a]Selection procedure: first, rank therapies by cost-effectiveness ratios, then add therapy options until budget is exhausted.
[b]Total QALYs for all patients benefiting.
[c]Total cost of treatment for all of targeted patient population.
[d]Cost per QALY.

or Accept" quadrant would be included in the health coverage.[4]

The World Bank health reform Web site goes into further detail about this quadrant approach and also discusses how one might consider using two or more drugs with different patient groups. Table 2 illustrates how some of these calculations are performed when one is using different therapy approaches. By establishing clinical protocols so that only high-risk patients receive the more expensive therapy, there are potential savings and better allocation of resources. As shown in Table 2, for a hypothetical 1,000 patients, it would be economically reasonable to use different drugs depending on the type of patient being treated. Thus, high-risk patients would receive the more expensive agent and low-risk patients would receive the less expensive agent. The incremental value in the fourth column is the slope of the line as discussed for the quadrant graph approach, with different drugs compared with each other and with a "selective" protocol.

Challenges and Opportunities

In this chapter, we have attempted to illustrate a few examples of how pharmacoeconomic concepts can be utilized in health policy and the allocation of scarce resources. Although

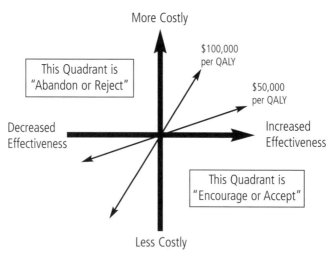

Figure 2. Quadrants and incremental cost-effectiveness. The center intercept is standard or baseline therapy.

pharmacoeconomics can be very useful, it is certainly not the panacea to answer all questions regarding the cost of pharmaceutical care and eliminate all disease, and there are still many challenges that must be faced now and in the future. Some of these problems include how to conduct long-range budgeting for predicted new biotechnologies, how to support research on new drugs, how to pay for appropriate use of new or unapproved uses of current drugs, and how to properly consider individual patient variation and patient preferences in drug treatment protocols.

The standard tools for pharmacoeconomic analyses make it possible to ask basic questions such as, "How much does illness cost in my population?" and "What is the more cost-beneficial way to treat an illness?" Yet final, conclusive answers can be difficult to discover when there is a need for continuing data collection on the cost and outcomes of treatment. Further research is required on how to fully consider issues such as willingness to pay, quality of life, and gene therapy.

We hope that this information will assist in cost-analysis and cost-justification efforts. There are encouraging reports in health economic and pharmacy literature that demonstrate that pharmaceutical therapy and interventions can have cost-beneficial effects in a number of areas. We must realize that, even though much of this pharmacoeconomic research has been positive, we need to continue to develop therapies and programs that maximize the benefits to society and global communities. Even though a pharmaceutical or pharmacy intervention can demon-

Table 2. Example of Incremental Analysis: Contrast Media

	Total Patients	Events	Contrast Cost	Incremental	
Ionic (100%)	1,000	47	$8,400		
Non-ionic (100%)	1,000	27	$200,000	$9,580	non-ionic vs ionic
Selective	1,000	30	$58,211	$47,263	non-ionic vs selective
				$2,930	selective vs ionic

Sample math:

$$\frac{(\$200{,}000 - \$58{,}211)}{(30-27 \text{ events})} = \frac{\$141{,}789}{3 \text{ events}} \quad \$47{,}263 \text{ per event avoided (non-ionic vs selective)}$$

strate cost-effectiveness, society and governments will ultimately invest their resources in the most needed programs that have the higher benefit or better incremental cost-effectiveness ratio. Healthcare decision-makers are encouraged to fully consider pharmacoeconomic tools so that their healthcare resources are used efficiently, fairly, and wisely.[5]

References

1. World Bank Health Economics. www.worldbank.org/hap/hsd/healtheconomics_index.asp (accessed 2004 Apr 16).
2. World Health Organization cost-effectiveness analysis. www3.whoint/whosis/cea (accessed 2004 Apr 16).
3. Hadorn DC. Setting health care priorities in Oregon: cost-effectiveness meets the rule of rescue. JAMA 1991;265:2218-25.
4. Canadian Coordinating Office for Health Technology Assessment. www.ccohta.ca (accessed 2004 Apr 16).
5. Drummond MF, Stoddart GL, Torrence GW. Methods for the economic evaluation of health care programs. Oxford: Oxford University Press, 1997.

Index